MORBIDITY OF URBAN POPULATIONS AND STANDARDS OF THERAPEUTIC-PROPHYLACTIC CARE

MORBIDITY OF URBAN POPULATIONS AND STANDARDS OF THERAPEUTIC-PROPHYLACTIC CARE

I. D. BOGATYREV, Editor

The American Public Health Association, Inc.

1740 Broadway, New York, N.Y. 10019

Prepared under the Special Foreign Currency Program of
The National Library of Medicine,
National Institutes of Health, Public Health Service,
U.S. Department of Health, Education, and Welfare,
and published for
THE NATIONAL LIBRARY OF MEDICINE
pursuant to an agreement with
THE NATIONAL SCIENCE FOUNDATION, WASHINGTON, D.C.
by
THE ISRAEL PROGRAM FOR SCIENTIFIC TRANSLATIONS,
JERUSALEM, ISRAEL

Translated from the Russian
Zabolevaemost' gorodskogo naseleniya i normativy
lechebno-profilakticheskoi pomoshchi
Izdatel'stvo "Meditsina," Moskva 1967
by E. ADELSON, M.D., and N. KANER

Library of Congress Catalog Card Number 72-92182
ISBN 0-87553-064-8

Composed and printed in Israel by Keter Press, Jerusalem

Table of Contents

Foreword to the English Edition

In making this English translation of a Russian book available to the American health profession, the American Public Health Association and the National Library of Medicine are providing an unusually thorough and massive statistical study of morbidity, hospital care and standards, and preventive health standards in the modern Union of Soviet Socialist Republics.

The view of Russian medicine and "capitalist countries" medical shortcomings is interwoven in the text to the extent that the American editors felt they could neither note nor remove some material that seemed to approach "propaganda" for the socialist way of giving universal health care. Consequently, the translation is presented literally, with only minor changes in word order and minimal editing for consistency in style.

Considerable effort has been made to check the "foreign" portions of the Bibliography and the contents of Chapter 3 for accuracy and consistency.

Foreword

The present monograph is the result of comprehensive work of the Public Health Organization Section of the Erisman Moscow Scientific Research Institute of Hygiene and nine scientific research clinical institutes of the Russian Soviet Federated Socialist Republic [RSFSR] Ministry of Health and of the Vladimirskii Clinical Institute of the Moscow Region, which was carried out in accordance with Directive No. 44 of the USSR Ministry of Health dated 31 January, 1962, and with Directive No. 86 of the RSFSR Ministry of Health dated 13 March, 1962. The work was carried out under the general organizational and scientific direction of Prof. I. D. Bogatyrev by the method that he worked out.

Among the workers of the Public Health Organization Section the following junior scientific workers participated in this work: T. A. Korol'kova, G. Ya. Ryumina, N. F. Burmistrova, A. Ya. Rzhevskaya, senior registrars N. V. Leont'eva, N. T. Potanina, K. I. Fomina, V. T. Anisimova and L. P. Stolpnik, as well as V. P. Grinavtseva, Chief Physician of the Stupino Hospital.

Workers of the foreign language public health group of the Public Health Organization Section—senior scientific workers E. N. Yakubova, Candidate of Biological Sciences, and V. Ya. Bereznev and V. I. Mushakov, junior scientific workers—collected and analyzed the foreign language material.

The sections *A Brief Outline of the Development of Methods for Working Out the Standards of Therapeutic-Prophylactic Care of the Population of the USSR; Organization and Methods of Scientific Research; Basic Patterns of Morbidity, Sickness Rate and Hospitalization and Composite Data on Therapeutic-Prophylactic Care Standards* were written by the Director of the Public Health Organization Section of the Erisman Moscow Scientific Research Institute of Hygiene, Prof. Bogatyrev.

The section *Methods of Studying the Morbidity and Determining the Hospital Bed Requirement of the Population in Capitalist Countries* was written by senior scientific worker E. N. Yakubova, Candidate of Biological Sciences, and junior scientific workers V. Ya. Bereznev and V. I. Mushakov (of the Public Health Organization Section of the Erisman Institute of Hygiene).

The section *Standards of Therapeutic-Prophylactic Care of the Urban Population in the Field of Internal Medicine* was written by R.A. Yarullina (Public Health Organization of the Erisman Institute of Hygiene).

The section *Standards of Therapeutic-Prophylactic Care of the Urban Population in the Field of Surgery* was written by E. I. Udintsov, Doctor of Medical Sciences (RSFSR Ministry of Health).

The section *Standards of Therapeutic-Prophylactic Care of the Urban Population in the Field of Pediatrics* was written by junior scientific worker M. A. Bogomol'skii (State Scientific Research Pediatric Institute of the RSFSR Ministry of Health).

The section *Standards of Therapeutic-Prophylactic Care of the Urban Population in the Field of Stomatology* was written by G. A. Novgorodtsev, Candidate of Medical Sciences (USSR Ministry of Health).

The section *Standards of Therapeutic-Prophylactic Care of the Urban Population in the Field of Orthodontics* was written by G. V. Baziyan (Central Scientific Research Institute of Dentistry).

The section *Standards of Therapeutic-Prophylactic Care of the Urban Population in the Field of Obstetrics and Gynecology* was written by junior scientific worker G. Ya. Ryumina (Public Health Organization Section of the Erisman Institute of Hygiene).

The section *Standards of Therapeutic-Prophylactic Care of the Urban Population in the Field of Otorhinolaryngology* was written by the Director of the Organizational Methods Section of the Institute of Ear, Nose and Throat Diseases of the RSFSR Ministry of Health, V. S. Kuznetsov, Candidate of Medical Sciences.

The section *Standards of Therapeutic-Prophylactic Care of the Urban Population in the Field of Ophthalmology* was written by A. I. Pocheikin, Candidate of Medical Sciences (Helmholtz State Scientific Research Institute of Eye Diseases).

The section *Standards of Therapeutic-Prophylactic Care of the Urban Population in the Field of Neurology* was written by G. V. Kovalevskaya (Chair of Neurology of the Moscow Region Scientific Research Clinical Institute).

The section *Standards of Therapeutic-Prophylactic Care of the Urban Population in the Field of Psychiatry* was written by T. I. Gol'dovskaya, Doctor of Medical Sciences, M. I. Rybal'skii, Candidate of Medical Sciences, and junior scientific workers E. S. Gur'yan and L. Ya. Guseva (of the State Scientific Research Institute of Psychiatry of the RSFSR Ministry of Health).

The section *Standards of Therapeutic-Prophylactic Care of the Urban Population in the Field of Tuberculosis* was written by N. S. Al'tshuller, R. G. Vinogradova, and B. A. Varsava, Candidates of Medical Sciences, as well as by V. S. Tekunov, V. P. Krashennikova, B. T. Lyubavina and R. Ya. Gaft (State Scientific Research Institute of Tuberculosis of the RSFSR Ministry of Health).

The section *Standards of Therapeutic-Prophylactic Care of the Urban Population in the Field of Dermatovenereology* was written by N. M. Turabov, R. S. Petrova, and K. V. Vozdvizhenskaya (Central Dermatovenereological Institute).

The section *Standards of Therapeutic-Prophylactic Care of the Urban Population in the Field of Logopedics* was written by V. B. Baranova, junior scientific worker (State Scientific Research Institute of Ear, Nose and Throat Diseases of the RSFSR Ministry of Health).

The section *Standards of Sanatorium-Health Resort Care of the Urban Population* was written by G. A. Rybinskii, Candidate of Medical Sciences (RSFSR Ministry of Health).

The section *Standards of Therapeutic-Prophylactic Care of the Urban Population in the Field of Physiotherapy* was written by T. A. Korol'kova, junior scientific worker (Public Health Organization Section of the Erisman Institute of Hygiene).

Scientific workers of the following scientific research clinical institutes participated in the comprehensive medical checkups on the population of the experimental section of the city of Stupino and in the evaluation of the patient sickness rate, hospitalization rate and outpatient attendance data: Central Dermatovenereological Institute, Institute of Obstetrics and Gynecology, Gertsen Oncological Institute, Helmholtz Institute of Eye Diseases, Pediatric Institute, Institute of Psychiatry, Institute of Ear, Nose and Throat Diseases, Institute of Tuberculosis, as well as the Vladimirskii Moscow Region Scientific Research Clinical Institute.

Prior to medical checkups, fluorographic examinations of the population were made by means of the apparatus and by the workers of the State Institute of Roentgenology and Radiology of the RSFSR Ministry of Health.

A Brief Outline of the Development of Methods for Working Out the Standards for Therapeutic-Prophylactic Care of the Population of the USSR

All branches of the national economy of the USSR, including public health, which is government-controlled under Soviet conditions, are developed on the basis of government plans. Planning of the economy is based on the deliberate utilization of known economic rules and regulations by the socialist government.

In contrast to the elementary economic development of capitalist countries, the economic laws of socialism manifest themselves as laws recognized and deliberately utilized in the practice of building socialism.

Engels wrote: "Here we have the same difference as between the destructive force of lightning from a thundercloud and electricity operating humbly in a telegraph apparatus or arc lamp, between a conflagration and a fire controlled by human hands" (Engels, *Anti-Dühring*, p. 229. 1938).

It should be said that, despite rich experience in the field of planning gained by Soviet public health, the problems of scientific-experimental rationalization of practical activity in this field have been inadequately worked out.

The problem of determining standards of the population requirement of hospital and outpatient-polyclinic care for concurrent and particularly for long-range planning is one of the most important and comparatively little studied.

The tremendous significance of the standards derives from the fact that by means of them a determination is made of the parameters of long-range plans for the development of all branches of public health, the interrelationship between these branches, the number of beds available for various types of patients, the distribution of visits to outpatient-polyclinic institutions according to the various medical specialties, the need for medical personnel, etc.

1

Since the initial years of the Soviet public health system, its agencies have given much attention to planning matters. Special importance was ascribed to planning, beginning with the First Five-Year Plan of development of the national economy of the USSR.

Problems of planning were analyzed at the Sixth Congress of Health Departments (1927), where Z. P. Solov'ev gave a report, as well as at the first special conference convoked by the Narkomzdrav [People's Commissariat of Health] of the RSFSR (1928). All-Union conferences on planning problems were also held in February and September, 1929. At these conferences problems of the methodology to be used in making up the public health plan of the First Five-Year Plan were analyzed. Planning problems remained on the agenda in subsequent years.

In May, 1932, a conference on planning problems was held by the Gosplan [State Planning Commission] of the USSR and the Narkomzdrav of the RSFSR; somewhat later (end of May, 1932) the Gosplan convoked the All-Union Conference on Public Health Planning and Rest for Workers.

It should be mentioned that at these conferences practical problems of compiling the plan were given more attention; not much light was thrown on problems of the methodology of determining standards. The scientific and statistical aspects of the standards recommended at these conferences were not adequately substantiated.

In the foreword to the book *Materialy k pyatiletnemu planu zdravookhraneniya RSFSR (Material on the Five-Year Public Health Plan of the RSFSR)* (Medgiz,1930), M. F. Vladimirskii, speaking of defects in the work of making up the second variant of the public health plan for the First Five-Year Plan, directed particular attention to the "absence of necessary basic statistical data both for the study of the morbidity and incidence of pathology and for keeping records of hospital activity."

The standards used as a basis for the parameters of the public health plans were usually the averages for the USSR, and in making them up inadequate account was taken of the morbidity rates of the various age, sex, and social groups of the population. At the same time, the standards recommended for practical utilization were not always properly correlated with the personnel and financial possibilities of public health organizations over the periods of time included in the plan or with the actual population requirements (particularly in the outpatient-polyclinic division), conditioned by the morbidity.

For example, in the First Five-Year Plan the average annual number of outpatient visits per city dweller planned was 11 (*Materialy k pyatiletnemu planu zdravookhraneniya RSFSR*, Medgiz. 1930); in the second, 12 (*Zdravookhranenie i rabochii otdykh vo vtoroe pyatiletie (Public Health and Rest for Workers in the Second Five-Year Plan)*), Vol. 1, Moscow. 1933). The standards of outpatient-polyclinic care for the urban population were set at the same level even later.

It should be noted that even in making up the second variant of the public health plan for the First Five-Year Plan, provision was made, even though inadequately substantiated scientifically, for differentiated standards of outpatient visits for workers of different branches of industry and their families. Specifically, 16.5 outpatient-polyclinic visits per year were planned per metallurgical worker, chemist or miner; 8 for the family members of this group of industrial workers; 13.5 and 7.4, respectively, for each worker of industrial enterprises in other fields; 10.2 and 6.8 for other insured workers and members of their families; and 3.4 visits a year for those not insured (*Materialy k pyatiletnemu planu zdravookhraneniya RSFSR,* Medgiz. 1930).

Despite the vigorous growth of the therapeutic-prophylactic network of institutions and the number of physicians involved, even in prewar years, the actual number of visits per city dweller (excluding visits of rural inhabitants to the cities) did not reach the standards mentioned and averaged 7.8 (according to records for the USSR in 1940). During the postwar years there was even a reduction in the average outpatient-polyclinic attendance per city dweller. While in 1950 this figure was 7.8, in 1955 it was 7.2.

It should be pointed out that in 1955 the number of physicians in the cities more than doubled compared with 1940 (in 1940 there were 104,000 physicians in the cities; in 1955, 233,000); the urban population during this period, however, rose by only one third (60,600,000 in 1940; 87,000,000 in 1955).

There has been no essential change in the frequency of outpatient-polyclinic visits in the cities even in recent years, despite the considerable increase in the number of physicians. For example, according to the records, there were 8.7 visits per city dweller in 1963 for the RSFSR, though the number of physicians increased by 77,900 from 1955 through 1963.

Evidently, many other factors besides the number of physicians have an influence in providing the population with adequate medical care equivalent to the number of outpatient-polyclinic visits by the population.

Standards for providing the urban population with beds were also set at different levels at various stages of development of Soviet public health.

At the Fifth Congress of Health Departments in 1924, a norm of 6.6 beds per 1,000 population was adopted. In 1932, the All-Union Conference on Public Health Planning proposed that 8.5 beds per 1,000 urban population be adopted as the standard for the Second Five-Year Plan. Actually, 6 beds per 1,000 population were made available in 1928, and 7.13 in 1937. In the prewar years (1940) the number of beds per 1,000 population in the cities was 7.92; in 1948, 9; in 1955, 9.5. In recent years the number of hospital beds has increased considerably; in 1963 there were 10.2 beds per 1,000 city inhabitants for the USSR as a whole.

The well-known work *Metodologiya razrabotki norm lechebnoi pomoshchi gorodskomu naseleniyu* (*Methodology for Working out Standards of Medical Care for the Urban Population*)(P. I. Kurkin, L. K. Khotsyanov, I. V. Novokhatnyi and others) should be considered the first serious attempt at scientific substantiation of standards for hospital and polyclinic care of the urban population after the October Revolution.

This work was performed on the basis of material on sickness rate, hospitalization, and patients' visits to institutions in a number of cities in the Moscow Region (Ore-khovo-Zuevo, Kolomna, Naro-Fominsk, Dmitrov), parallel to a study of the sanitary-hygienic state of these cities. The work is of considerable value even today.

It envisages, for the first time, a methodical approach to the determination of standards on the basis of sickness rate data.

In the prewar years elaboration of standards of medical care of the population occupied a number of authors (L. S. Kaminskii, Ya. O. Rodov, I. L. Gurevich and L. V. Nepomnyashchii, A. M. Efman and others). After World War II standards of hospital and polyclinic care were elaborated by V. A. Goryushin, D. G. Oppengeim, A. M. Dvorkin, S. S. Ostroumov, V. I. Fershtudt, V. S. Nikitskii and others).

In determining standards of therapeutic-prophylactic care of the urban population, the various authors in most cases based their work on current data on the sickness rate, hospitalization and patients' visits to institutions (V. A. Goryushin, S. S. Ostroumov, V. I. Fershtudt, D. G. Oppengeim, A. M. Dvorkin, L. S. Kaminskii and others). In some cases the data of records were supplemented by material of a special, more detailed study of sickness rate and visits to various institutions (V. S. Nikitskii). Some authors, in addition, resorted to the medical examination method (V. A. Goryushin, I. L. Gurevich and L. V. Nepomnyashchii), using physicians of different specialties in this work.

M. Mazur and T. I. Dobrovol'skaya, working at the medical institutions of Stupino, made use of the initial records (outpatient chart, hospital case history, etc.), copying from them the essential data on sickness rate, hospitalization and visits of the urban population.

In connection with the workup of long-range plans of public health development in the last 10 years, wider use has been made of scientific research for determining standards of therapeutic-prophylactic care requirements by various urban population groups. The authors of these works usually made use of the initial records of therapeutic-prophylactic institutions as a source of information on morbidity, patients' visits and hospitalization rate (I. D. Bogatyrev, O. A. Aleksandrov, A. E. Shakhgel'dyants, M. S. Brilliantova, I. V. Pustovoi, K. A. Gashimova, N. S. Nazarova and E. V. Abramova, A. P. Zhuk, F. M. Ilupina, V. D. Dubrovina, L. G. Lekarev, F. S. Ryukhov, V. I. Tyshetskii, V. A. Minyaev and others).

On the basis of the essential information they copied from the initial records they determined standards of medical care of the rural population also (P. I. Kal'yu, E. A. Loginova, B. M. Matsko, E. D. Zagorskaya, S. E. Il'in, O. N. Stel'makh, L. G. Lekarev and coworkers, and others).

The medical examination method began to be used more widely in scientific research work on standard-planning topics. Experienced clinicians were generally used as experts. However, this method was in many cases applied without proper caution, which sometimes ultimately led to figures for hospital care requirements which were definitely too high for the immediate future. This may be illustrated in quite a striking manner through the examples of the work of V. A. Minyaev ("Nekotorye voprosy planirovaniya statsionarnoi meditsinskoi pomoshchi vzroslomu naseleniyu v bol'nitsakh goroda" (Some Problems in the Planning of Medical Care for the Adult Population in City Hospitals), *Sovetskoe Zdravookhranenie*, No. 7. 1957), L. G. Lekarev, F. S. Ryukhov, and V. I. Tyshetskii ("Potrebnost' naseleniya Vinnitsy v statsionarnoi pomoshchi i metodika ee opredeleniya" (Hospital Care Requirement of the Population of Vinnitsa and Means of Determining It), *Vrachebnoe Delo*, No. 6. 1951), and F. M. Ilupina, V. D. Dubrovina and L. I. Gribkova ("Opredelenie potrebnosti gorodskogo naseleniya v statsionarnoi pomoshchi" (Determination of the Hospital Care Requirement of the Urban Population), *Sovetskoe Zdravookhranenie*, No. 1. 1961).

Despite the considerable value of the basic data analyzed, a defect common to these studies was the fact that the authors, after determining the number of persons needing hospital care, which in most cases was almost twice as great as the actual number hospitalized, continued to use the actual average length of the patient's stay in bed for calculations of the bed requirement.

When there is a comparatively high hospitalization rate, mild cases of disease are seen in even greater proportion, which, as experience shows, leads to a substantial reduction in the average length of the patient's stay in bed. Quite convincing evidence of this is the tendency toward reduction of average hospital stay noted in recent years. The appearance of new, more effective treatment facilities and methods also contributes to this. By using the actual figures for the average length of the patient's stay in bed for the calculations without appropriate correction the authors inevitably overestimate the bed requirement.

A number of authors (F. M. Ilupina, V. D. Dubrovina and L. I. Gribkova ("Opredelenie potrebnosti gorodskogo naseleniya v statsionarnoi pomoshchi" (Determination of the Hospital Care Requirement of the Urban Population), *Sovetskoe Zdravookhranenie*, No. 1. 1961), I. V. Pustovoi ("Izuchenie potrebnosti v lechebno-profilakticheskom obsluzhivanii na promyshlennom predpriyatii" (Study of the Therapeutic-Prophylactic Care Needs of an Industrial Enterprise), *Sovetskoe Zdravookhranenie*, No. 6. 1956) and others, were not entirely correct in the tasks they set before clinical experts. An experienced expert can with sufficient reliability determine the hospitalization requirement for a given patient only (with consideration of sex and age) and for a given form and stage of disease; the expert can also determine the degree to which a certain patient needs outpatient care (number of visits to the polyclinic and house calls, their distribution among various specialists, etc.) and attention from therapeutic-diagnostic departments and laboratories.

Even the most experienced expert cannot, however, determine the average number of outpatient visits necessary as a whole for the fields of internal medicine, surgery, etc., per city dweller per year, because this figure is an average statistical one and is made up of a tremendous number of visits by persons of different sex and age for different diseases. Nor can the expert be given the task of determining the average periods of hospital treatment in the majority of nosologic entities, because these figures are also derived, and they must be determined by the investigator himself on the basis of the objective data at appropriate centers rather than by the expert. The latter can correctly determine the average periods of hospital treatment for only a limited group of hospitalized cases (operations for abortion, chronic tonsillitis, nonstrangulated hernia, appendicitis, etc.). The expert clinician cannot introduce any corrective factors into the total rate or distribution of the morbidity.

A defect common to the work based on the study of records is a discrepancy in the parameters for standards not due to differences in the rate or distribution of the morbidity.

D. G. Oppengeim and A. M. Dvorkin, for example, proposed making calculations on the basis of seven outpatient-polyclinic visits per city dweller per year (excluding dental visits); V. A. Goryushin, S. E. Ostroumov and V. M. Fershtudt, from 7 to 9 visits (for cities of different sizes); Ya. O. Rodov, 10; V. S. Nikitskii, 11.8; L. S. Kaminskii, 12.55, etc.

It should be stated that in the majority of these studies visits for prophylactic purposes were not separated out of the total number of outpatient visits, while the standards themselves were inadequately correlated with the morbidity of the population and the actual number of outpatient visits needed for the treatment of the various diseases, particularly those with a high incidence.

This may be the explanation of the fact that the standards for outpatient-polyclinic care of the urban population proposed even at the time of creation of the first five-year plans of public health development in the Soviet Union have not been fulfilled even today, although the availability of medical care has been increased substantially, and the number of physicians has risen many times during this period.

One of the most important parameters which make it possible to establish an interrelationship between the population morbidity and the visits to therapeutic institutions for treatment purposes is the number of visits to outpatient-polyclinic institutions according to the various nosologic entities and groups of diseases which are ordinarily referred to certain medical specialists (those working in certain departments).

The number of visits for therapeutic purposes according to each nosologic entity and class of disease should also be determined at centers with a well-developed system of therapeutic-prophylactic institutions. Only under these conditions and with a sufficient number of observations at the various therapeutic institutions can we detect the quantitative relationships between the disease and the number of visits needed in practice, which have been determined over many years of medical experience. The greater the number of observations of these relationships at well-selected centers, the more reliably will the average figures obtained reflect the actual need for treatment visits, which is determined primarily by the duration of the pathological process and the available treatment facilities and methods.

Certain organizational principles of public health organs and primarily the established procedure of mandatory notice to patients to come to the polyclinic to extend their sick-leave certificates every three days (for those on an outpatient routine) also have an essential influence on the number of outpatient-polyclinic visits.

Differences in the rate and distribution (according to the nosologic entities) of the morbidity of different age, sex and social groups of the urban population are also reflected in the number of outpatient-polyclinic visits by the population, and therefore in the evaluation of the number of visits consideration should be given to the composition of the population of various inhabited places selected as centers for the study.

Finally, the availability of hospital care affects the rate and distribution of visits (particularly house calls).

The more persons in a group of patients who enter the hospital during the year, the smaller will be the total number of polyclinic visits (for therapeutic purposes) and the number of visits for certain groups of diseases for which the patients are usually admitted to the hospital.

As for visits for prophylactic purposes, they should be considered separately from those for therapeutic purposes, because their frequency in various population groups and their relative proportions among the visits in the various medical specialties are essentially determined by the directives and principles of public health organizations (occupational checkups of various industrial workers, of pregnant women, adolescent workers, etc.).

Here the extensive application of the medical experts' evaluation of the level of prophylactic care and determination of its optimum level are possible by consideration of the medical staff available and a number of other factors.

In recent years a number of studies have been made of the attendance at outpatient-polyclinic institutions and its relationship with total population morbidity (as judged by patient turnover). These studies have permitted the establishment of quite distinct rules and regulations for the attendance for therapeutic purposes and the number of outpatient visits needed for different diseases as well as the demonstration of the age and sex characteristics of this attendance. It was shown that in recent years the frequency of outpatient visits for treatment did not increase essentially and that it was considerably less than had appeared from the records.

A. P. Zhuk, F. M. Ilupina and V. D. Dubrovina have determined that there were 3,856.7 visits for therapeutic purposes per 1,000 of the adult population in

Ivanovo for the year (the average number of visits per disease was 2.7); in Saratov these figures were, respectively, 4,237.7 and 2.7 (A. P. Zhuk, F. M. Ilupina and V. D. Dubrovina, "Opredelenie potrebnosti vzroslogo gorodskogo naseleniya v poliklinicheskom obsluzhivanii" (Determination of the Requirements of Polyclinical Service by Adult Urban Population), *Sovetskoe Zdravookhranenie*, No. 10. 1962).

According to O. V. Grinina's data, there were 6.6 outpatient visits (for therapeutic and prophylactic purposes) per Moscow inhabitant, while the average number of visits for therapeutic purposes per disease was 3.3; this figure was 3 and 3.2 in various groups studied (O. V. Grinina, "Lechebno-profilakticheskoe obsluzhivanie semei trudyashchikhsya (po dannym nepreryvnogo nablyudeniya)" (Therapeutic-Prophylactic Care of Workers' Families (According to Continuous Observation Data)), *Zdravookhranenie Rossiiskoi Federatsii*, No. 7. 1964).

In Kiev N. V. Maslenkova found through special research that the average number of visits by a patient per disease was 3.1 (excluding dental and oral diseases). It is of some interest to note that during the year of this study, according to the records, there were 9.7 outpatient visits per inhabitant of Kiev, and the number of conditions treated* was 1,193.6 per 1,000 adult population (N. V. Maslenkova, "Ispol'zovanie materialov zabolevaemosti i poseshchaemosti vzroslogo naseleniya v praktike planirovaniya raboty bol'nitsy" (Utilization of Morbidity and Visit Rate Data of the Adult Population in the Practice of Planning Hospital Work), *Sovetskoe Zdravo-okhranenie*, No. 3. 1964).

According to I. D. Bogatyrev's data, the average number of outpatient visits per disease was 2.7 (for treatment purposes) (I. D. Bogatyrev, "Materialy po normativam potrebnosti gorodskogo naseleniya v lechebno-profilakticheskom obsluzhivanii" (Data on Standards for the Urban Population Requirement of Therapeutic-Prophylactic Care), *Zdravookhranenie*, No. 1. 1959). In the city of Stupino in 1949 M. M. Mazur and T. I. Dobrovol'skaya established the fact that the average number of visits per disease was 2.1 (M. M. Mazur and T. I. Dobrovol'skaya, "Kontingenty bol'nykh i zabolevaemost' naseleniya g. Stupino v 1949 g." (Patient Groups and Population Morbidity in Stupino in 1949) in the book *Voprosy izucheniya zabolevae-mosti* (*Problems of Studying Morbidity*), Medgiz. 1956).

The comparison of figures for the attendance at outpatient-polyclinic institutions in the USSR with the data of special studies in other countries is interesting.

In such a comparison consideration should be given to the fundamental differences in public health organization of the population in the USSR and capitalist countries. The high cost of private practitioners' services keeps a portion of the population in capitalist countries from visiting the physicians when they have comparatively mild illnesses. It should also be noted that the great majority of visits in capitalist

---

* [*Translator's note:* the actual word used here is *obrashchenie*, which indicates the patient's coming to the physician for a single disease, but it does not indicate how many visits he made per disease; for this reason it is translated as the number of conditions treated rather than the number of visits.]

countries is to general practitioners. This renders the data published in the majority of capitalist countries not fully comparable with similar material of Soviet authors, because in the USSR medical care is free of charge and is completely available with a high degree of specialization.

For comparison, the data of English authors, published after the creation of a national health service with free medical care in Britain, are of the greatest value. According to survey data (Logan and Brooke), the average per person in England was 4.8 outpatient visits in 1947; 5 in 1948; 5.5 in 1950 (including 3.1 visits to the office of a general practitioner, 1.7 house calls to the patient and 0.7 visits to outpatient departments of hospitals, where specialists attended them) (Logan, W. P. D. and E. Brooke, *The Survey of Sickness, 1943 to 1952.* London. 1957).

Approaching these figures are data published by a general practitioner (Fry), in whose area (4,000 persons) the numbers of visits per inhabitant averaged: 3.7 in 1949; 3.8 in 1950; and 3.28 in 1951 (*Brit. Med. J.* p. 249, 2 August 1952.)

According to the data of 106 general practitioners in England and Wales there were 3,751 visits per 1,000 population in 1955–1956 (Studies on Medical and Population Subjects, No. 14, *Morbidity Statistics from General Practice,* Vol. 1 (General). London. 1958).

In the U.S.A. the average number of outpatient visits per inhabitant was 5.3 in 1957–1958; 4.7 in 1958–1959 (Health, Education, and Welfare. *Trends,* 1961, p. 19. Washington D.C., 1962).

A communication has also been published showing that the average number of general practitioner visits ranges from 2.75 (Sweden) to 8.46 (Israel) in different countries, and on the average for the majority of countries it is 4.5 per inhabitant per year (*Medical World,* Vol. 98, No. 1. 1963).

The figures for the frequency of outpatient visits in capitalist countries are related essentially to the diseases in the population which compel the patient to seek medical treatment.

The relative importance of prophylactic visits is very small, because only very well-to-do persons can afford periodic health checkups by a physician.

In the USSR and other socialist countries where all types of medical care are free and available, the frequency of outpatient-polyclinic visits for prophylactic purposes is very high.

Studies made and published in different years on determination of standards of therapeutic-prophylactic care of the urban population on the basis of records are, at present, essentially of historical interest only. In their day they played a definite beneficial part and were useful in working out long-range plans of public health development.

The majority of these studies were based on records of public health organs, which did not enable their authors to suggest adequately substantiated standards based on practical experience.

It should be pointed out that even the best records did not afford the opportunity of determining the following:

a) total patient sickness rate, attendance at outpatient-polyclinic institutions, and hospitalization rate of the population from social, age and sex aspects;

b) characteristics of the sickness rate, hospitalization and outpatient-polyclinic attendance of various population groups associated with certain working conditions (workers of enterprises in various branches of industry, etc.);

c) the frequency of prophylactic visits for the various age-sex groups of the population, distributed according to the various medical specialties;

d) which population groups (social position, sex, age) constitute the greatest load on the therapeutic-prophylactic institutions and for what reasons.

A no less serious error was the fact that the record data used as the basis for working out the standards were collected by certain authors in cities where the therapeutic-prophylactic network was not fully available and did not completely satisfy the needs of the population for medical care, particularly in the matter of hospital treatment.

This fact undoubtedly had an influence on the level and distribution of the morbidity, hospitalization and attendance at outpatient-polyclinic institutions, and in a definite way distorted them.

Of greater value was the scientific research work done on the basis of the initial records and with the use of expert clinicians.

The data collected in this way, however, reflected only the amount of work due to the existing sickness rate in the population and the capacity of the medical institutions at the given stage.

The experts were able to introduce corrective factors into the data obtained, which increased their reliability. However, even in this case the data could serve only as a sufficiently dependable basis for working out standards of therapeutic-prophylactic care for the immediate future.

For the purpose of long-range planning it was necessary to detect all cases, those for which the population came in by themselves, as well as the chronic cases, which do not attain a degree of clinical expression sufficient to force the patient to seek the physician immediately, but ultimately require medical care.

This fact also made it necessary to seek out new methodological approaches to working out standards for therapeutic-prophylactic care of the urban population when this task was given to us by Directive No. 44 of the USSR Ministry of Health dated January 31, 1962, and Directive No. 86 of the RSFSR Ministry of Health dated March 13, 1962.

The characteristics of the methods used in the current study are given in the next section.

Organization and Methods
of Scientific Research

For the purpose of working out scientifically substantiated standards for the urban population requirement of therapeutic-prophylactic care it was necessary first of all to determine objectively the existing patterns of the total morbidity of various age-sex and social groups of the population as well as the extent of hospitalization and attendance at outpatient polyclinic institutions.

The main source of information on the morbidity under Soviet conditions is the sickness incidence rate of the population.

Numerous studies of the total morbidity rate and distribution in the population made in the Soviet Union in the first decade after the Revolution and particularly in recent years in connection with the 1959 census have shown in a convincing manner that it is possible to obtain quite a complete idea of the so-called "exhaustive" morbidity for the majority of nosologic entities by the sickness rate of the population coming to therapeutic-prophylactic institutions and that the initial records of medical therapeutic-prophylactic institutions are a fully reliable basis for obtaining information on the total population morbidity.

S. M. Bogoslovskii wrote that the "outpatient data for a sufficiently concentrated system of medical institutions (we may say this quite definitely) is a reflection of the actual incidence of disease of the population and therefore is reliable and quite suitable material for its statistics" (S. M. Bogoslovskii, *Statistika professional'noi zabolevaemosti (Statistics of Occupational Diseases)*, Izdatel'stvo TsSU [Central Statistical Administration] USSR, Moscow. 1926).

Somewhat later, approximately the same idea was expressed by B. Ya. Smulevich ("K mezhdunarodnoi diskussii o statistike zabolevaemosti i o zadachakh statisticheskogo issledovaniya SSSR v etoi oblasti" (An International Discussion on Morbidity Statistics and Tasks of Statistical Investigation in the USSR in this Field), *Vestnik statistiki*, No. 4. 1928), M. M. Mazur ("Ob istochnikakh izucheniya zabolevaemosti" (Sources for Studying Morbidity), *Sovetskoe Zdravookhranenie*, No. 10, 1960), and others.

It is also well known that the first large-scale study of problems of planning standards, the results of which were published in 1930 in the book *Metodologiya razrabotki norm lechebnoi pomoshchi gorodskomu naseleniyu* was made under the direction and with the direct participation of P. P. Kurkin on the basis of sickness rate data.

A very important condition for obtaining satisfactory data for the population sickness rate, however, is the choice of centers for making the study. All types of highly specialized outpatient and hospital medical care should be fully available to the population, and medical records should be kept in a well-organized manner in the various therapeutic-prophylactic institutions at the experimental centers.

Cities comparatively well provided with all types of medical care—Chelyabinsk, Kopeisk, Dneprodzerzhinsk, Rubezhnoe and Stupino, with total populations up to 1,500,000 persons—were selected as experimental centers for the present study.

These centers were deliberately chosen in different climato-geographic regions of the country. The study of the sickness rate of the population was undertaken at each of them for a full year, which permitted the detection of its seasonal fluctuations.

The sickness rate data, hospitalization rate, and attendance at outpatient poly-clinic institutions were obtained by copying the necessary information from the initial records of all types of therapeutic-prophylactic institutions.

Experience has shown that in the initial records of medical institutions adequate information is contained on acute diseases requiring immediate outpatient or hospital care and on chronic diseases with definite clinical manifestations com-pelling the patient to seek medical care.

There is quite a considerable number of diseases, however, which do not produce any serious difficulties for those afflicted, do not interfere with the usual rhythm of life and work, and therefore the current sickness rate does not reflect the actual incidence of such types and forms of disease.

The fact that not all these patients come to the physician in the case of mild illnesses contributes to errors in the organization of care of the population in the therapeutic-prophylactic institutions and in health education work.

In working out standards for the population requirement of therapeutic-pro-phylactic care for the next few years, and particularly in perspective, all diseases needing therapeutic-prophylactic care must be considered.

The availability of all types of medical care is improving every year. The level of health education of the population is also rising, which obviously will contribute to some increase in the parameters of the sickness incidence rate for mild and occult types and forms of diseases.

In general perspective, when dispensary care of the whole population is achieved in accordance with the tenets of the CPSU* program, provision should be made for additional therapeutic-prophylactic care for this group of diseases.

In consideration of these facts we have made provision for mass comprehensive medical checkups of the population along with a detailed study of the data of sickness rate, hospitalization, outpatient attendance and the subsidiary therapeutic-diagnostic departments (X-ray study, functional diagnosis, and physiotherapy) and laboratories.

Therefore, the primary characteristic of the method of this investigation (and its distinction from those of a number of previous studies) is the combination of the sickness rate data in therapeutic-prophylactic institutions with the data of comprehensive medical checkups of the population.

The main aim of these checkups is the detection of previously unknown, chronic cases for making the appropriate corrections in the total morbidity rate and distribution in the population in accordance with the sickness rates determined in therapeutic-prophylactic institutions.

The data of medical checkups also permit the correction of data on hospitalization, outpatient attendance, and dispensary care, and make it possible better to define the need for sanatorium-health resort treatment and the use of night preventoria, as well as service of therapeutic-prophylactic departments and laboratories.

The workup of the data of medical checkups simultaneously with sickness rate data of the same persons makes it possible to determine the incidence of chronic diseases for which the patients came to the physician but which were not confirmed on examination by virtue of the patient's recovery or correction of the diagnosis. These are very important data for determining the groups which need dispensary care.

Comprehensive medical checkups of the population are a very laborious task; therefore they were organized at only one experimental center, in the city of Stupino, where a detailed investigation of 10,000 persons was made by physicians in all the main specialties.

Experienced clinicians in all the main specialties from Moscow research clinical institutes of different categories participated in the checkups: The Institute of Obstetrics and Gynecology, the Central Dermatovenereological Institute, the Gertsen State Oncological Institute, the Helmholtz State Institute of Eye Diseases, the State Scientific Research Pediatric Institute of the RSFSR Ministry of Health, the Institute of Psychiatry, the Institute of Ear, Nose and Throat Diseases, the Tuberculosis Institute, as well as the Vladimirskii Moscow Region Clinical Institute.

Fluorography on every person, conducted with the apparatus and by the workers of the State Institute of Roentgenology and Radiology of the RSFSR Ministry of Health, preceded the clinicians' examinations.

---

* [Communist Party of the Soviet Union.]

For the purpose of clarifying the diagnosis during the examinations at Stupino Hospital, laboratory, X-ray, and other studies were made in all cases.

Therefore, the second characteristic of the method of our investigation is the correlation of the work of the Public Health Organization Section with that of a number of scientific research clinical institutes of different categories.

Stupino was selected as a center not only for making comprehensive medical checkups of the population but also for the purpose of determining many other corrective factors for the mass data collected in other cities.

Here the typical distribution of outpatient therapeutic visits, connected with the various nosologic entities among physicians of different specialties, was determined; experienced clinicians rendered expert opinions on the degree to which the thera-peutic-diagnostic departments (X-ray and physiotherapy) and laboratories (clinical and biochemical) were used; the need for sanatorium-health resort treatment, for dispensary care and for being kept in night preventoria was determined, and a study was made of the influence of the degree to which dental offices were outfitted with technical equipment on the work of the dentists.

Before all this work was done, the medical staff was increased and the medical institutions of Stupino were furnished with modern dental and other equipment.

Therefore, preliminary increase in the technical equipment of the medical insti-tutions of one of the centers with the aim of working out corrective factors for mass data and extensive utilization of experts, for which experienced clinicians of all the basic specialties were invited, should be considered the third characteristic of the method of the present study.

Above we have already pointed out that the study of the total morbidity of the population (by the sickness rate) in all cities selected was made on the basis of the initial records of all types of therapeutic-prophylactic institutions. An exception was Chelyabinsk, where the study was made on the basis of the form No. 25-c slips, which were completely alphabetized within the city limits, and this made it possible to eliminate duplication of diagnosis. In addition, the morbidity data were supplemented and clarified by special extracts of the necessary data in all special dispensaries as well as by the charts of those discharged from hospitals and extracts from death certificates.

In Stupino, Chelyabinsk and Dneprodzerzhinsk the study was made by the survey method; in Kopeisk and Rubezhnoe, by complete coverage.

The method of studying the total population morbidity (by the sickness rate) was uniform in all cities; therefore, as an example, we are describing the organi-zation of this work and the record forms for Stupino only.

In 1962 notes were made from the initial records of the therapeutic-prophylactic institutions of Stupino, of all cases of disease (admissions for disease), hospitalization, outpatient visits, prophylactic checkups and examinations in therapeutic-diagnostic departments on the population of four experimental therapeutic districts of Stupino

(Nos. 1, 2, 6 and 7), where over 22,000 persons lived (half of the city's inhabitants).

This was preceded by obtaining the entire population census within these districts from the house record books of the housing operation offices.

For each person who had lived in these districts in 1961 and had visited therapeutic institutions that year a special statistical card (see form No. 1) was filled out, in which all the necessary data provided by the study program were entered from all the types of initial records.

Among the initial records from which the information had to be taken were the following:

1. Outpatient chart of polyclinic for adults.
2. Developmental history of children.
3. Chart of pregnant women.
4. Hospital case history.
5. Fluorography record book.
6. Chart of tuberculosis dispensary department.
7. Lists of occupational checkups (of workers, draftees, schoolchildren).
8. Individual adolescent worker's card.
9. Records of nurseries, kindergartens and schools.

Specially instructed nurses of the therapeutic-prophylactic institutions in which this work was done were responsible for the copying of the material. At the same time, instructions on methods of copying the data from the initial records were prepared which were issued to all those taking part in this work. The nurses are usually well acquainted with the handwriting and signatures of the physicians working in a given institution, which permits them to read the record correctly and, most important, to determine each physician's specialty accurately. The completeness with which the copying was done was checked for each outpatient chart, case history, developmental history of the child, etc., by the scientific workers participating in this work.

In each of the medical institutions (or departments of the same institution) in which special medical records were kept a separate statistical record card was filled out.

The personal identification data of the statistical record card were filled in on the basis of the existing medical records with subsequent more exact determination of age and population group from census cards.

In the personal identification section of the statistical record card the following were indicated: last name, first name and middle name of the patient (in full), sex, age, population group and address.

The number of years completed at the end of 1961 and, for children under one year, the number of months completed were indicated in the column "Age."

For indicating the sex the appropriate letter (M or F) was underlined.

Form No.1

STATISTICAL RECORD CARD

No. of district _____

Sex $\frac{M}{F}$

Last name, first name, middle name _____ (in full)

Age _____ Address _____

Number of years or months completed

Social group–laborer, white-collar worker, pre-school child, schoolchild, pensioner, housewife, other (underline)

1	2	Date of visit and hospitalization		Hospital		7	Date of examination		Examinations			In physiotherapy			Expert's opinion			
Serial No.	Diagnosis (if the visit was prophylactic indicate its type)	Polyclinics	Home	Date of admission	Date of discharge	Specialty of polyclinic physician or name of hospital department	Date of appointment	Date accomplished	In functional diagnosis department	In the laboratory	In X-ray room	Name of procedures	Number of procedures prescribed	Number of procedures carried out	Name of unnecessary procedures and their number	Name of additional procedures and their number	Number of unnecessary or additional visits for this disease	Number of cases of unnecessary or additional hospitalization
1	2	3	4	5	6	7	8	9	10	11	12	13	14	15	16	17	18	19

The population group was indicated by underlining one of these groups—laborer, white-collar worker, pensioner, housewife, pre-school child, schoolchild, etc. If there were difficulties in determining the social group the instructions of the TsSU in the 1959 population census were used.

All diagnoses of consultations for disease and outpatient visits associated with them, cases of hospitalization and those sent to therapeutic-diagnostic departments and laboratories as well as prophylactic checkups from January 1, 1961, through January 1, 1962, were entered in the special section of the card.

In column 2 of the statistical record card and in the chronological order recorded in the initial records the diagnosis (or group of diagnosis) was indicated when the consultation was for disease, as well as the name of the type of prophylactic visits.

Of all the prophylactic visits the following were distinguished for analysis:

1. Physicians' regular house calls to child patients.
2. Checkups of pre-school children.
3. Dispensary check of seven-year-old children entering school.
4. Checkups of schoolchildren.
5. Checkups of adolescent workers.
6. Prophylactic checkups of workers.
7. Checkups of pregnant women.
8. Checkups of workers in the public dining room system and children's institutions.
9. The various certificates issued and examinations made when the patients were sent to the Medical Commission for Determining Disability and for sanatorium-health resort treatment.
10. Periodic checks of patients under dispensary care.
11. Other prophylactic visits.

In columns 3 and 4, on the same line on which the diagnosis made in the polyclinic or the name of the type of prophylactic visit was written, its date was inserted (and an indication was made whether it was at home or at the polyclinic).

The date of admission to the hospital (column 5) and the date of discharge (column 6) were written on the line on which the diagnosis was recorded.

If several visits were made for a certain disease, the date of each of them was put on the same line as the diagnosis and on the unused lines below it.

Subsequent records in column 2 were placed below the others, on the next unused line.

In column 7 the polyclinic physician's specialty or the name of the hospital department was indicated. In the polyclinic the following specialties were distinguished: 1) internal medicine; 2) surgery; 3) otorhinolaryngology; 4) ophthalmology; 5) psychiatry; 6) pediatrics; 7) dentistry; 8) obstetrics and gynecology; 9) phthisiology; 10) neuropathology; 11) dermatovenereology; 12) urology; 13) logopedics.

The date of an appointment by the therapist for some examination (X-ray, laboratory, functional diagnosis department) or treatment (physiotherapy, therapeutic physical culture) was written in column 8.

The appointment dates were determined from the physician's notes in the outpatient chart, developmental history of children, case history, etc.

In column 9 was written the date on which the procedure prescribed by the physician was actually carried out (for physiotherapy and therapeutic physical culture, the date on which begun), as determined from notes in the outpatient chart, case history, developmental history of children, etc. (X-ray examination, ECG examination) or from attached records (laboratory analyses, physiotherapy records).

In column 10 was noted the type of examination, which was conducted in the functional diagnosis department (electrocardiography, plethysmography, oscillography, etc.).

In column 11 the type of laboratory examination was indicated.

After completion of the copying work all the filled-out statistical record cards were arranged alphabetically. All record cards filled out on a particular person in different therapeutic-prophylactic institutions were collected and attached to the census card of that person. This made it possible, when coding the material, to eliminate duplication of diagnosis and simultaneously to determine which portion of the population had not sought medical care during the year.

After this, experienced clinicians, scientific workers of all the research institutes participating in this work, made an expert evaluation. Instructions on methods were also worked out for the clinician experts on the procedure to be used for the evaluation.

Each of the expert clinicians gave an opinion in his own specialty on whether or not there were sufficient laboratory or X-ray examinations, outpatient visits, examinations in the functional diagnosis department for the given person and for the given disease. An evaluation was also made of the degree to which hospital treatment and treatment in the physiotherapy department had been used.

In column 17 the expert indicated what additional examination in the functional diagnosis department, X-ray, laboratory (clinical or biochemical), fluorography or therapeutic physical culture department should have been carried out for the disease or at the time of the prophylactic visit, in his opinion. In the same column the number of additional examinations or appointments made for treatment were indicated.

The type of additional examination or treatment was also noted on the line on which the disease diagnosis or the type of prophylactic checkup for which the examination was made was recorded.

The number of additional outpatient visits was indicated in column 18; the number of unnecessary or additional cases of hospitalization, in column 19.

After completion of the evaluation the collected data were coded and then the coded record cards were sent to a computing center for statistical workup.

CARD FOR CODING

Last name, first name, middle name—————————————————————————

Personal identification data		For this patient the total number of										Prophylactic procedures				
				visits											laboratory	
					to the poly-clinic											
sex	age	population group	diseases for which patient consulted physician	total	therapeutic	prophylactic	house calls	cases of hospitalization	laboratory examinations	X-ray examinations	number of physiotherapy appointments made	physician's specialty (dept.)	type of visits	number of visits	type of examination	number of examinations
1	2	3	4	5	6	7	8	9	10	11	12	13	14	15	16	17

Prophylactic procedures													Visits			
X-ray room		functional diagnosis department		physiotherapy										total	including house calls	
type of examination	number of examinations	type of examination	number of examinations	type of treatment	number of appointments	number of procedures		Name of disease	Specialty of physician making the diagnosis	Date of first visit for this disease	specialty of physician	number	specialty of physician	number		
18	19	20	21	22	23	24	25	26	27	28	29	30	31	32		

Hospital			Functional diagnosis department			X-ray room			Laboratory			Physiotherapy				
				number			number			number			polyclinic		hospital	
name of department	number of hospitalizations	number of days in hospital	type of examination	in polyclinic	in hospital	type of examination	in polyclinic	in hospital	type of examination	in polyclinic	in hospital	type of treatment	number of appointments	number of procedures	number of appointments	number of procedures
33	34	35	36	37	38	39	40	41	42	43	44	45	46	47	48	49

Form No.2 (continued)

							Expert's opinion										
functional diagnosis department						laboratory						X-ray room					
unnecessary examinations			additional examinations			unnecessary examinations			additional examinations			unnecessary examinations			additional examinations		
type of examination	number		type of examination	number		type of examination	number		type of examination	number		type of examination	number		type of examination	number	
type of examination	in polyclinic	in hospital	type of examination	in polyclinic	in hospital	type of examination	in polyclinic	in hospital	type of examination	in polyclinic	in hospital	type of examination	in polyclinic	in hospital	type of examination	in polyclinic	in hospital
50	51	52	53	54	55	56	57	58	59	60	61	62	63	64	65	66	67

Form No. 2 (continued)

Physiotherapy											Outpatient visits		Hospital-ization
unnecessary procedures prescribed					additional procedures prescribed								
	polyclinic		hospital			polyclinic		hospital					
type of treatment	number of appointments	number of procedures	number of appointments	number of procedures	type of treatment	number of appointments	number of procedures	number of appointments	number of procedures		physician's specialty	additional visits	name of department	additional hospitalizations
68	69	70	71	72	73	74	75	76	77		78	79	80	81

The data were coded by experienced physicians.

A separate code card (see form No. 2) was filled out for each inhabitant of the experimental districts who had or who had not visited a medical institution in 1961 for therapeutic or prophylactic purposes.

All physicians participating in the coding of the data were first given instructions. In addition, each of them received written instructions in which a detailed description was given of how to fill in each column of the code card, and code designations were assigned to various items.

Aside from the code cards and code systems a set of analytical tables was sent to the computing center at the time of coding; these made it possible to obtain both the absolute numerical data and the necessary relative figures for all material copied down.

In copying the data special attention was paid to accurate determination of the nature of each outpatient visit.

First of all, it was essential to divide all visits into therapeutic and prophylactic. The frequency of the former was determined essentially by the morbidity rate and distribution for the population; that of the latter, by the official instructions of public health organizations and the degree of activity of the staff of physicians in the medical institution in the field of prophylactic work.

The visits for therapeutic purposes in turn showed substantial qualitative differences. Physicians in the appropriate specialties receive all patients coming for the first time with complaints of disease to the city outpatient polyclinic institutions. However, the same patients do not always make repeat visits to the physicians who first saw them. Some of them go to therapeutic-diagnostic departments (X-ray, functional diagnosis, physiotherapy) and laboratories (clinical and biochemical).

The patients are not always seen by physicians in these departments and laboratories. In physiotherapy departments the physiotherapist, a physician, usually sees the patient at the time of the first visit and at the end of the course of treatment, but the majority of visits by the patient are for therapeutic procedures which are always carried out under a nurse's supervision. The same situation is often observed for visits to laboratories and functional diagnosis departments.

It should be said that the frequency with which patients are sent to the therapeutic-diagnostic departments and laboratories depends to a considerable degree on the qualifications of the physicians in different specialties, who are immediately responsible for receiving the patients, as well as on the technical equipment and capacity of these institutions.

The planning of the duties of physicians and nurses engaged in the therapeutic-diagnostic departments and laboratories is usually connected with the capacity of the medical institution rather than the population census or morbidity. Therefore, in studying the volume and distribution of outpatient care for the population it is important to distinguish all visits (polyclinic and house visits) to and by the physicians who receive the patients directly after being sent from the registrar's office. This will provide the possibility of determining the relative proportion of therapeutic visits to physicians in different specialties within the total number of visits to physicians for treatment purposes, which will permit the determination of the correct proportions among them as well as the number of repeat visits for different diseases. Both will be connected, to a considerable degree, with the total morbidity rate and distribution and will thus show the objective pattern.

Above we have pointed out that the comprehensive medical checkups of the population were made in Stupino by sufficiently experienced physicians working in scientific research clinical institutes of different categories.

Checkups were made of half of the inhabitants of the experimental districts in which the total morbidity was studied according to the sickness rates determined in therapeutic-prophylactic institutions. Considerable work in explaining the significance and purposes of the checkups to the population preceded them. An article was published in the local paper by the chief physician of the city hospital, and he spoke on the radio. At the same time, district physicians and district nurses were entrusted with the task of giving talks in the apartment houses on the same topic and of giving out specially printed invitations for checkups.

The medical checkups were conducted on the premises of the city polyclinic, where a whole floor with the requisite number of departments for physicians was set apart for this purpose. The registrar's office was placed in the hall of this floor; the fluorographic unit was also set up here.

The results of the medical examinations were recorded on special medical examination cards (see form No. 3) by physicians in all specialties participating in this work. Beforehand, all the statistical record cards of the person, including records of the number of his visits to physicians, hospitalization and outpatient attendance for the previous year (1961), were attached. This made it possible for each physician making a checkup of a given person to acquaint himself with his state of health in the previous year.

Also appended to the medical record card were records with notes of the results of the preliminary fluorography and examinations in diagnostic departments (X-ray, functional diagnosis) and laboratories (clinical and biochemical).

Before beginning the medical checkups a series of conferences was held with all the participants for the purpose of giving them instructions; here, the methodological approaches to evaluation of disease and health were clarified and standardized. It was agreed that all physicians doing the checkups would consider only the forms of disease which required some kind of medical care.

During the course of the checkups and following them the need of each person examined for treatment in a hospital, sanatorium, night preventorium, or for being put on a dispensary record was determined by expert evaluation.

For the purpose of creating a definite degree of standardization in the evaluation and in the recording of it, instructions on methods for conducting the evaluation of the data obtained from the medical checkups of the population were specially formulated. All the data were then coded and analyzed at the computing centers.

It should be pointed out that the participants in this work were unable to get the entire population of the experimental districts to come in for the checkups. For the most part, perfectly healthy young persons and very old and sick persons were the ones who failed to come in for checkups.

In order to avoid distorting the normal age-sex distribution of the population we had to omit from the workup all members of a family in which at least one person had not had a medical checkup. For this reason, only 10,000 persons out of 13,000 examined were used in the statistical analysis.

Utilization of the data of mass comprehensive medical checkups of the population

M/F   Form No.3

MEDICAL EXAMINATION CARD

—   District No.

1. Last name, first name, middle name————————— 2. Age————————
                                                                     (No. of completed years)

3. Address————————————————————————————
                             (street, No. of house, apartment)

4. Population group: laborer, white-collar worker, pensioner, housewife, preschool child, schoolchild, other (underline)

5. Whether treated at a sanatorium during the current year

Specialty	Initial diagnosis	Additional examinations prescribed	Results of additional examinations (indicate abnormalities)	Final diagnosis	Conclusion of the board (underline which)
1	2	3	4	5	6

1. Internist			1. Healthy
			2. Needs outpatient treatment
2. Surgeon			a) by an internist
			b) by a surgeon
3. Pediatrician			c) by a pediatrician
			d) by a phthisiologist
4. Phthisiologist			e) by an obstetrician- gynecologist
			f) by a neuropathologist
5. Obstetrician-gynecologist			g) by a psychiatrist
			h) by an otorhinolaryngologist
			i) by an ophthalmologist
6. Neuro-pathologist			j) by a dermatovenereologist
			k) by an oncologist
			l) by a logopedist
7. Psychiatrist			3. Needs hospital treatment in the following department:
8. Otorhino-laryngologist			a) internal medicine
			b) surgery
			c) pediatrics
9. Ophthalmo-logist			d) tuberculosis
			e) obstetrics-gynecology
			f) neurology
			g) psychiatry
			h) otology
			i) ophthalmology
			j) dermatovenereology
			k) oncology
			l) logopedics
			4. Needs treatment in the following kind of sanatorium:
			a) general

Specialty	Initial diagnosis	Additional examinations prescribed	Results of additional examinations (indicate abnormalities)	Final diagnosis	Conclusion of the board (underline which)
1	2	3	4	5	6
10. Dermato-venereo-logist					b) tuberculosis c) neurology d) other 5. Needs dispensary care by:
11. Oncologist					a) internist b) surgeon
12. Logopedist					c) pediatrician d) phthisiologist e) obstetrician-gynecologist f) neuropathologist g) psychiatrist h) otorhinolaryngologist i) ophthalmologist j) dermatovenereologist k) oncologist l) logopedist 6. Needs hospital and sanatorium treatment 7. Needs outpatient and sanatorium treatment 8. Needs to be sent to: a) a home for invalids b) a hospital for chronic diseases

for working out standards of the need for therapeutic-prophylactic care by the population should be made with the greatest caution. The main errors which the investigator can make in using these data are the following:

a) the thoughtless addition of all cases of disease and pathological conditions found on examination, including those for which the population does not usually come to the physician, to the sickness incidence rate data, which unavoidably leads to a serious exaggeration of the figures for outpatient polyclinic and hospital care requirement.

b) the thoughtless addition of all corresponding diseases detected in the examinations and which had accumulated over a period of years to the figures for the sickness rate of the population for various chronic diseases calculated for a single calendar year. This can also lead to a definite increase in the figures for the standards, which may be sound enough for one year but are definitely too high for subsequent years.

For the purpose of clarifying the principles stated above we had to resort to illustrations, using data of the comprehensive medical checkups of the population collected in Stupino.

Statistical treatment of the comprehensive medical checkups of the population of the experimental districts of Stupino permitted us to demonstrate a number of very interesting characteristics of this type of information, characterizing the state of health of the groups studied.

For every 1,000 persons examined, 839.5 cases of different chronic diseases and abnormalities were detected which had not been recognized previously.

Through a detailed evaluation by experts it was determined that only 596.7 cases of chronic disease or abnormality per 1,000 persons examined require some form of therapeutic-prophylactic care. In 195.3 cases per 1,000 population the checkups failed to confirm the presence of chronic disease which had been recorded in the same persons during the previous year in their sickness rate data.

A study of the checkup data convinced us of the fact that among the newly detected chronic cases there was a predominance of comparatively mild illnesses, which did not lead to incapacity and did not cause any serious bodily disorders.

For example, 178.1 cases of different chronic ear, nose and throat diseases, including 39.4 cases of chronic pharyngitis, 48 of chronic tonsillitis, and 23.5 of chronic rhinitis, were detected per 1,000 persons examined.

These figures were approximately twice those of the sickness rates for the same diseases, which included acute and chronic forms of the disease.

The figure for the sickness incidence rate because of varicose veins was 1.6 per 1,000 population in the experimental districts, whereas in the checkups 26.7 previously unrecognized cases, mostly in the incipient stage, were detected.

From the checkup data the prevalence of benign tumors, thyroid disease, eczema and menopausal neurosis was found to be about twice as high as from the sickness rate data; hemorrhoids were found eight times as often in the checkups. A considerable number of cases of stammering and other forms of speech disorders (dyslalia and others) were detected.

The differences between the sickness rate data and those of the comprehensive medical checkups among the population for the incidence of dental and oral diseases were quite considerable. The figure for the sickness rate of the population for dental and oral diseases in Stupino was comparatively high and amounted to 340.8 per 1,000 population per year; however, it was demonstrated that 87.2% of the population examined had caries. In addition, 5.8% of the population suffers from various forms of periodontosis, according to the data of the checkups.

We have already pointed out that the main purpose of the comprehensive medical checkups was the determination of the prevalence of chronic diseases for which the population does not come spontaneously to the therapeutic-prophylactic institutions, in order to introduce corrective factors in the work load of the outpatient polyclinic and hospital institutions and to determine the additional number of those needing dispensary care, sanatorium-health resort treatment and admission to night preventoria.

From the initial records we determined the average number of outpatient visits per consultation for disease. [As mentioned previously, the term "consultation" used here refers to the total number of visits made for a single condition.] This objective index may be utilized for determining the additional volume of outpatient work required for the group of cases newly detected in the examinations. However, it would be an error mechanically to add to the sickness rate figures all the chronic cases newly detected in the checkups and calculate the additional outpatient visits from them. It is necessary, first of all, to determine the number of additional cases of disease in which the services of a physician are actually needed.

Above we have pointed out that in the checkups a considerable number of persons suffering from speech disorders was found. Of these it was necessary to distinguish only those who needed the care of medical logopedists or neuropathologists and to determine the additional number of outpatient visits by physicians from them alone. The great majority of patients with speech disorders should be cared for by teachers of speech correction, and they should be excluded from the calculations for additional outpatient service by a physician.

There are also many others, detected by medical checkups of the population, who do not need the full volume of outpatient care as determined by the average figures for the number of visits made for disease.

The forms of fungus disease (epidermophytosis and others) without allergic aggravation which are not clinically overt will hardly, in the future, require much outpatient work, because they can apparently be successfully eliminated by improving the living conditions of the population, extending dispensary care and developing health education.

Posture disorders in schoolchildren, *pes planus*, and rickets in infants can be eliminated through the development of prophylactic work with children and improvement of physical training in the schools.

In the medical checkups a considerable number of persons with hypermetropia was detected, including some in the groups of children. However, far-sightedness in children is well compensated by the inner reserves of the eye, and glasses are usually not prescribed for them. In middle-aged and older persons this power is lost, and for this reason glasses have to be prescribed for them and periodically changed (once every three to four years). However, in the future the degree to which the glasses prescribed correct the error of refraction may be checked through annual prophylactic checkups of the population of this age, and for this reason no special visits are needed for the selection of glasses.

It would hardly be correct to provide a full volume of dental care for the year for all the existing dental and oral diseases detected in the checkups.

These diseases have accumulated over many years, and if the entire work of treating the mass of carious teeth were planned for a single calendar year, the work volume of dentists determined in this way for the years to come would be definitely too high.

It would be better to distribute the additional outpatient work load for dentists over several years and thereby consider the average duration of usefulness of the fillings as well as the fact that the expansion of the outpatient dental service would contribute to reducing the frequency of complicated forms of caries requiring more work than the simple forms.

The fact should also be taken into account that many diseases detected during the checkups require chiefly hospital treatment with surgery, after which complete recovery usually occurs (benign tumors, chronic tonsillitis, cataract, and others).

A smaller volume of outpatient care should be provided for this group of cases.

The evaluation of the additional load presented to hospital care for the chronic cases newly detected in the medical checkups also requires considerable caution.

In Stupino the number of cases hospitalized for cataract per 1,000 population was 0.2; for chronic tonsillitis, 3.2, and for benign tumors, 1.8; the figures for those needing hospitalization, as determined by the experts from the group of cases detected, were, respectively, 0.8, 16.3, and 6.4.

Therefore the amount of hospitalization required for just the newly detected cases is increased four times over the actual amount; for chronic tonsillitis, more than five times; and for benign tumors, more than three times.

It would be a definite error to provide annually an additional amount of hospitalization equal to that determined from a single medical checkup.

Above we have already pointed out that patients with chronic diseases needing hospital treatment have been accumulating in the population for years because of a certain shortage of beds.

Because of an exacerbation of the disease some of these patients may be sent for hospital treatment every year or even several times a year, while others recover almost completely after being in hospital only once (usually after surgery).

The great majority of patients hospitalized for cataracts, chronic tonsillitis and benign tumors are in the second group.

In determining the amount of additional hospitalization needed, evidently it is necessary to adopt a different approach to different groups of diseases. For the group of diseases with a chronic course and those which recur frequently (peptic ulcer, hypertension, chronic gastritis, and others) annual hospitalization of all patients with adequately manifest clinical symptoms should be provided.

It is well known that even now many leading medical institutions hospitalize certain patients kept on dispensary records not only when they have an exacerbation of the disease process but also to prevent possible exacerbations, usually in the spring and fall.

Those suffering from diseases that are usually reliably cured after a single hospitalization should, evidently for calculation of standards, be distributed over several years in order not to increase sharply the need for beds, which they may not need in such numbers subsequently. Consideration should also be given to the clinical form of the disease and the age of the patients.

Of considerable interest for calculation of standards are data on the incidence of chronic diseases, unconfirmed in the comprehensive medical checkups, for which visits for medical care had been recorded in the previous year.

As we have already mentioned, the medical checkups of the population of the experimental districts of Stupino have shown that 195.3 cases of disease were not confirmed per 1,000 population. Usually there was failure to confirm chronic disease in which some kind of symptom of a temporary nature was masked under a serious diagnosis, or where there were diseases completely cured, usually by operation.

In the checkups there was failure to confirm 9.2 cases of peripheral nervous disease, 15.2 of neurosis, 15.4 of chronic gastritis, 15.8 of bone, muscle and joint diseases, 4.2 of skin diseases, 9.5 of chronic tonsillitis, 1.7 of hemorrhoids, all per 1,000.

In determining the work load for the dispensary service to patients with chronic diseases, evidently there should be an appropriate reduction in the groups of those under dispensary care, but outpatient care of these patients should be maintained at the current level.

It should also be pointed out that in determining the amount of hospital care for the remote future, consideration should be given to expanding sanatorium-health resort care, which will be free, as provided by the CPSU Program. Evidently, sanatorium treatment will be the natural continuation of hospital treatment, although these types of medical care will be interchangeable to a considerable degree.

In conclusion, we should discuss the problem of utilization of data on chronic cases, unknown from visits of the previous year, during the medical checkups for working out standards for the various planning stages.

In working out the standards of therapeutic-prophylactic care of the population for the next few years (1966–1970), apparently we cannot automatically add all the chronic cases detected in the medical checkups of the whole population to the sickness rate data and thereby determine the additional number of outpatient visits and cases needing hospitalization. The situation is such that during these years the public health organizations cannot provide medical checkups for the entire urban population by physicians of 12 specialties (as was done during the investigation), and therefore the majority of occult conditions remain unknown.

Even now, however, various population groups are undergoing medical checkups (children under 15, adolescents, those to be drafted, various occupational groups of workers, etc.) and for this reason it is possible to detect in these persons the early and clinically occult forms of disease requiring medical care and determine the additional volume of this care (hospital and outpatient).

In the distant future, when dispensary care covers the entire population, in accordance with the CPSU Program, during the course of which the early and clinically occult forms of disease will be detected in the entire population, it will be possible to utilize more fully the data of medical checkups for determining the additional amount of outpatient and hospital care required.

Methods of Studying the Morbidity and Determining the Hospital Bed Requirement of the Population in Capitalist Countries

In capitalist countries the planning of public health organization became the subject of discussion only after World War II.

Through a 1946 decree but actually starting with 1948, a national system of medical care was introduced in Great Britain. This matter began to be quite actively discussed in France. In the United States an investigation was made of the activity of local public health organizations for purposes of evaluating the efficiency of the American "health system," and plans were even drawn up for a system of regional medical care embracing the entire territory of the country and financed to a certain degree by government agencies.

All these measures required an exact determination of the economic practicality of the public health organization systems being planned and a clear-cut plan of medical care facilities for the population, and its financial and material basis by means of clarifying the actual medical care requirement by the population. In solving the latter problem public health organizers and planning economists ran into difficulties stemming from the very nature of the capitalist system.

In capitalist countries, because of the absence of a government medical system, the statistics of morbidity and attendance at medical institutions and hospitalization rate cannot be of a nationwide character. Almost everywhere to date the only criterion and measure for judging the population morbidity is constituted by the statistics for causes of death. The statistics for mental disease and tuberculosis, which are recorded by the corresponding medical institutions, as well as the statistics for epidemic and infectious diseases, recorded on the basis of obligatory reports, are exceptions. These data are published, by international agreement, in monthly bulletins and annual national statistical references and are sent to the World Health

Organization for official publication as part of the general procedure for all countries.

The degree to which statistics of causes of death fulfills its purpose may be judged by the following statement of one of the greatest medical scientists of France, the cardiologist Lenègre, which he gave to the press: "Unfortunately, in France statistics from records of civil documents do not offer any guarantee of reliability. At present, there are no statistics of the exact causes of death from cardiovascular disease. Practicing physicians, on the one hand, and physicians of the departments recording civil documents, on the other, should be required to bend their efforts to clarifying diagnoses of the causes of death and to a thorough review of the records in civil documents. They should be given the necessary instructions so that these records become a reliable basis for exact information about causes of death." (Lenègre, J., "Le dépistage, la prévention et la recherche dans les maladies cardio-vasculaires," Chapter V of *La Politique de la Prévention,* by J.A.Huet and J.Rivière, pp. 121–122, Paris, 1964).

The study of the population morbidity is being made to a progressively greater extent in all countries by government and public health officials and men of science. This has led to a search for methods of studying morbidity that are available to capitalist medicine.

The technique of direct interrogation of the population about all diseases occurring during a certain period was primarily such a method.

This very costly method, which requires suitably trained clerks and competent supervision by physicians, was widely used in the United States.

The abundance of public, private, insurance and welfare organizations, which now cooperate, now compete with one another, does not provide the requisite uniform basis for statistical records. (In the U.S. there is no compulsory insurance established by legislation; 70% of the population are covered by voluntary insurance, complete or partial (with certain strictly limited functions—for surgical operations, medical examination for diagnostic purposes, etc.), in various organizations— Blue Cross, Blue Shield, and others.) The President's Commission (1951), created for purposes of introducing order into the medical care of the American population, came to this conclusion (*Building American Health*. A Report to the President's Commission on the Health Needs of the Nation, Vol. 1, p. 29, Washington, D.C., 1952–1953.)

Therefore, the anamnestic method is the only way to obtain the morbidity data needed for various kinds of economic calculations.

It was first used for calculating economic losses from disease with incapacity, for which purpose the 1880 census was utilized. The interviews included questions and answers on diseases of the group surveyed.

Life insurance companies (1915) in cooperation with the Bureau of Labor Statistics, various sociologists (Sydenstricker, 1921–1924) (Sydenstricker, E., "Illness Rate among Males and Females," *Public Health Reports,* Vol. 42, 1939–1957, 1927), health departments of certain states and, finally, beginning with 1955, the U.S. Department of Health, took up the study of the morbidity by interviewing the population by the survey method. Study of the morbidity was made by the Federal Service Department in 1935–1937 in 81 cities with a population of 2,500,000.

In January, 1949, the U.S. National Committee on Vital and Health Statistics was created; this, in turn, created the Subcommittee on National Morbidity Survey in February, 1951.

In 1954 surveys were made of the cities of San Jose, Pittsburgh, Baltimore, Kansas City and others. They had the aim of checking the efficacy of methods used in previous investigations studying the morbidity.

Actually, there were weak points in both the organization and methods of this work in the United States and Great Britain.

First of all, the questioning was not often done by physicians. The person questioned was himself supposed to judge whether or not he had been sick, because those making the investigation suggested that "disease" be considered to mean what the "person reporting means by this in the ordinary, generally accepted sense." (Logan W.P.D. and E.M. Brooke, "General Registrar's Office, Studies on Medical and Population Subjects," No. 12, *The Survey of Sickness 1945–1952,* pp. 4–10. London, 1957.) Therefore subjectiveness actually played the principal part in this. Errors of memory led to errors in the date, in the duration of the disease, and to forgetting the doctor's diagnosis; for the most part, the patients remembered only the acuteness of one symptom or another. The time of the interview also contributed to this. Some investigations were made for two weeks; others, for months, and some dragged on up to $3\frac{1}{2}$ years with repeated questioning of the population. (Sydenstricker, E., "The Illness Rate among Males and Females", *Public Health Reports,* Vol. 42, No. 33,1927.) It was determined that the greater the interval between interviews, the more errors there were. This also had an influence on the morbidity figures derived subsequently.

In some investigations, chronic illnesses were not considered if there had been no exacerbation of them during the interview period. In cases that included several diseases, consideration was given to only one. All this gave rise to the need for careful checking, sometimes very prolonged. The clerks determined the last name of the physician who treated the patient or the name of the hospital where the patient had been hospitalized. Many patients had not come for medical care at all, though they mentioned a hospital. The records of the hospitals very frequently failed to confirm the reports of the persons questioned; there were also considerable discrepancies in diagnoses.

The laboriousness and time needed for checking were so great that in generalizing on the results of the study of morbidity in the six investigations made in 1928–1943, Collins, the well-known American medical statistician, was able to publish them only

Table 1

Investigation	Period	Coverage: number of man-years of observations	Total morbidity per 1,000 population (for a year)
of 18 states	12 months between 1928 and 1931	38,544	983
of 18 states	Not a full year between 1928 and 1931	4,236	850
Syracuse (N.Y.)	January, 1930–July, 1931	6,341	865
Cattaraugus county (N.Y.)	October, 1929–June, 1932	10,142	1,362
Baltimore	June, 1938–May, 1943	21,505	1,379
Hagerstown	December, 1921–May, 1924	16,517	1,081
	Total	97,285	

Table 2

COMPARISON OF THE AVERAGE MONTHLY MORBIDITY FIGURES OBTAINED IN SAN JOSE BY INTERVIEW AND DIARY METHODS

Diseases	Diseases associated with medical care			Diseases unassociated with medical care		
	number of cases per 100 persons per month		ratio of diary to interview data	number of cases per 100 persons per month		ratio of diary to interview data
	from diaries	from interviews		from diaries	from interviews	
All cases	14.5	11.9	1.2	54.4	23.7	2.3
Traumatism	2.5	2.2	1.2	5.4	2.2	2.5
Diseases and symptoms, total	12.0	9.7	1.2	49.0	21.5	2.3
Infectious and parasitic diseases	0.6	0.6	1.0	1.3	1.1	1.2
Mental disorders (including "neuroses" and "headache")	0.6	0.2	3.0	6.0	1.0	6.0
Eye diseases	0.3	0.2	1.5	0.5	0.2	2.5
Ear diseases and mastoiditis	a*	0.5	–	0.5	a*	–
Arthritis, rheumatic fever, sciatica, etc.	0.4	0.6	0.7	1.2	0.5	2.4
Circulatory diseases	1.2	0.9	1.3	0.8	0.7	1.1
Acute respiratory diseases	2.6	1.6	1.6	20.6	10.5	2.0
Other respiratory diseases	0.8	1.4	0.6	3.1	1.5	2.1
Dental diseases	0.6	0.3	2.0	0.7	0.2	3.5
Diseases of the upper G.I. tract	0.3	0.3	1.0	2.9	0.6	4.8
Diseases of the lower G.I. tract	0.8	0.5	1.6	2.0	0.7	1.7
Diseases of the G.U. tract	1.2	1.6	0.8	3.0	3.2	0.9
Diseases of the skin and skeletal system, anomalies	0.4	0.3	1.3	0.8	0.5	1.6
Other diseases and symptoms	2.1	0.8	2.6	6.8	0.6	11.3

a*—less than 0.05.

in 1955 (Collins, S.D., "Sickness Experience in Selected Areas of the United States", *Public Health Monographs,* No. 25. 1955).

In this work the following investigations, made in various cities and states, at various periods and by various methods, were included (Table 1).

For the purpose of checking the degree of reliability of the data obtained by the interview method in a special study in San Jose, the older members of the households investigated kept diary notes parallel to interview records. These data were compared (Table 2).

As is evident from Table 2, the morbidity data from the diaries are in all cases higher than the data derived from interviews. However, the analysis of both these methods, made by the physicians Allen and Breslow, showed that the additional information obtainable from the diaries pertained largely to "mild" illnesses. The authors write that such illnesses are of particular interest when they can be found to be the early manifestations of serious diseases, but this determination cannot be made in the short investigation period which has the general purpose of studying morbidity. (Allen, G.I., Breslow, L. and others, "Interviewing Versus Diary Keeping in Eliciting Information in a Morbidity Survey", *American Journal of Public Health and the Nation's Health,* 44, 917–927, 1954.)

The method of keeping diaries was not widely used because it is much more expensive than the house-to-house interview method.

In October, 1953, the U.S. National Committee on Vital and Health Statistics presented a report to the Surgeon General of the U.S. Public Health Service, *Suggestions for Collecting Data on Diseases and Health Disorders among the Population of the United States.* The report was prepared by the Subcommittee on National Morbidity Survey. This document was the basis of the principles and methods for subsequent investigations of the state of health of the U.S. population. The subcommittee recommended making a number of surveys rather than a single investigation of the whole country. It was pointed out that the interview method for determining morbidity is the main one; however, it must be supplemented by selected data from medical records or a complete medical examination, or a combination of these sources for obtaining reliable information on morbidity. (Woolsey, T.D., "The Concept of Illness in the Household Interview for the U.S. National Health Survey", *American Journal of Public Health and the Nation's Health,* 48, 703–712, 1958.)

In 1956, on the basis of a report of the Subcommittee on National Morbidity Survey of the National Committee of Vital and Health Statistics, Congress passed a law permitting the Surgeon General to conduct a long study of morbidity on a countrywide scale. In May, 1957, a study of the population morbidity for the whole U.S. was begun. The investigation is being made by the Department of Public Health Methods of the National Public Health Service and by all interested institutions. It is proposed to cover the 48 states and the District of Columbia in the study. In

1958–1959, a study was made of the morbidity of the members of 38,000 households, that is, about 125,000 persons; in 1959–1960, 37,000 households, that is, about 120,000 persons.

A study of the morbidity is being made by the household survey method. The entire country has been divided into 1,900 geographic regions. Of these 500 have been designated primary survey units. Each region is divided into smaller units, "segments," each with six households. The survey will be continued as follows: of the primary units under survey it is planned to use several segments in each for the study.

In this way, it is assumed, the sampling will be representative for the whole country (*National Health Survey Interviewer's Manual*, U.S. Department of Commerce, Bureau of the Census).

The interview method has been worked out by the U.S. Public Health Service. Specially instructed persons who are being trained by the Bureau of the Census are making the interviews.

The data obtained by the interview method are coded and processed in computers in the Bureau of the Census, after which they are analyzed by the Public Health Service. Appropriate correction factors are introduced to correct the survey errors. The intensive indexes are calculated for the population covered by the Bureau of the Census in any given year.

The reliability of data obtained in this way, however, continues to evoke doubt in the minds of some American authors. The physicians Allen and Breslow, and others mentioned above, write that the tremendous difficulty in interpreting the morbidity data obtained by the interview method, as Collins and many others have already pointed out, lies in eliminating the influence of memory errors on the analysis. The interviews were conducted personally, but there were cases where relatives living together answered for a member of the family, because the latter was absent at the time of the interview. Here, memory errors were simply unavoidable (Allen, *op. cit.*).

Therefore the results of the investigations made constitute the basis for annual reports by the U.S. Public Health Service (*Health Statistics,* Series B, No. 29, from the *U.S. National Health Survey* ("Disability Days"), Washington, 1961) and publications of data on morbidity in the official publications of the Department of Health, Education, and Welfare (see the annual publication, *Trends*) (U.S. Department of Health, Education and Welfare, *Trends,* 14, Washington, 1961).

Information on the activity of all hospitals published annually by the American Hospital Association and the Public Health Service serves as the source for the study of hospitalization in the U.S. It includes data on the number of patients admitted and discharged, the number of cases of death, as well as the average duration of stay in bed and the bed turnover. However, in these publications there is no information on diagnoses of diseases for which the treatment was given. The latter is given only in the hospital reports sent to the public health departments, from which they were obtained by various investigators who published these data in their works (Belloc, N.B., "Validation of Morbidity Survey Data by Comparison with Hospital Records", *Amer. Stat. Assn.,* 49, 832–846, 1954; McGibony, J.R., "Hospitals— Retrospect and Prospect," *Hospitals,* 38, 77–81, 1964).

Therefore, the data on hospitalization were included in the questionnaires when the morbidity studies were made.

Comparison of the interview data with those of the hospital records showed comparatively minor differences, both with respect to the dates and number of days of hospitalization and with respect to diagnoses (Table 3).

Table 3

	According to interview data	According to hospital data
Number of cases of hospitalization per 1,000 population per year	65.5	67.9
Number of days spent in bed per person per year	0.609	0.655

The investigators, in validating the data, concluded that the "information on hospitalizations obtained through the survey interview method is sufficiently accurate to use instead of the similar hospital data." (Belloc, N.B., *op. cit*).

Probably the authors came to this conclusion after considering all the difficulties of working with official reports. It should be recognized that the forms of hospital reports are better suited to determining economic practicability of hospital care than for satisfying scientific and public interest in the study of the population morbidity.

Problems of the quality of hospital activity are not reflected in the reports either. Various investigators are doing work according to their own programs, trying to derive the necessary criteria through personal direct contact with the hospital selected and its data.

Such is the work of the American physician, Block, done with the aim of analyzing various elements of care of patients in hospitals. (Block, L., "Analysis of Elements of Patient Care", *Mod. Hosp.,* 86, 72–4, 1956.) From his data certain indexes may be derived, for example, on therapeutic-diagnostic care per patient.

English sanitary inspectors, public officials, and scientists have also used the method of interviewing the population for study, first of the incidence of pathology (in 1851) and then of various types of morbidity (infectious disease with incapacity) and, finally, of total morbidity, gradually perfecting the interview and survey method. Data obtained from a number of such investigations were given timely publication, but they succeeded only partly and with various assumptions in clarifying the morbidity picture in certain population groups of England (Smith, Calpin and Farmer, *A Study of Telegraphists' Cramp,* Industrial Research Board, 1927).

This gave the medical statisticians Logan and Brooke reason to state that prior to the war in 1939 there was not a single source through which one might get a complete picture of the population morbidity in the country. (W.P.D. Logan, and Brooke, E.M., *The Survey of Sickness, London, 1943–1052,* p. 4, 1957.)

The most extensive survey of morbidity in England was made during the years of World War II. This investigation was entrusted to the Ministry of Information, which carried it out with personnel of an organization, Wartime Social Survey, which they created especially in 1941. The survey included 14 areas of England and Wales, where 2,500 persons were interviewed each month. At the end of the war the work was continued until 1951. Its data were processed in the Bureau of General Statistics of England and Wales from age-sex and occupational aspects and published periodically in the series *Studies on Problems of Medicine and Population,* as well as in the reports of the Chief Medical Inspector (1939–1948) (Ministry of Health, *Reports of the Chief Medical Officer for the Years 1939–1945* (p. 229), *1946* (102), *1947* ((141), *1948* (193), London).

In these tables the following data are given:

1) the number of patients per 100 interviewed who had had sickness or injury, regardless of the time;

2) the number of diseases and injuries per 100 interviewed;

3) the number of days of incapacity for workers and the number of days of outpatient treatment per 100 persons interviewed, for nonworkers;

4) the number of visits per month per 100 persons questioned (this includes visits to specialists but not dentists).

The analysis by diagnosis was made according to the International Disease Nomenclature and Causes of Death, as revised in 1948.

The Bureau of General Statistics workers themselves, who analyzed the data collected, declared, however, that they were insufficiently reliable, because they had not been collected by medical workers, and it was very difficult to check them. Therefore, when the need for planning free and generally available medical care for the entire population arose in the United Kingdom in accordance with the 1946 law creating the National Health Service, these data could no longer be used for determining the medical care requirement of the population.

The British National Health Service organized a permanent record of the population morbidity according to the sickness rate data and consultation rate at the offices of general practitioners in government service.

Such a record and workup were first made in eight medical districts over a period of three years beginning with April 1, 1951. Afterward, the scale of the study was increased. In 1956, 106 medical districts in various parts of England and Wales were included in the work of recording and analyzing the morbidity. In all, 382,829 persons were covered by the record. The population structure in these districts with regard to age and sex was not much different from that of the population as a whole.

At the present time this work is supervised by an occupational association of physicians, the College of General Practitioners, in cooperation with the Bureau of General Statistics. Even now some English data are of great interest for comparison. For example, the number of visits in 1951–1952 amounted to 3.36 per man; in 1955–1956, 3.38; these figures were 4.2 and 4.07, respectively, per woman.

The morbidity statistics according to sick rate data determined by general practitioners, however, do not cover the entire population needing outpatient care. A general practitioner takes care of his patients within the limits of so-called general medicine. Specialized care is given by the hospital. A general practitioner usually sends the patient to the hospital, where he is seen by a consultant in a general ward for incoming patients or in his own specialized department, where outpatient reception is provided.

In the past decade the number of visits to hospital consultants has increased by 32.1%. Initial visits have increased by 15.9%; checkups by specialists, by 134.8% (*Public Health Reports*, Vol. 77, 9, 735–744. 1962).

Hospital consultants are giving special attention to hospitalized patients, for whom they are completely responsible. In the outpatient departments they receive patients for whom they must make the diagnosis at the request of the general practitioner, at certain strictly defined hours. The physician who has sent the patient must often personally obtain the information about the diagnosis made by the specialist by phone or in writing or through a personal visit to the hospital. In general, there is a gap between the general practitioner's work and that of the hospital.

Nationalization of the hospitals made it possible for the public health service in Britain to utilize and analyze the annual reports of the hospitals. These data can also be used for obtaining at least tentative information needed for the planning of hospital construction.

In England in the 1950s many studies appeared on the determination of standards for the hospital bed requirement by the population (Brooke, E.M., "Factors Affecting the Demand for Psychiatric Beds", *Lancet,* II, 1211–13, 1962; "Children in Hospital. Studies in Planning," *A Report of Studies Made by the Division for Architectural Studies of the Nuffield Foundation,* London—New York. 1963; "Estimating Future Needs," *Hospital,* 56, 341–3, 1960; Farrer-Brown, L., "Hospital for Today and Tomorrow," *Brit. Med. J.,* 5126, 18, 1959; "Health and Welfare Services, The 10 Years Plan," *Hospital,* 59, 254, 1963; Hay, M.A., Tutor, M.A., "Bed Occupancy in the General Hospital," *Hospital,* 50, 145, 1954; "Hospital Needs and Population Trends," *Brit. Med. J.,* 5201, 789–791, 1960; *A Hospital Plan for England and Wales,* London. 1962; "How Many Beds the Hospital Needs," *Hospital,* 58, 581, 1962; "How Many Hospital Beds Are Needed?", *Hosp. Soc. Serv. J.,* 66, 1111, 1956; "Planning for Psychiatric Services," *Hospital,* 59, 123–125, 1963; Spence, J., "Hospital Beds for Children: An Estimate of Needs", *Lancet,* 68, 719–721, 1954). They are all based on the groups awaiting hospitalization. In the data of the Manchester Regional Hospital Council such a calculation was made by the director of its medical service, Mr. Marshall. The standard he determined was 10.5 per thousand.

The National Hospital Association has made the most careful methodological approach to the determination of the population hospitalization requirement; for this purpose it has made a special study in four different hospitals of the North-ampton district.

For any year the number of patients sent in for hospitalization multiplied by the average duration of stay in bed of the patients discharged from the hospital gives the number of bed-days which would be recorded if all those sent for hospitalization were put in bed. If this figure for bed-days is divided by the number of days in a year, the critical number of beds with one hundred percent occupancy may be obtained. From this the norm for the population bed requirement may be obtained with different degrees of occupancy (80, 85, 90, 95 and 100%).

In this investigation, 85% occupancy was used for the calculation of the norms. In addition, corrections were made in determining the norms with consideration of the season and the reserve. However, many English public health workers have warned that the norms obtained by the critical number method are too high.

In 1962, the Porritt Committee was created, which proposed specifically the following norms for hospital care (*Brit. Med. J.,* 53, 1178–1186, 1962).

Psychiatric beds	1.8 per thousand
Beds for patients with acute forms of disease	3.4 per thousand
Lying-in beds	0.6 per thousand
Geriatric beds	2.0 per thousand
Other (including infectious-disease) beds	0.2 per thousand

In all, the Committee provided eight beds per 1,000 population; that is, this figure was close to the norm adopted after two years in making up the hospital construction plan.

Being guided by all these calculations, the British Ministry of Health worked out a 10–year plan of hospital construction (1962–1971); however, an 11.5% reduc-tion in the number of beds through a shortening of the average length of stay in bed by patients with acute diseases and transferring a considerable number of mental and senile patients to home care was envisaged, after assuming a general norm of 8.48 per 1,000 population (including special beds) for the country.

The same situation occurred in the U.S., where in the preparation of the well-known Hill-Burton Act on Hospital Construction (1946) standard norms were needed for the whole country. In 1944, the government of the U.S. appointed a special board for the study of hospital care of the population of the country, which also analyzed the problem of norms. The commission did not consider it possible to use as a basis the data on morbidity obtained by interview.

The commission proposed a method for calculating the bed requirement on the basis of data on the number of cases of death in the hospital and the number of deliveries. The morbidity and mortality, it says in the report, are interrelated. A certain number of diseases precede the majority of cases of death; each disease exerts an influence on the mortality rate and the life expectancy. Therefore, the number of cases of death can be used as a basis for determining the hospital care requirement.

On the basis of the data on the number of cases of death in the hospitals and days of hospitalization the commisssion found that there are about 250 days of hospital care per case of death in the hospital. On this basis, they calculated that 0.7 of a bed (250:365) per year is used for each case of death per day. In order to determine the number of beds needed that would be occupied per year, the figure of 0.7 must be multiplied by the assumed number of cases of death in the hospital (*Hospital Care in the United States,* Commission on Hospital Care, New York. 1947).

On the average for the period from 1939 through 1943, the overall mortality rate figure was 10.6 per 1,000 population.

For the calculation, 50% of this number is used, amounting to 5.3; from this figure bed occupancy per 1,000 population would be (5.3 × 0.7 = 3.71 beds). Based on the fact that in 1944 the hospital beds were 74.8% used on the average per year, this would amount to (3.71:74.8 × 100) or 4.96 beds per 1,000 population.

This figure was also used as a norm for planning the construction of general hospitals over the whole country. Depending on the population density, it varied from 4.5 to 5.5 per thousand in various states and was adopted in 1946 (*Public Health Regulations,* Part 53, Public Health Service Publication, No. 93–A–1, Washington. 1962).

The commission also proposed the use of a figure derived from the birthrate as a norm for the requirement of obstetric beds. In the report, it was mentioned that if the average duration of stay in bed during delivery is assumed to be 11 days, then 11:365 = 0.03 of a bed is needed per year for one delivery. This figure will vary in accordance with the duration of hospitalization. If the bed index, derived from the birthrate, is used, then the figure derived from the death rate must be reduced by an amount corresponding to the proportion of all obstetric beds to be set up.

For patients with mental illnesses it is considered essential to have five beds per 1,000 population; for patients with chronic diseases, two beds; and for patients with tuberculosis, 2.5 beds.

The number of tuberculosis beds, according to this reasoning, should be $1\frac{1}{2}$ times the average number of patients with active tuberculosis per year shown by morbidity figures for the previous two years, or $2\frac{1}{2}$ times the number of cases of death from tuberculosis, according to the average data for the last five years.

On the basis of these norms the capacity of the hospital system and the bed supply for the population of different states were estimated. In states where the supply was less than the norm, a special subsidy from the Federal government was provided.

At the same time, the need for beds which had to be set up in the whole country, an additional 908,000, was also determined.

In 1951, for the purpose of "evaluating the effectiveness of measures taken for satisfying the immediate public health requirements of the population," the Presidents's Commission on Health of the United States was created, consisting of 14 members under the chairmanship of the eminent public health and medical education worker, Professor Magnuson.

The Commission attracted a multitude of physicians, lawyers, teachers, workers in insurance organizations and others to its work as experts.

The American Hospital Association's Committee on Hospital Planning in 1935, in a special report, had made critical comments about the practice of planning hospital beds on the basis of the existing public health agency recommendations: ". . . For many years the number of hospital beds has been calculated by two generally accepted formulas. . . first, from 2 to 3% of the population are sick at any time, and of these about 10% need hospitalization; secondly, in the cities five beds are needed per 1,000 population; in the rural areas, from 1 to 3 beds . . ." *(Report of the Committee on Hospital Planning and Equipment,* 740–752, Chicago, 1935.) At present, these formulas and methods of using them need revision.

Based on the experience of utilizing hospital beds in the country, the Committee recommended the following norms:

1) for cities with a large population and extensive suburbs, 5 beds per 1,000 population (according to the census);

2) for cities which serve as medical centers for large suburban areas, 4 to 5 beds per 1,000 population;

3) for larger cities, 3 to 4 beds;

4) for rural areas, one bed per 1,000 population.

After this, in 1938, 1943, and 1945, a number of interdepartmental commissions made studies of the hospital activities and worked out norms which usually were equal to 4–5.5 beds per 1,000 population. The most used method for calculating the norms for the hospital care requirement was as follows. The following were determined: 1) the percentage of persons hospitalized in the entire population of a given city or state; 2) the average length of stay in bed, considering the established interval needed for sanitizing the bed. The required number of beds was determined from the following formula:

$$\frac{\text{Population} \times \% \text{ of those needing hospitalization} \times \text{the average length of stay}}{\text{Average number of days of bed utilization}} \times 1,000.$$

In 1961 the combined commission of the American Hospital Association and the Department of Health, Education, and Welfare of the United States released a report "Area-Wide Planning of Hospital Beds" *(Area-Wide Planning for Hospitals and Related Health Facilities, Public Health Service Publication,* No. 855,

Washington 1961), in which a prospective method for calculating beds was recommended.

First, the average daily number of patients who will be hospitalized in a certain year (in prospect) is determined. For this, the actual total number of bed-days of hospitalization in a given year is multiplied by the ratio of the population census calculated for a certain year in prospect to the actual population census in the given year.

Keeping in mind all the calculations made in the previous studies and statements of the participants of the meeting, the Magnuson Commission approved the norms established by the Hill-Burton Act, but recommended that they be reviewed periodically in connection with the rapid progress of the treatment method and change in the morbidity rate structure (reduction of the mortality from tuberculosis, elimination of some infectious diseases, a possible reduction of traumatism, etc.).

Wishing to avoid a future increase in expenditures for hospital building, the U.S. public health workers recommended that the bed turnover be increased by reducing the length of hospitalization. Not wishing to lag behind the U.S. and Britain, France had published its plan for the reorganization of hospital care in 1946. It was recommended that hospital centers be created in various areas of the country (with 800 to 1,000 beds in each), with a system of subordinate smaller regional and rural hospitals around them (Thoillier, H., *L'hôpital français,* Paris. 1948).

It should be noted that in France not only the general norm for the hospital care requirement but also the distribution of beds in the basic specialties were almost identical with those in the UK, probably because of the same method of calculation (Table 4).

Table 4

Specialty	Country	
	UK	France
	Number of beds per 1,000 population	
Internal medicine	2.7	2.7
Surgery	2.2	2.3
Obstetrics	0.6	0.6
Infectious diseases	0.5	1.2
Phthisiology	1.0	1.0
Otorhinolaryngology	—	0.5
Beds for chronic patients and convalescents	1.4	0.5
Psychiatry	1.5	—
Oncology	0.04	0.04
Neurosurgery	0.03	0.03
Total	9.97	8.87

The "plan of hospital reform" published in the press, however, to date continues to exist only on paper.

With respect to the formulation of morbidity statistics, France constitutes no exception among the other capitalist countries; although, having a public charity organization independent of the government, which has 1,834 hospitals with 198,000 hospital beds and outpatient departments in its system, it would be able to organize sufficiently reliable morbidity statistics for certain population groups (the needy, the relatively poor, insured, etc.) on the basis of attendance and hospitalization at these institutions.

In 1960, the Institut National de Statistique et des Etudes Economiques, Centre de Recherches et de Documentation sur la Consommation, and the Caisse Nationale de la Sécurité Sociale started an investigation of the degree to which the entire population of the country needed medical care. It should be noted that it is the first investigation of this kind in Europe ("La consommation médicale des Français", *La Presse Médicale,* 70, 1329–1330, 1962.)

In the conclusions of the investigators officially presented at the press conference of May 21, 1962, in Paris, among the factors primarily determining the need for medical care, mention was made of the population morbidity for those of different ages and sex. (Even earlier, they were published in the press: Bosch, J., Rampp, J. M., Magdelaine, M., *Consommation*, 1, 3–84, 1962v Rampp, "Premiers resultats d'une enquête sur les dépenses de santé," *Etudes Statistiques*, Nos. 1–13, 71–97, 1962.) However, because of the absence of morbidity data it will be necessary to resort to mortality figures, adequately worked out.

In the investigation extensive use was made of the survey method. During the year a study was made of one family in each 4,000, and, in all, 3,239 families throughout the country (with the exception of Corsica) were included in the investigations. The data collected by the investigators constitute a list of all the medical services for the month preceding the investigation and the amounts paid out for bills, also for a month.

The medical services and expenditures were grouped as follows:
1) hospitalization;
2) visits and consultations of physicians;
3) electrocardiographic study and treatment;
4) laboratory examinations;
5) auxiliary facilities;
6) dental care; glasses and prostheses;
7) regular medical examinations (medical care in industry, etc.);
8) medical care of schoolchildren and students, draft boards;
9) drugs.

Consideration was also given to interruptions of work for disease and for confinement to bed.

The following were also determined: the social category and occupation of the head of the family, the number of members in the family and the type (city or rural), economic condition of the commune and the region.

The population reacted positively to the study: 92.9% of the families selected answered the questions completely, questionnaires about the payment for medical care were filled out completely in 90.1% of the cases.

The results of the study: the average number of visits and consultations per person per year was 3.54; 17.6% of the population saw their physician at least once a month. Almost four-fifths of all visits were cared for by general practitioners. The medical specialists saw the patients usually in consultations. Ophthalmologists and oto-rhinolaryngologists were responsible for the major portion of the consultations.

For each 100 persons per year there were 40.3 laboratory examinations; 2.7 out of 100 persons had at least one examination per month; 1.6 persons out of 100 received care from a nurse, mainly for injections.

Friends, relatives, acquaintances or neighbors gave a considerable number of injections to the patients.

The number of visits for dental treatment was quite high—1.8 per person per year. Finally, an average of one person per 100 buys glasses (for the correction of vision) once a month, and the number of purchases of other orthopedic appliances or prostheses is small.

Private physicians take care of all visits and most of the consultations. More than half of the vaccinations are given by private physicians also. The distribution of medical services according to age has shown that it is comparatively high in children under two and minimal at the age of 10 to 20; in the older groups it increases to a certain limit and drops in the population of advanced age.

Women resort to medical aid more often than men, particularly at the age of 20–30.

The volume of medical care as a whole is less in the rural communes. The effect of social-occupational position on incapacity because of disease is quite striking: it is equal to an average of 13.5 days a year for laborers, younger and older students. The degree to which various persons and groups participated in payment for medical care was determined.

Only 12% of the number of all visits, 8% of dental visits, 25% of consultations and half of all X-ray examinations were free.

Professor Péquignot, the well-known teacher of medical graduate studies in France and head of the Department of General Medicine of the Hôtel Dieu Hospital, and his assistants made a study of patients in public charity hospitals and their morbidity. To acquaint the reader with them, we are presenting, as an example, the work of Dr. Magdelaine, pupil and coworker of Professor Péquignot (Magdelaine, M. *Techniques d'étude de la fonction hospitalière* (Methods of Studying Hospital Activity). Paris, 1959).

To collect the necessary material the author worked out a questionnaire which the departmental treating physicians filled out while questioning the patients. In total, 5,500 questionnaires were filled out and processed. The processing was done with computers. The study was made only in the so-called general medical departments, that is, internal medical departments in the broad sense.

Patients treated in the general medical departments *(médecine générale)* of the public charity hospitals are among the poorest strata of the population. They are usually persons who have no fixed residence, inhabitants of slums, furnished rooms and attics, single old persons, illegitimate children, the unemployed and those having no means of support. They constitute two-thirds of the total number of patients. Very poor immigrants from North Africa, chiefly students, are in this group also.

In the hospitals there are beginning to be more elderly and chronic patients. The duration of stay in bed is increasing yearly. Half of the patients were hospitalized several times over the two years during which the study was made. Only 26% of the patients can be considered cured; 10% die; all the others are chronic cases, of which only one-third return temporarily to work; half of them need a repeat hospitalization.

A pamphlet of the French Ministry of Health, published May 28, 1963, suggests making the calculation of the bed requirement on the basis of data on hospital activity. As is pointed out in this pamphlet, the determination of the bed requirement depends on the population census and composition, its economic status, geographic characteristics, population morbidity, amount of medical equipment and the attitude of the population itself toward hospital treatment. Considering that some of these elements can be fully determined, while some are hard to estimate (economic status of the population, attitude of the population toward the hospital), those who wrote the pamphlet suggest calculating only three important indexes *(Techniques hospitalières médico-sociales et sanitaires*, No. 218. 1963): 1) the number of cases hospitalized; 2) the average duration of the patient's stay in bed; 3) the average occupancy of beds and departments rendering medical services.

These three types of indexes, which are interrelated, permit the calculation of the population requirement of hospital beds (general and special) in a certain area.

In 1959 in France the number of cases hospitalized in public and private hospitals was 7.91 per 100 inhabitants, as follows:

Internal medicine	1.57
Pediatrics	0.33
Other internal specialties	0.69
Surgery	3.04
Other surgical specialties	0.54
Gynecology and obstetrics	1.31
Other specialties	0.43
Total	7.91

(In the public hospitals there were 5.34 cases hospitalized per 100 inhabitants; in the private hospitals, 2.57. Quoted from *Techniques Hospitalières*, No. 218. 1963.)

The patients hospitalized in tuberculosis and mental hospitals and sanatoria are not included here.

It is thought that during the period 1959–1980 the average number of days in bed will be reduced to 10–20.

The chief sanitary inspector and assistant chief of the Seine Department of Public Health Problems, Bridgman, published the generally used method for calculating norms with all the preliminary calculations, and including in it the population of adjacent areas which gravitates to the same hospital because of certain conditions. (Bridgman, R.F., *L'Hôpital rural. La structure et son organisation.* Genève, 1954.)

Actually, when the hospitals are located near one another, the locality is thickly populated and transportation is convenient, the patients go to the hospital they prefer.

Table 5
AVERAGE DURATION OF STAY IN HOSPITAL BED IN FRANCE
IN DIFFERENT YEARS

Specialty	Total, 1954	1959		
		total	in public hospitals	in private hospitals
Internal medicine and related specialties		30.7	30.8	31.2
In this group:				
general medicine only	30.8	26.6	25.8	30.3
General surgery and related specialties		13.9	15.8	11.8
In this group:				
general surgery only	16.8	13.9	16.4	11.8
Obstetrics and gynecology	10.5	9.1	9.2	9.0

The sizes of the districts easily permit hospitalization in any hospital, so that the concept of a health district completely disappears.

How are we to calculate the population needing hospitalization?

For this the following calculation is made.

1. Each hospital is asked for information about the number of patients hospitalized during the year from other administrative districts.

2. The initial data which come in are distributed according to types of hospital (regional hospital center, auxiliary hospital center, branch hospital, local hospital, or rural hospital), which affords the opportunity of determining the number of patients living in the various districts and hospitalized in each of the types of hospital.

After determining, in this way, the total number of patients hospitalized in any institution of one district or another, the initial data are regrouped according to hospitals, and the ratio of patients hospitalized in a given hospital to those hospitalized in others is obtained; from this the population needing hospitalization in each hospital is calculated (see Table 6).

Table 6

POPULATION NEEDING HOSPITALIZATION IN REGIONAL HOSPITAL CENTER A

District	Population	No. of patients hospitalized in regional hospital center	Total No. of patients hospitalized in all the hospitals	Ratio of column 3 to column 4	Population needing hospitalization
1	150,000	8,500	10,000	0.85	1,275
2	40,000	800	1,000	0.80	32
3	50,000	600	1,500	0.40	20
4	—	—	—	—	—
—	—	—	—	—	—
			11,900		190

The figures in column 5 represent the ratio of all patients hospitalized in their own districts to those who selected a regional hospital center. Multiplication of each of these ratios by the population of each district gives the number of the population which can, if necessary, be hospitalized in the regional hospital center.

If the average occupancy is close to 70–80% and if the average length of stay in bed approaches the figure which is the norm for the given country, the index is regarded as acceptable and the hospitals are considered to fulfill their purposes and accomplish their tasks.

If the average occupancy reaches 90%, and the average duration of the patient's stay in bed is particularly low, evidently the degree to which the hospital is equipped is too low, and an additional number of beds needs to be set up.

Conversely, if the average occupancy is lower than 60% and the average duration is too high, the index is too high, and the number of beds in the hospital is too high.

After selecting the optimum figures for the average occupancy and the average length of stay in bed, one can calculate the number of beds needed for hospitalization of the population during the year.

In West Germany specialists in hospital care believe that it is essential to have the following data for proper planning of hospital beds (Gerfeldt, E. and R. Trub, *Das Krankenhaus und seine Betriebsfuhrung* Stuttgart. 1959).

1) the morbidity of the population and the number needing hospital treatment;
2) the average duration of hospital treatment;
3) the number of days the bed is utilized during the year.

The authors mentioned adhere to the opinion that 20% of the number of calendar days in the year must be set apart for sanitization, disinfection and repair of the bed.

In East Germany 15% of the population was hospitalized in the course of a year in 1953–1958; the average length of stay in bed was 30 days.

Based on these data, the population requirement of hospital beds is determined in the following way. Each bed can be set up 10 times during the year; therefore the bed requirement per 100 inhabitants will be 15/10, or 1.5, which will amount to 15 per 1,000 population.

If the number of days the bed is used is reduced to 18 %, as was done during periods of very great demand for hospital care, and the average length of stay in bed is reduced to 21 days, then 10.7 beds will be needed per 1,000 inhabitants.

For rural localities, where the population morbidity is lower and only 10 % of the population is hospitalized, 7 beds per 1,000 population are needed. In the industrial areas this figure reaches 14 beds per 1,000 population. At the same time, provision is made for the addition of 10 % of the beds for the hospitalization of infectious disease patients and 12 % for the hospitalization of patients with tuberculosis (i.e., of the total number of beds).

The data for calculation of the hospital bed requirement are taken from the hospital records regularly received in the public health departments of East Germany.

Therefore, in the capitalist countries which are best developed economically, the need for having data on the population morbidity for determining its norms of hospital care is fully realized. However, the tremendous complexity of the task of obtaining such data in a capitalist system compels the hospital organizers to resort to more readily available data on the number of admissions and discharges obtained from the yearly hospital records.

Therefore the Commission on Hospital Care which we mentioned previously, which worked in the U.S. in 1944–1947, had to formulate the principle that it is necessary to refrain from using data on population morbidity when determining the hospital care requirement (*Hospital Care in the United States,* Commission on Hospital Care, p.290, New York. 1947).

This Commission wrote: "The use of morbidity data for calculation of the norms for the hospitalization requirement simplifies the problem. However, study of the morbidity on a countrywide scale is very costly, laborious and lengthy. The study made over a number of years is not suited to present conditions. Moreover, even if the data on morbidity were exhaustive and fully suitable it would still be difficult to determine the need for hospital care by means of them. Opinion and judgement play a major part in the interpretation of the data."

Essentially the same has been said in the pamphlet of the French Ministry of Health and Population in its recommendations to use "practically significant" calculations without utilization of the morbidity.

The absence of overall morbidity statistics in capitalist countries is to be expected. It reflects the characteristics of their public health system.

In this respect the speech of the Minister of Health of East Germany, Elizabeth Schwartzhaupt, at the Third Session of the State Medical Council on March 21, 1963 is very characteristic; she noted the absence of overall morbidity statistics in the country and suggested the study of foreign experience in those countries where the appropriate attempts had been made (*Bundesgesundheitsblatt,* No. 7, p. 68. 1963).

Therefore we can speak here only of attempts, sometimes ingenious and costly; but proceeding from the attempts to introduce a nationwide system of medical statistics would interfere with the private nature of medicine in the capitalist countries.

Without having a reliable statistical basis, public health officials of capitalist countries must, in planning hospital and outpatient care for the population, limit themselves to imperfect methods, which reflect only the actual state of affairs at a given time, and which they try more or less successfully to adapt to the future by calculating for the population expected.

Standards of Therapeutic-Prophylactic Care of the Urban Population in the Field of Internal Medicine

The internal medical service occupies a leading place in the amount of work, its a group of diseases chiefly under the care of internists are shown in Table 7.

A group of diseases chiefly cared for by internists were analyzed according to the overall morbidity (as judged by the sickness rate and medical checkup data), hospitalization rates and attendance at therapeutic-prophylactic institutions as bases for determining the standards.

Incidence of Diseases Cared for Chiefly by Internists in the Adult Urban Population

The average intensive morbidity indexes (judged by sickness rate) for five cities of a group of diseases under the care chiefly of internists are shown in Table 7.

This shows the standardized indexes with the aim of eliminating the influence of differences in the age structure of the population in the cities being compared. As a standard the age distribution of the adult urban population of the USSR according to the 1959 census was used. The standardized indexes are somewhat lower than usual for this group of internal diseases, chieflly because of a reduction in the incidence of sore throats and colds.

As is evident from Table 7, the overall morbidity (sickness rate) of the adult population for this group of diseases is 486.2 per thousand.

Infectious diseases, whose study we emphasized, are the most prevalent—126.8 per 1,000 adult population (24.0% of the total number of diseases under the care of internists).

If to this figure we add colds, which are put in the category "ENT diseases" according to disease nomenclature (fourth edition, 1952), and infectious hepatitis,

50

Table 7

INTENSIVE AND STANDARDIZED MORBIDITY INDEXES OF THE ADULT POPULATION FOR DISEASES CHIEFLY UNDER THE CARE OF INTERNISTS

(averages for 5 cities)

Disease	Number of cases (sickness rate) per 1,000 adult population			Standardized indexes		
	men	women	both sexes	men	women	both sexes
Infectious hepatitis	1.8	1.5	1.7	1.9	1.4	1.6
Sore throat	51.0	45.9	48.1	49.8	40.6	44.3
Influenza	92.8	68.3	78.8	89.5	65.9	76.1
Colds	171.1	109.8	135.4	161.7	93.9	102.7
(Helminthic) infestations	1.5	2.8	2.2	1.5	2.9	2.3
Rheumatic fever	7.2	14.3	11.4	7.3	13.6	10.8
Metabolic diseases and allergic disorders	3.5	5.5	4.8	3.2	4.8	4.2
These include :						
Diabetes mellitus	0.5	0.6	0.6	0.5	0.6	0.6
Bronchial asthma	1.0	1.6	1.4	1.0	1.5	1.3
Respiratory diseases	50.4	34.8	41.6	51.2	33.6	41.3
These include :						
Acute bronchitis	8.5	9.0	8.8	8.4	8.5	8.4
Chronic bronchitis	13.8	7.9	10.5	14.3	8.0	10.9
Bronchopneumonia	11.6	8.4	9.7	11.6	8.0	9.5
Pulmonary fibrosis and emphysema	5.7	2.5	3.9	6.2	2.8	4.3
Circulatory diseases	44.6	70.0	59.1	44.5	71.1	59.7
These include :						
Cardiac valvular defects	2.1	3.3	2.8	1.7	3.2	2.5
Myocardial fibrosis from myocarditis	4.5	6.6	5.6	4.5	6.8	5.8
Angina pectoris	1.1	0.8	1.0	1.2	0.8	1.0
Myocardial infarction	0.6	0.4	0.5	0.6	0.4	0.5
Myocardial fibrosis from atherosclerosis	14.3	21.6	18.5	14.6	22.9	19.3
Essential hypertension	15.3	26.3	21.5	15.4	26.9	22.0
Digestive diseases	83.8	66.4	74.0	80.3	60.7	68.6
These include :						
Acute gastritis	15.4	13.5	14.3	15.3	12.2	13.3
Chronic gastritis	30.8	26.8	28.5	30.1	25.1	27.1
Enteritis and colitis	12.6	7.6	9.7	11.5	7.0	9.0
Chronic hepatitis and cirrhosis	1.6	1.8	1.8	1.5	1.7	1.6
Gastric and duodenal ulcer	13.5	1.9	6.9	13.0	1.7	6.5
Cholelithiasis	0.3	1.1	0.8	0.3	1.0	0.7
Renal and urinary tract diseases	6.7	17.8	13.1	6.7	17.3	12.7
Thyroid diseases	0.9	9.2	5.7	0.9	8.4	5.2
Other diseases	12.1	9.6	10.3	11.4	8.9	9.9
Total	527.4	455.9	486.2	509.9	423.1	457.4

which is included among "Digestive diseases," the sickness rate for infectious diseases is increased to 263.0 per thousand, and their proportion rises to 54.1%.

In second place are the digestive diseases, a sickness rate of 74 per 1,000 adult population (15.2%).

In third place are the diseases of the circulatory organs, 59.1 per 1,000 adult population (12.2%).

Essential hypertension (36.9%) and myocardial fibrosis (32.3%) are the most common in this group.

Respiratory diseases (sickness rate of 41.6 per 1,000 adult population) are in fourth place; of these bronchitis (46.7%) and bronchopneumonia (23%) are most important.

Renal and urinary diseases and rheumatic fever are in fifth and sixth places. They are followed by metabolic diseases and allergic disorders.

Industrial and occupational diseases, vitamin deficiency diseases and diseases of the hematopoietic system, intoxications and others are combined under the heading "Other diseases."

In the group of diseases chiefly under the care of internists, an increase, on the whole, was noted for the sickness rate with increase in age and the associated physiological changes of the body (Figure 1).

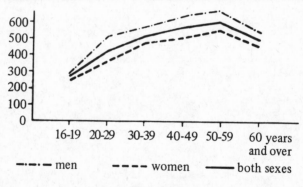

Figure 1

Average age morbidity indexes of the adult urban population for the group of diseases chiefly under the care of internists (number of cases per 1,000 population of the corresponding age and sex)

Reduction of the morbidity (477.5) at the age of 60 or more is evidently connected with a decrease in the sickness rate for sore throats, influenza, colds and other infectious diseases (except infectious hepatitis).

The sickness rate in men is higher than in women.

Study of the sickness rate for various nosologic entities (Table 8) shows that their prevalence is determined to a considerable degree by age and sex.

In the analysis of this table the uniformity of dynamics of the age indexes for such prevalent diseases as influenza and colds is also demonstrated.

It should be noted that the difficulty of differential diagnosis of these diseases does not permit a sufficiently exact calculation of the number of cases separately. Therefore, these two diseases are considered together here.

The highest incidence of influenza and colds is noted at the age of 30–39 (247.8 per thousand). Beginning with 40–49 the sickness rate for these diseases begins to drop, reaching 90.7 per thousand in the age group 60 and over.

The age indexes for the incidence of rheumatic fever (Figure 2) show a different appearance.

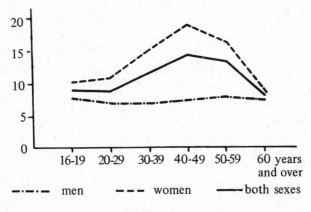

Figure 2

Average morbidity indexes according to age of the adult population for rheumatic fever (number of cases of disease per 1,000 population of the corresponding age and sex)

In adolescents (16–19) the incidence of rheumatic fever is 9 per 1,000 population. There is approximately the same incidence at the ages of 20–29. In subsequent age groups the sickness rate for rheumatic fever gradually increases, reaching a maximum in the 40–49 age group (14.5 per thousand). Rheumatic fever is observed more often in women. In the middle and older age groups the incidence of rheumatic fever in women is $2\frac{1}{2}$ times as high as in men.

The significance of rheumatic fever is determined not only by the sickness rate. Rheumatic fever leads to serious, irreversible cardiac lesions and is one of the main causes of invalidism in the youngest and most productive age groups. Over 50% of rheumatic fever cases have definite cardiac valvular defects (the data pertain to the population over age 16).

The rheumatic fever data must be supplemented, however, by cases of acquired cardiac valvular defects included in the category of circulatory diseases (2.8 per 1,000 adult population), because most of them are also the result of rheumatic lesions.

Table 8
AVERAGE AGE INCIDENCE OF DISEASES IN THE ADULT POPULATION
(number of cases per thousand of the adult

Disease	16–19			20–29		
	men	women	both sexes	men	women	both sexes
Infectious hepatitis	2.2	1.7	2.0	2.6	1.5	1.9
Sore throat	57.6	59.0	58.2	66.7	57.6	61.2
Influenza	61.6	46.8	54.3	82.1	73.5	77.3
Colds	74.6	66.9	70.6	192.9	103.7	141.3
Helminthic infestations	2.4	4.2	3.3	1.3	3.3	2.3
Rheumatic fever	7.8	10.1	9.0	7.0	10.8	8.9
Metabolic diseases and allergic disorders	1.8	1.7	1.6	2.8	2.3	2.6
These include						
Diabetes mellitus	—	0.1	—	0.3	0.1	0.2
Bronchial asthma	0.1	0.2	0.1	0.4	0.7	0.6
Respiratory diseases	21.7	15.5	18.6	31.6	18.9	24.6
These include :						
Acute bronchitis	5.7	4.3	5.0	8.2	5.8	6.8
Chronic bronchitis	2.1	1.7	1.9	6.0	2.9	4.4
Bronchopneumonia	8.5	4.7	6.6	9.1	5.0	6.9
Pulmonary fibrosis and emphysema	—	0.1	0.1	0.2	0.1	0.2
Circulatory diseases	7.2	7.5	7.4	13.8	15.7	14.8
These include :						
Cardiac valvular defects	1.1	1.3	1.2	2.2	2.9	2.6
Myocardial fibrosis from myocarditis	0.1	0.3	0.2	0.8	0.9	0.8
Angina pectoris	—	—	—	0.2	0.3	0.2
Myocardial infarction	—	—	—	—	—	—
Myocardial fibrosis from atherosclerosis	—	—	—	0.8	0.6	0.7
Essential hypertension	3.0	2.3	2.7	5.0	2.7	3.8
Digestive diseases	28.9	25.5	27.0	80.8	44.6	60.8
These include:						
Acute gastritis	8.6	8.7	8.7	21.8	11.5	15.9
Chronic gastritis	6.7	6.0	6.4	26.2	14.2	19.7
Enteritis and colitis	8.3	6.1	7.1	13.3	7.8	10.3
Chronic hepatitis and cirrhosis	0.4	—	0.2	0.9	0.8	1.1
Gastric and duodenal ulcer	2.3	0.6	1.4	10.5	0.8	5.1
Cholelithiasis	—	0.1	0.1	0.2	0.1	0.2
Renal and urinary tract diseases	3.7	5.3	4.4	6.2	16.9	11.7
Thyroid diseases	0.3	3.8	2.1	1.0	9.7	5.6
Other diseases	8.6	8.4	8.7	12.1	8.1	9.9
Total	278.4	256.6	267.2	500.9	366.6	422.9

CHIEFLY UNDER THE CARE OF INTERNISTS IN FIVE CITIES
population of the corresponding age and sex)

	Age groups										
30–39			40–49			50–59			60 and over		
men	women	both sexes	men	women	both sexes	men	women	both sexes	men	women	both sexes
1.1	1.5	1.3	1.8	1.0	1.2	1.6	0.6	1.0	2.1	2.2	2.2
57.7	48.8	52.4	36.9	30.3	32.9	21.3	21.1	21.1	9.0	11.3	10.7
110.5	83.2	95.2	110.9	69.3	86.3	104.6	60.9	77.8	49.7	37.6	41.1
192.0	125.1	152.6	181.3	111.3	138.7	143.0	78.1	104.1	75.7	36.9	49.6
1.6	3.0	2.4	1.6	2.7	2.2	1.3	2.7	2.2	0.6	1.5	1.2
7.1	15.3	11.7	7.5	19.2	14.5	8.1	16.4	13.2	7.6	8.7	8.4
3.1	4.0	3.7	5.8	8.1	7.2	6.1	10.5	8.8	7.0	8.1	7.7
0.4	0.2	0.3	1.3	0.3	0.7	0.5	1.5	1.1	1.1	2.2	1.8
0.6	1.1	0.9	1.2	2.7	2.1	2.4	3.2	2.9	3.3	1.9	2.5
43.3	31.4	37.0	72.8	37.9	52.0	98.2	50.6	68.9	100.9	57.6	71.0
9.2	11.3	10.4	10.7	10.1	10.3	8.6	11.6	10.4	8.4	6.6	7.0
10.0	6.4	8.1	22.7	9.0	14.6	35.7	14.3	22.5	36.3	18.1	23.8
10.7	7.1	8.7	14.0	8.4	10.7	16.9	11.8	13.8	17.3	13.5	14.8
1.9	0.4	1.1	9.3	1.6	4.7	21.5	6.1	11.9	27.3	12.7	17.2
26.2	37.0	32.3	65.4	87.7	78.8	132.4	179.6	161.2	183.5	203.3	197.4
1.6	3.9	2.9	1.9	3.7	3.1	1.4	3.5	2.7	0.8	3.7	2.7
3.0	3.7	3.4	8.9	12.6	11.1	12.4	18.0	15.8	12.3	10.1	10.8
0.8	0.6	0.7	2.1	1.6	1.7	3.9	1.7	2.5	2.8	1.2	1.7
0.2	0.1	0.2	0.6	0.2	0.3	2.5	0.4	1.2	3.0	2.2	2.3
1.1	2.3	1.8	16.5	17.4	17.0	49.6	65.0	59.0	81.1	84.7	84.3
9.3	10.4	9.9	21.8	33.2	28.6	40.2	69.4	58.0	50.2	72.4	65.3
92.7	68.4	78.5	111.7	89.0	98.1	107.9	87.9	95.8	68.1	60.9	63.0
14.6	13.3	13.7	12.9	15.5	14.5	15.1	12.4	13.5	7.8	9.9	9.2
33.9	25.1	28.8	43.4	38.4	40.3	44.5	42.1	43.1	31.6	27.0	28.3
11.5	7.2	9.1	16.1	7.0	10.7	13.6	7.4	9.9	7.8	6.2	6.7
1.5	2.7	2.1	3.0	2.4	2.6	2.9	2.5	2.6	1.5	1.8	1.7
19.8	2.4	9.8	19.6	3.1	9.7	17.6	2.1	8.1	5.5	0.9	2.4
0.1	1.0	0.7	0.2	1.5	1.0	0.8	2.1	1.6	1.0	1.5	1.4
7.6	19.9	14.5	7.5	21.2	15.6	7.3	19.5	14.9	13.9	9.7	15.6
1.3	14.4	8.7	0.7	9.4	5.9	1.3	4.7	3.4	0.7	1.8	1.4
12.6	9.4	10.9	15.3	10.8	12.6	12.5	9.4	10.6	9.6	7.2	8.2
556.8	461.4	501.1	619.2	497.9	546.0	645.6	542.0	583.0	528.4	446.8	477.5

In making up the population morbidity indexes for diseases of the circulatory organs the age factor is of decisive importance. While at the age of 16–19 the sickness rate for these diseases is 7.4 per 1,000 population, at 60 and over this figure increases by 28 times, reaching 197.4 per thousand. Many of the nosologic entities included in this class of diseases (coronary insufficiency, myocardial infarction, myocardial fibrosis) are not at all characteristic of younger persons.

Essential hypertension is the most prevalent of circulatory diseases. At the age of 16–19 the sickness rate for essential hypertension is 2.7 per thousand; at 20–29, 3.8 per thousand. Essential hypertension begins to acquire particular importance beginning with the 30–39 age group. At this age the sickness rate increases $2\frac{1}{2}$ times over that of the previous group. In the older age groups the incidence of essential hypertension reaches its maximum in persons aged 60 and over (65.3 per thousand).

The prevalence of essential hypertension among the population of various age groups and persons of different sexes is shown in Figure 3.

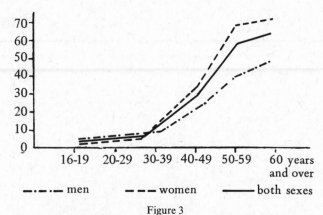

Figure 3

Average figures for the incidence of essential hypertension in the adult population by age groups (number of cases per 1,000 population of the corresponding age and sex)

As is evident from Figure 3, the relationships of the figures for essential hypertension in persons of different sexes in the various age groups are different.

In the 16–29 age group essential hypertension is found more often in men (3–5 per 1,000 men; 2.3–2.7 per 1,000 women). In the older age groups essential hypertension involves many more women. Thus, at the age of 40–49 the sickness rate is 33.2 per 1,000 women; for men it is 21.8 per thousand. The morbidity of women 50–60 and over is about $1\frac{1}{2}$ times higher (64.4–72.4 per thousand; in men, 40.2–50.2 per thousand).

It should be emphasized that the other cardiovascular diseases predominate in the female part of the population. Only coronary insufficiency and myocardial infarction, which are more often encountered in men, are exceptions.

In contrast to diseases of the cardiovascular system, respiratory diseases are comparatively often found in young persons. At the age of 16–19 the sickness rate noted for these diseases was 18.6 per 1,000 population. This figure, rising uniformly in every successive age group, increases by four times in persons aged 60 and over (71 per thousand).

The indexes in the category of respiratory diseases, particularly in the young and middle-aged groups, are determined to a considerable extent by acute bronchitis and bronchopneumonia. At the age of 19–29 the latter constitute 65–60% of the sickness incidence rate for this category of disease; at 30–39, 50%. At the age of 40–49 the proportion of acute bronchitis and bronchopneumonia decreases, but at the same time there is an increase in the proportion of chronic bronchial and pulmonary diseases (chronic bronchitis, pulmonary fibrosis, and emphysema). All forms of respiratory disease are prevalent chiefly in men of all ages.

Diseases of the digestive organs are widespread in all groups of the population, and their incidence increases with increase in the age of the population. Thus, at 16–19 the sickness rate for digestive diseases is 27 per thousand; at the age of 20–29, 60.8 per thousand. The highest morbidity is noted in the age groups 40–59 (98.1–95.8 per thousand). At the age of 60 and over the sickness rate figure drops to 63 per thousand, that is, it reaches about the same figure as at 20–29 years.

In adolescents and young adults about 50–60% of the sickness rate is from acute gastritis and enterocolitis. In the older age groups the proportion of these diseases drops, and those with a chronic course—chronic gastritis, gastric and duodenal ulcer, chronic hepatitis and cirrhosis—are encountered more often.

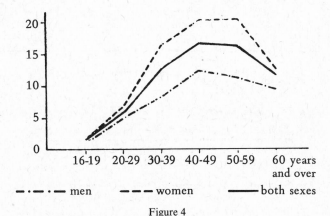

Figure 4

Average age incidence of hepatic and biliary diseases in the adult population (number of cases per 1,000 population of the corresponding age and sex)

Essential differences in the morbidity indexes of persons of different sex for the various nosologic entities included in the category of digestive diseases attract attention. Hepatic and biliary tract diseases are much more often found in women (Figure 4).

Gastric and duodenal ulcers, on the other hand, are more common in men (Figure 5).

The intensive indexes for renal and urinary diseases and thyroid diseases are higher in women (Figures 6 and 7).

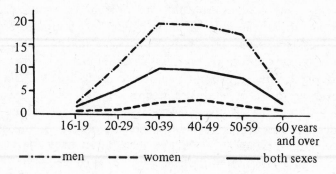

Figure 5
Average incidence of peptic ulcer in the adult population by age groups (number of cases per 1,000 population of the corresponding age and sex)

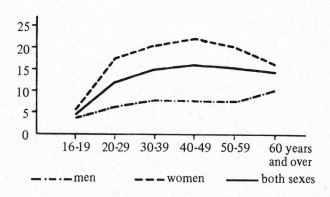

Figure 6
Average age indexes of renal and urinary tract diseases for the adult population with the exception of nephrolithiasis (number of cases per 1,000 population of the corresponding age and sex)

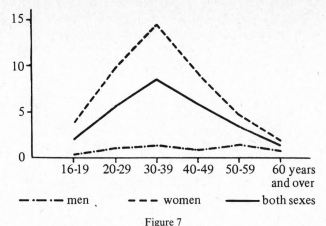

Figure 7

Average age incidence of thyroid diseases in the adult population (number of cases per 1,000 population of the corresponding age and sex)

Attendance at Outpatient-Polyclinic Institutions by the Adult Population

The average intensive indexes for attendance at outpatient-polyclinic institutions for therapeutic purposes for diseases chiefly under the care of internists are shown in Table 9.

In Table 9 data are given on the amount of outpatient medical aid actually rendered and the corrective factors made by clinical physicians on the basis of current clinical concepts of methods and times of treatment of the various diseases.

The number of therapeutic visits for diseases actually made under the care chiefly of internists is 1,198 per 1,000 population of both sexes over 16.

The rules and regulations for attendance according to age groups are about the same as for sickness rates.

Men visit outpatient-polyclinic institutions somewhat more often than women. Thus, per 1,000 men at the age of 16 there are 1,354.1 visits; per 1,000 women, 1,093.

The relationship between the composition of the attendance and sickness rate for persons of both sexes for various groups of diseases and nosologic entities (Table 10) shows that the highest number of visits was made for colds and influenza. In the group of diseases under analysis these conditions accounted for 39.9% of the total number of visits. Circulatory diseases occupy second place (17.7% of the visits) in attendance structure, third place in the sickness rate distribution.

As in the sickness rate structure respiratory diseases are in fourth place.

It should be noted that rheumatic fever is in fifth place with respect to proportion of attendance, sixth for sickness rate.

These relationships are explained by the comparatively high number of visits for

Table 9

ATTENDANCE OF THE ADULT POPULATION AT OUTPATIENT-POLYCLINIC INSTITUTIONS FOR TREATMENT PURPOSES FOR DISEASES CHIEFLY UNDER THE CARE OF INTERNISTS (number of visits per thousand of the adult population)

Disease	Average morbidity (by sickness rate) per 1,000 adult population	Number of treatment visits					
		total			including those of internists		
		actually made	added by experts	total	actually made	added by experts	total
Infectious hepatitis	1.7	6.1	0.2	6.3	6.1	0.2	6.3
Sore throat	48.1	89.9	14.3	104.2	68.4	7.8	76.2
Influenza	78.8	137.3	62.0	199.3	134.7	56.6	191.3
Colds	135.4	340.4	41.8	382.2	330.6	33.3	363.9
Helminthic infestations	2.2	3.0	1.0	4.0	2.9	0.7	3.6
Rheumatic fever	11.4	45.8	6.8	52.6	44.0	3.3	47.3
Metabolic diseases and allergic disorders	4.8	14.6	3.2	17.8	11.6	0.9	12.5
These include:							
Diabetes mellitus	0.6	1.9	0.2	2.1	1.7	0.1	1.8
Bronchial asthma	1.4	5.0	0.2	5.2	4.8	0.2	5.0
Respiratory diseases	41.6	88.0	9.1	97.1	82.7	6.8	89.5
These include:							
Acute bronchitis	8.8	16.5	3.4	19.9	15.9	2.4	18.3
Chronic bronchitis	10.5	16.4	1.1	17.5	15.5	1.1	16.6
Bronchopneumonia	9.7	24.5	0.8	25.3	23.0	0.6	23.6
Pulmonary fibrosis, emphysema	3.9	9.0	0.3	9.3	9.0	0.3	9.3
Circulatory diseases	59.1	211.9	58.8	270.7	193.3	19.7	213.0
These include:							
Cardiac valvular defects	2.8	12.8	0.1	12.9	11.7	0.1	11.8
Myocardial fibrosis from myocarditis	5.6	16.6	1.1	17.7	16.3	0.6	16.9
Angina pectoris	1.0	2.6	0.6	3.2	2.6	0.2	2.8
Myocardial infarction	0.5	3.4	0.2	3.6	3.1	0.2	3.3
Myocardial fibrosis from atherosclerosis	18.5	54.4	13.9	68.3	52.9	7.0	59.9
Essential hypertension	21.5	91.9	27.5	119.4	83.3	6.9	90.2
Digestive diseases	74.0	199.1	21.3	220.4	184.8	16.3	201.1
These include:							
Acute gastritis	14.3	31.1	3.7	34.8	29.9	3.0	32.9
Chronic gastritis	28.5	75.2	7.7	82.9	72.7	5.8	78.5
Enteritis and colitis	9.7	13.8	1.3	15.1	13.0	0.9	13.9
Chronic hepatitis and cirrhosis	1.8	6.9	0.3	7.2	6.8	0.2	7.0
Gastric and duodenal ulcer	6.9	34.5	1.9	36.4	29.6	1.7	31.3
Cholelithiasis	0.8	3.3	0.6	3.9	2.6	0.4	3.0
Renal and urinary tract diseases	13.1	33.0	6.7	39.7	22.2	2.3	24.5
Thyroid diseases	5.7	15.2	7.5	22.7	12.8	4.6	17.4
Other internal diseases	10.3	13.7	1.0	14.7	11.8	0.4	12.2
Total	486.2	1,198.0	233.7	1,431.7	1,105.9	152.9	1,258.8
In addition, for other diseases					350.7	33.0	385.8
Total per 1,000 adult population					1,456.6	185.9	1,642.5
per 1,000 population of all ages					1,126.0	143.7	1,269.7

Table 10

STRUCTURE OF THE SICKNESS RATE AND ATTENDANCE
FOR DISEASES CHIEFLY UNDER THE CARE OF INTERNISTS

Disease	Proportion of the sickness rate in % of total	Proportion of visits in % of total
Colds	27.8	28.4
Influenza	16.2	11.5
Digestive diseases	15.2	16.6
Circulatory diseases	12.2	17.7
Respiratory diseases	8.6	7.4
Renal and urinary tract diseases	2.6	2.7
Rheumatic fever	2.4	3.8
Thyroid diseases	1.2	1.3
Metabolic diseases and allergic disorders	1.0	1.2
Other internal diseases	12.8	9.4
Total	100.0	100.0

circulatory diseases and rheumatic fever, which are distinguished by a chronic and severe course.

The outpatient-polyclinic attendance for the population of the various age groups shows essential differences conditioned chiefly by corresponding variations in the sickness rate level.

The average age indexes of attendance of the urban population for diseases chiefly cared for by internists are shown in Table 11 and in Figure 8.

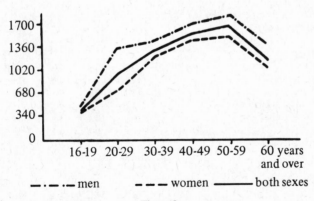

Figure 8

Average age indexes for outpatient attendance of the adult urban population for the group of diseases chiefly cared for by internists (number of visits per 1,000 population of the corresponding age and sex)

Table 11

AVERAGE AGE INDEXES OF OUTPATIENT ATTENDANCE OF THE ADULT
CHIEFLY UNDER THE CARE
(number of visits per 1,000 population

Disease	16–19			20–29		
	men	women	both sexes	men	women	both sexes
Infectious hepatitis	3.2	3.3	3.3	11.4	5.7	8.1
Sore throat	97.5	102.7	99.7	149.0	103.2	121.7
Influenza	63.0	48.4	55.9	133.2	155.5	122.7
Colds	139.6	135.6	137.7	565.2	259.3	384.0
Helminthic infestations	4.2	8.0	6.1	1.4	4.0	3.2
Rheumatic fever	17.7	34.2	26.1	27.5	37.2	32.8
Metabolic diseases and allergic disorders	3.5	4.3	4.0	10.6	4.7	7.3
Diabetes mellitus	—	—	—	0.6	0.5	0.6
Bronchial asthma	—	—	—	3.6	1.6	2.5
Respiratory diseases	37.6	25.2	31.1	77.6	32.6	51.4
These include:						
Acute bronchitis	9.3	6.7	8.0	15.3	8.3	11.3
Chronic bronchitis	3.2	2.1	2.6	11.8	2.9	6.9
Bronchopneumonia	14.8	7.7	11.1	28.4	9.9	17.2
Pulmonary fibrosis emphysema	—	—	—	—	0.1	0.1
Circulatory diseases	14.1	22.2	18.4	48.9	33.6	40.0
These include:						
Cardiac valvular defects	3.0	3.2	3.0	11.0	11.5	11.0
Myocardial fibrosis from myocarditis	0.2	0.4	0.3	1.3	2.0	1.6
Angina pectoris	—	—	—	0.2	0.4	0.3
Myocardial infarction	—	—	—	—	—	—
Myocardial fibrosis from atherosclerosis	0.8	—	0.4	2.2	1.8	2.0
Essential hypertension	6.8	12.9	10.2	20.9	4.4	11.7
Digestive diseases	53.7	33.7	43.4	243.9	86.1	152.6
These include:						
Acute gastritis	12.6	13.5	13.1	50.0	23.0	34.1
Chronic gastritis	12.2	6.1	9.0	78.0	27.7	49.6
Enteritis and colitis	11.5	8.0	9.8	24.9	8.2	15.1
Chronic hepatitis and cirrhosis	1.0	—	0.5	5.8	3.3	4.5
Gastric and duodenal ulcer	10.0	0.4	4.9	64.0	2.6	28.3
Cholelithiasis	—	0.2	0.1	3.6	0.1	1.6
Renal and urinary tract diseases	13.8	8.4	11.0	17.5	35.0	27.0
Thyroid diseases	0.4	6.1	3.3	2.2	19.5	11.9
Other diseases	10.0	6.9	8.2	15.4	19.5	12.8
Total	458.3	439.0	447.8	1,303.8	746.9	975.5

POPULATION FOR THERAPEUTIC PURPOSES IN GROUPS OF DISEASES OF INTERNISTS IN FIVE CITIES

of the corresponding age and sex)

Age group											
30–39			40–49			50–59			60 years and over		
men	women	both sexes	men	women	both sexes	men	women	both sexes	men	women	both sexes
7.2	7.2	7.2	3.0	3.5	3.3	8.8	0.7	4.1	22.8	5.1	11.6
129.7	118.3	122.1	86.1	57.5	68.6	45.4	43.8	44.4	24.3	22.1	22.6
191.8	169.2	179.2	211.4	132.7	164.1	225.0	102.4	151.4	79.7	30.3	45.7
553.2	355.0	433.8	521.6	331.4	404.1	433.4	220.2	307.1	206.9	84.1	124.6
2.8	4.0	3.5	1.6	3.8	2.9	1.1	3.5	2.5	0'9	1.1	1.0
23.6	57.7	43.0	31.0	91.6	68.0	69.7	80.0	75.4	14.9	30.8	25.8
7.3	12.8	9.7	17.6	31.2	22.5	17.5	42.2	29.3	11.6	30.6	22.0
1.3	0.5	0.8	6.5	1.2	3.3	1.8	4.9	3.7	0.4	7.7	5.6
1.0	2.2	1.7	3.2	10.7	7.7	9.6	18.7	15.0	6.2	7.4	6.9
82.6	72.3	76.4	168.1	96.1	124.2	253.8	89.2	155.9	176.4	101.9	128.0
14.9	24.1	20.1	19.6	26.6	23.9	16.4	20.7	19.0	16.7	15.9	16.0
13.6	12.3	12.6	34.9	18.3	24.7	65.2	16.3	36.1	42.9	17.3	26.2
23.1	19.3	20.9	40.5	26.0	31.7	54.8	32.7	41.7	57.8	29.5	39.4
1.5	0.1	0.7	26.8	1.0	11.2	67.0	7.9	31.9	32.3	26.7	29.9
82.2	126.1	106.7	212.0	317.1	275.5	437.5	605.0	537.2	651.6	589.8	609.6
7.1	19.1	14.3	11.6	19.0	16.1	7.0	30.3	20.8	1.1	17.5	11.7
8.2	9.4	8.8	33.6	38.0	36.3	34.8	50.1	44.0	37.1	32.3	34.1
4.0	1.5	2.5	4.1	5.3	4.8	8.1	2.7	4.9	1.6	4.2	3.2
0.2	3.8	2.4	3.1	0.1	1.3	10.8	0.3	4.7	45.0	12.0	21.7
3.9	7.2	5.8	54.8	56.6	56.0	166.3	180.4	174.3	229.3	206.5	216.7
36.9	49.1	44.0	69.6	154.7	120.7	156.6	298.1	241.1	253.5	263.4	259.5
301.9	180.8	229.6	351.1	255.2	292.0	338.0	224.1	270.1	146.6	129.8	136.4
30.5	29.9	29.9	30.1	45.2	39.4	39.0	34.5	36.4	16.3	24.2	21.5
100.7	67.0	80.9	135.0	102.7	114.9	134.0	109.9	119.4	64.5	54.1	57.5
11.6	9.9	10.6	27.0	12.3	18.0	23.8	9.0	15.0	11.5	9.8	10.6
3.4	10.9	7.6	12.9	10.9	12.0	8.9	10.8	10.0	1.7	3.8	3.0
110.2	10.9	51.8	93.3	16.2	46.0	90.0	9.3	41.9	25.1	6.7	13.9
0.5	7.5	4.5	0.8	4.0	2.7	2.0	10.5	7.1	4.8	2.7	3.3
30.1	42.2	36.7	34.2	58.0	64.2	17.2	45.7	34.5	17.7	34.1	38.9
1.8	42.7	25.0	1.0	32.9	20.2	12.5	10.5	11.3	1.7	3.1	2.6
16.2	13.3	14.5	15.8	22.0	19.6	16.2	11.0	13.1	10.0	6.8	8.1
1,428.4	1,202.2	1,287.4	1,654.5	1,433.0	1,529.1	1,875.9	1,478.3	1,636.3	1,363.1	1,069.6	1,166.9

From Table 11 and Figure 8 it is evident that the frequency of visits increases from the youngest to the oldest age groups of the population. Thus, per 1,000 population at the age of 16–19 there are 447.8 visits for therapeutic purposes; even at the age of 20–29 the attendance level increases by more than $2\frac{1}{2}$ times and reaches 975 per thousand.

The highest number of visits for therapeutic purposes is noted in the age group 50–59 (1,636.3 per thousand). At the age of 60 years and over this figure drops to 1,116.9 per thousand. For men of all age groups the attendance figures are higher than for women (except between 16 and 19 years, when the differences are slight).

In each age group of the population there are more visits for therapeutic purposes for the diseases that affect it most often.

In young persons therapeutic visits for acute diseases are predominant (colds, influenza, sore throat). In middle-aged and older persons there are more visits for the group of diseases of the circulatory organs and other chronic diseases.

For the purpose of determining the work load of internists it is essential to know the degree of their participitation in the care of patients suffering from infectious and other diseases requiring internal medical aid (Table 12 and Figure 9).

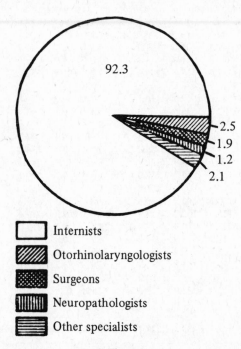

Figure 9

Distribution of therapeutic visits associated with diseases chiefly under the care of internists according to physicians' specialties (in percentages of the total)

DISTRIBUTION OF OUTPATIENT VISITS ACTUALLY MADE FOR THERAPEUTIC PURPOSES AMONG PHYSICIANS OF DIFFERENT SPECIALTIES IN THE GROUP OF DISEASES CHIEFLY UNDER THE CARE OF INTERNISTS

Name of disease	Proportion (in %) of visits to appropriate specialists						Number of visits per 1,000 adult population						
	internists	surgeons	otorhinolaryngologists	phthisiologists	neuropathologists	other specialists	Total	internists	surgeons	otorhinolaryngologists	phthisiologists	neuropathologists	other specialists
Infectious hepatitis	100.0	—	—	—	—	0.7	6.1	6.1	—	—	—	—	0.5
Sore throat	75.9	—	23.4	—	—	0.4	89.9	68.6	—	21.0	—	0.3	0.5
Influenza	98.1	0.3	0.7	0.3	—	0.2	137.3	134.7	0.4	1.0	0.4	0.3	0.5
Colds	97.1	0.2	1.5	0.9	—	—	340.4	330.6	0.7	5.2	3.1	0.1	0.1
Helminthic infestations	97.4	—	—	—	2.6	1.3	3.0	2.9	—	—	—	0.1	0.6
Rheumatic fever	96.0	0.3	0.3	—	6.7	8.8	45.8	44.0	0.1	0.1	—	0.6	1.9
Metabolic diseases and allergic disorders	80.3	4.2	—	—	—	—	14.6	11.6	0.5	—	—	—	0.2
These include:													
Diabetes mellitus	90.0	—	—	—	2.3	10.0	1.9	1.7	—	—	—	0.1	0.1
Bronchial asthma	95.3	0.2	—	—	—	2.4	5.0	4.8	0.3	—	—	—	0.1
Respiratory diseases	94.1	—	1.5	4.1	—	0.1	88.0	82.7	0.3	1.4	3.5	—	—
These include:													
Acute bronchitis	96.5	—	3.2	0.3	—	—	16.5	15.9	—	0.5	0.1	—	—
Chronic bronchitis	94.1	0.7	2.9	2.1	—	0.3	16.4	15.5	0.1	0.5	0.3	—	—
Bronchopneumonia	93.9	—	1.2	4.6	—	—	24.5	23.0	—	0.3	1.1	—	—
Pulmonary fibrosis, emphysema	100.0	—	—	—	—	—	9.0	9.0	—	—	—	—	—
Circulatory diseases	82.5	—	0.4	—	5.7	2.6	211.9	193.3	2.0	0.8	—	10.3	5.5
These include:													
Cardiac valvular defects	91.3	—	—	—	1.0	8.7	12.8	11.7	—	—	—	0.1	1.1
Myocardial fibrosis from myocarditis	98.0	1.0	—	—	—	—	16.6	16.3	0.2	—	—	—	—
Angina pectoris	100.0	—	—	—	—	—	2.6	2.6	—	—	—	—	—
Myocardial infarction	92.4	3.8	0.3	—	3.8	3.3	3.4	3.1	0.1	0.3	—	0.2	—
Essential hypertension	90.5	0.6	0.5	—	5.3	0.6	91.9	83.3	0.4	0.3	—	4.9	3.0
Myocardial fibrosis from atherosclerosis	97.2	—	—	—	1.7	1.1	54.4	52.9	—	—	—	0.9	1.6
Digestive diseases	83.2	15.5	—	—	0.2	—	199.1	184.8	12.4	—	—	0.3	0.2
These include:													
Acute gastritis	96.2	3.0	—	—	—	0.8	31.1	29.9	1.0	—	—	—	—
Chronic gastritis	96.8	1.7	—	—	0.1	1.4	75.2	72.7	1.4	—	—	0.1	1.0
Enteritis and colitis	94.6	4.6	—	—	—	0.8	13.8	13.8	0.7	—	—	—	0.1
Chronic hepatitis, cirrhosis	99.3	0.7	—	—	—	—	6.9	6.8	0.1	—	—	—	—
Gastric and duodenal ulcer	85.8	14.2	—	—	—	—	34.5	29.6	4.9	—	—	—	—
Cholelithiasis	78.9	21.1	—	—	0.7	—	3.3	2.6	0.7	—	—	0.1	—
Renal and urinary tract diseases	61.5	20.4	1.5	—	3.6	17.4	33.8	22.2	4.6	0.2	—	0.5	6.1
Thyroid diseases	83.6	8.8	1.5	—	—	2.5	15.2	12.8	1.3	—	—	—	0.4
Other internal diseases	82.6	6.3	—	—	11.1	—	13.7	11.6	0.4	—	—	0.7	0.3
Total	92.3	1.9	2.5	0.6	1.2	1.5	1,198.0	1,105.9	23.2	29.7	7.0	14.2	18.0

The great majority of patients' visits are under the care of internists (92.3%). Physicians in other specialities do not participate much (7.7%) in therapeutic-consultation work. As might have been expected, surgeons participate most often in taking care of patients suffering from digestive diseases. Thus surgeons take care of 21.1% of visits for cholelithiasis, 14.2% for gastric and duodenal ulcers, 20.4% for renal and urinary tract diseases. The otorhinolaryngologist receives 23.4% of the visits for sore throat. Neuropathologists take care of 5.3% of the visits for essential hypertension.

The work load of internists in outpatient-polyclinic care of the adult population is not determined solely by the therapeutic-prophylactic care given for the diseases listed.

It is known that frequently patients with diseases which do not always correspond to the internist's specialty are seen by internists. Usually these are patients with diseases of the nervous system, nasopharynx and pharynx, muscles, bones and joints. For determination of the work load of internists we also took into account all the outpatient visits which they accepted, even those for diseases outside their specialty.

Therefore the total number of visits actually made by internists with the existing morbidity level (judged by sickness rate) is 1,456.6 per 1,000 population over 16, including 1,105.9 for the group of diseases chiefly under the care of internists and 350.7 for other diseases. Of the total number of all visits to internists for therapeutic purposes, 77% were in the group chiefly under their care, 23% for other diseases.

In calculating per 1,000 population (including children), the total number of internists' visits for all diseases is 1,126.

While the indexes for visits to internists for internal diseases may be considered relatively constant, the indexes for visits for other diseases depend largely on the degree of specialization of the medical care and its availability.

At the same time, it would be incorrect to suppose that further development of specialized care would free district physicians from having to receive patients of a category other than internal medical.

Consultations by internists are often needed also for giving regular treatment to patients consulting physicians in other specialties.

Through the evaluation of the data of outpatient care of the population by experts it was determined that the number of therapeutic visits for almost all diseases chiefly under the care of district internists is too low.

The experts recommended that 233.7 visits be added for every 1,000 of the adult population, of which 152.9 should be under the care of internists and 80.8 under the care of physicians in other specialties.

The highest number of additional visits by district physicians is recommended for cases of influenza; by other specialists, for essential hypertension, renal and urinary tract diseases, thyroid diseases and sore throat (consultations).

DISTRIBUTION OF OUTPATIENT VISITS FOR THERAPEUTIC PURPOSES AMONG PHYSICIANS OF VARIOUS SPECIALTIES (actually made plus those added by the experts) FOR THE GROUP OF DISEASES CHIEFLY UNDER THE CARE OF INTERNISTS

Name of disease	Proportion (in %) of visits to appropriate specialists						Number of visits per 1,000 adult population						
	internists	surgeons	otorhinolaryngologists	phthisiologists	neuropathologists	other specialists	Total	internists	surgeons	otorhinolaryngologists	phthisiologists	neuropathologists	other specialists
Infectious hepatitis	100.0	—	—	—	—	—	6.3	6.3	—	—	—	—	—
Sore throat	73.2	—	25.5	—	—	1.3	104.2	76.2	—	26.6	—	—	1.4
Influenza	96.0	0.3	1.4	0.3	0.8	1.2	199.3	191.3	0.6	2.8	0.5	1.7	2.4
Colds	95.2	0.2	2.4	1.0	0.3	0.9	382.2	363.9	0.7	9.2	3.7	1.4	3.3
Helminthic infestations	90.0	—	—	—	7.5	2.5	4.0	3.6	—	—	—	0.3	0.1
Rheumatic fever	89.9	0.2	1.0	—	4.1	4.8	52.6	47.3	0.1	0.5	—	2.2	2.5
Metabolic diseases and allergic disorders	70.8	3.9	—	—	10.1	15.2	17.8	12.5	0.6	—	—	1.4	3.3
These include:													
Diabetes mellitus	85.7	—	—	—	4.8	9.5	2.1	1.8	—	—	—	0.1	0.1
Bronchial asthma	96.2	—	—	—	1.9	1.9	5.2	5.0	—	—	—	0.1	0.1
Respiratory diseases	92.3	0.3	2.2	0.4	0.4	0.5	97.1	89.5	0.3	2.2	4.1	0.4	0.6
These include:													
Acute bronchitis	92.0	—	6.0	0.5	0.5	1.0	19.9	18.3	—	1.2	0.1	0.1	0.2
Chronic bronchitis	94.8	0.6	2.9	1.7	—	—	17.5	16.6	0.1	0.5	0.3	—	—
Bronchopneumonia	93.3	—	1.6	4.3	—	0.8	25.3	23.6	—	0.4	1.1	—	0.2
Pulmonary fibrosis, emphysema	100.0	—	—	—	—	—	9.3	9.3	—	—	—	—	—
Circulatory diseases	78.6	1.0	0.5	0.1	8.6	11.2	270.7	213.0	2.7	1.2	0.2	23.4	30.2
These include:													
Cardiac valvular defects	95.1	1.1	—	—	1.7	8.5	12.9	11.8	0.2	—	—	0.3	1.1
Myocardial fibrosis from myocarditis	95.5	—	—	—	3.1	1.7	17.7	16.9	—	—	—	0.1	0.3
Angina pectoris	87.5	—	3.1	—	5.5	6.3	3.2	2.8	—	0.1	—	0.2	0.2
Myocardial infarction	91.7	2.8	—	0.2	0.5	—	3.6	3.3	0.1	—	0.2	—	—
Essential hypertension	75.5	0.3	0.3	—	7.3	16.4	119.4	90.2	0.4	0.3	—	8.7	19.6
Myocardial fibrosis from atherosclerosis	87.7	0.1	0.7	—	5.4	6.1	68.3	59.9	0.1	0.5	—	3.7	4.1
Digestive diseases	91.2	6.0	—	—	0.5	2.3	220.4	201.1	13.3	—	—	1.0	5.0
These include:													
Acute gastritis	94.5	3.2	—	—	0.6	2.3	34.8	32.9	1.1	—	—	—	0.8
Chronic gastritis	94.7	1.9	—	—	0.7	2.8	82.9	78.5	1.6	—	—	0.6	2.3
Enteritis and colitis	92.0	5.3	—	—	—	2.0	15.1	13.9	0.8	—	—	—	0.3
Chronic hepatitis, cirrhosis	97.2	1.4	—	—	—	1.4	7.0	7.0	0.1	—	—	—	0.1
Gastric and duodenal ulcer	86.0	14.0	—	—	0.8	—	36.4	31.3	5.1	—	—	0.3	—
Cholelithiasis	76.9	20.5	—	—	—	2.6	3.9	3.0	0.8	—	—	—	0.1
Renal and urinary tract	61.7	16.9	—	—	10.0	20.6	39.7	24.5	6.7	—	—	0.3	8.2
Thyroid diseases	76.6	9.7	0.9	—	5.3	7.5	22.7	17.4	2.2	0.2	—	1.2	1.7
Other diseases	75.7	8.6	1.4	—	—	4.3	14.7	12.2	1.3	0.1	—	0.7	0.4
Total	87.9	2.0	3.0	0.6	2.4	4.1	1,431.1	1,258.8	28.3	42.8	8.5	34.0	59.3

Table 14

AVERAGE NUMBER OF THERAPEUTIC VISITS PER DISEASE ACCORDING TO
THE VARIOUS NOSOLOGIC ENTITIES

Disease	Average number of therapeutic visits per disease			
	actually accomplished		according to expert evaluation	
	by all specialists	of these, the number by the internist	by all specialists	of these, the number by the internist
Infectious hepatitis	3.6	3.6	3.7	3.7
Sore throat	1.9	1.4	2.2	1.6
Influenza	1.7	1.7	2.5	2.4
Colds	2.5	2.4	2.8	2.7
Helminthic infestations	1.4	1.3	1.8	1.6
Rheumatic fever	4.2	3.9	4.6	4.2
Metabolic diseases and allergic disorders	3.0	2.4	3.7	2.6
These include:				
Diabetes mellitus	3.2	2.8	3.5	3.0
Bronchial asthma	3.6	3.4	3.7	3.6
Respiratory diseases	2.1	2.0	2.3	2.2
These include:				
Acute bronchitis	1.9	1.8	2.3	2.1
Chronic bronchitis	1.6	1.5	1.7	1.6
Bronchopneumonia	2.5	2.4	2.6	2.4
Pulmonary fibrosis, emphysema	2.3	2.3	2.4	2.4
Circulatory diseases	3.6	3.3	4.6	3.6
These include:				
Cardiac valvular defects	4.6	4.2	4.6	4.2
Myocardial fibrosis from myocarditis	3.2	2.9	3.2	3.0
Angina pectoris	2.6	2.5	3.2	2.8
Myocardial infarction	6.8	6.2	7.2	6.6
Essential hypertension	4.3	3.9	5.6	4.2
Myocardial fibrosis from atherosclerosis	2.9	2.8	3.7	3.2
Digestive diseases	2.7	2.5	3.0	2.7
Acute gastritis	2.2	2.1	2.4	2.3
Chronic gastritis	2.6	2.5	2.9	2.7
Enteritis and colitis	1.4	1.3	1.6	1.4
Chronic hepatitis and cirrhosis	3.8	3.7	4.0	3.9
Gastric and duodenal ulcers	5.0	4.3	5.3	4.5
Cholelithiasis	4.1	3.3	4.9	3.7
Renal and urinary tract diseases	2.5	1.7	3.0	1.9
Thyroid diseases	2.7	2.2	4.0	3.0
Average for the whole group of diseases	2.5	2.3	2.9	2.6

The distribution of outpatient visits among physicians in the various specialties with consideration of the corrective factors introduced by the experts is shown in Table 13.

The proportion of visits by internists after the corrections made by the experts dropped from 92.3 to 87.9%; on the other hand, the proportion of visits by physicians in other specialties increased. The proportion of neuropathologists' visits increased from 1.2 to 2.4%; otorhinolaryngologists' visits, from 2.5 to 3%, etc.

Aside from the 152.9 per thousand additional therapeutic visits by internists the experts added 33 per thousand consultation visits for diseases cared for by other specialists. After the corrections made by the experts the total number of visits by internists for therapeutic purposes is 1,642.5 per 1,000 population over 16. The index of visits by internists is 1,269.7 per 1,000 of the whole population.

The average number of visits actually made per disease in the group chiefly under the care of the district internist is 2.5; this includes 2.3 internists' visits and, with consideration of the corrections, 2.9 and 2.6, respectively (Table 14).

The highest number of visits to internists per disease was noted for myocardial infarction (6.6), essential hypertension (4.2), cardiac valvular defects (4.2), rheumatic fever (4.2), gastric and duodenal ulcers (4.5).

Hospitalization of the Adult Urban Population for Diseases Chiefly under the Care of Internists

The average intensive indexes of the hospitalization rate of the adult urban population of the five cities are shown in Table 15.

Among those hospitalized for the diseases listed patients with digestive diseases are in first place (31.1%).

Then come those with respiratory diseases (15%), half of which are from bronchopneumonia; then come the circulatory diseases (14%). In almost half of all cases the reason for hospitalization in the group of circulatory diseases is essential hypertension.

The hospitalization rate for almost all diseases is higher in men than in women.

In comparing the morbidity and hospitalization rate indexes (Table 16) it is evident that the ratio of hospitalization to the total number of cases is highest in lobar pneumonia (75%).

Of those with all respiratory diseases 21.6% were hospitalized, circulatory diseases, 14.2%.

The proportion of those hospitalized with digestive diseases is 25.3% (without counting appendicitis, hernia, rectal diseases and acute intestinal obstruction).

Of the total number of all those hospitalized for diseases chiefly under the care of internists, 37.6 per 1,000 population over 16 (62.6%) were sent to the internal medicine department (Table 17).

Table 15
AVERAGE INTENSIVE INDEXES OF THE HOSPITALIZATION RATE OF THE POPULATION OF FIVE CITIES
(number of hospitalizations per 1,000 population over 16)

Disease	Men	Women	Both sexes
Infectious hepatitis	1.4	1.0	1.1
Sore throat	1.8	1.4	1.6
Influenza	4.8	2.5	3.5
Colds	1.8	1.4	1.6
Rheumatic fever	2.8	3.8	3.5
Metabolic diseases and allergic disorders	1.0	1.2	1.1
These include:			
Diabetes mellitus	0.3	0.3	0.3
Bronchial asthma	0.4	0.6	0.5
Respiratory diseases	11.8	6.9	9.0
These include:			
Acute bronchitis	0.2	0.2	0.2
Chronic bronchitis	1.1	0.5	0.6
Bronchopneumonia	6.3	4.3	5.2
Pulmonary fibrosis, emphysema	1.1	0.4	0.7
Circulatory diseases	8.8	7.9	8.4
These include:			
Cardiac valvular defects	0.5	1.0	0.8
Angina pectoris	0.3	0.2	0.3
Myocardial infarction	0.5	0.2	0.3
Essential hypertension	3.6	3.6	3.6
Myocardial fibrosis	2.4	1.6	2.0
Digestive diseases			
Acute gastritis	1.6	1.7	1.6
Enterocolitis	5.1	2.5	3.7
Chronic gastritis	6.1	2.9	4.3
Gastric and duodenal ulcers	7.9	0.7	3.8
Chronic hepatitis, cirrhosis	1.1	0.5	0.8
Cholelithiasis	0.4	0.6	0.5
Renal and urinary tract diseases	2.6	2.5	2.6
Thyroid diseases	0.2	1.5	0.9
Other internal diseases	9.1	7.2	8.1
Total	72.0	50.2	60.1

As a rule, patients with cardiovascular disease, respiratory disease, metabolic disease and allergic disorders (Figure 10) are sent to the internal medicine department.

The great majority of those with acute gastritis and enterocolitis, put in the class of digestive diseases, are hospitalized in the infectious disease department, in addition to those with diseases included in the category of infectious diseases.

Of the group of those hospitalized for digestive diseases 59.6 % were sent to the internal medicine department, 28.3 % to the infectious disease department, and 11.8 %

Table 16

COMPARISON OF THE MORBIDITY (by sickness rate) AND HOSPITALIZATION
RATES FOR SEPARATE DISEASES

Disease	No. of cases of disease (by sickness rate) per 1,000 population over 16	No. of cases of hospitalization per 1,000 population over 16	Cases of hospitalization in % of the number of corresponding diseases
Infectious hepatitis	1.7	1.1	64.7
Sore throat	48.1	1.6	3.3
Influenza	78.8	3.5	4.4
Colds	135.4	1.6	1.2
Rheumatic fever	11.4	3.5	30.7
Metabolic diseases and allergic disorders	4.8	1.1	22.9
These include:			
Diabetes mellitus	0.6	0.3	50
Bronchial asthma	1.4	0.5	35.7
Respiratory diseases	41.6	9.0	21.6
These include:			
Acute bronchitis	8.8	0.2	2.3
Chronic bronchitis	10.5	0.6	5.7
Bronchopneumonia	9.7	5.2	53.6
Lobar pneumonia	0.8	0.6	75
Pulmonary fibrosis, emphysema	3.9	0.7	17.9
Suppurative diseases of the lungs	0.9	0.4	44.4
Circulatory diseases	59.1	8.4	14.2
These include:			
Cardiac valvular defects	2.8	0.8	28.6
Angina pectoris	1.0	0.3	30
Myocardial infarction	0.5	0.3	60
Essential hypertension	21.5	3.6	16.7
Myocardial fibrosis	24.1	2.0	7.9
Digestive diseases	74.0	18.7	25.3
These include:			
Enterocolitis	9.7	3.7	38.1
Chronic gastritis	28.5	4.3	15.1
Gastric and duodenal ulcers	6.9	3.8	55.1
Chronic hepatitis and cirrhosis	1.8	0.8	44.4
Cholelithiasis	0.8	0.5	62.5
Renal and urinary tract diseases	13.1	2.6	19.8
Thyroid diseases	5.7	0.9	15.8
Other internal diseases	12.5	8.1	48.3
Total	486.2	60.1	12.4

Table 17

DISTRIBUTION OF PATIENTS HOSPITALIZED ACCORDING TO HOSPITAL DEPARTMENTS

Disease	No. of cases hospitalized per 1,000 population over 16				Hospitalization according to departments (in % of total)			
	internal	infectious disease	surgical	other departments	internal	infectious disease	surgical	other departments
Infectious hepatitis	—	1.1	—	—	—	100.0	—	—
Sore throat	—	0.2	—	1.4	14.3	—	—	85.7
Influenza	0.7	2.8	—	—	23.8	76.2	—	—
Colds	0.6	1.0	—	—	37.5	62.5	—	—
Rheumatic fever	3.3	—	—	0.2	94.3	—	—	5.7
Metabolic diseases and allergic disorders	1.1	—	—	—	100.0	—	—	—
These include:								
Diabetes mellitus	0.3	—	—	—	100.0	—	—	—
Bronchial asthma	0.5	—	—	—	100.0	—	—	—
Respiratory diseases	8.6	0.4	—	—	95.6	4.4	—	—
These include:								
Acute bronchitis	—	0.2	—	—	—	100.0	—	—
Chronic bronchitis	0.6	—	—	—	100.0	—	—	—
Bronchopneumonia	5.0	0.2	—	—	96.2	3.8	—	—
Pulmonary fibrosis, emphysema	0.7	—	—	—	100.0	—	—	—
Circulatory diseases	8.1	—	0.2	0.1	96.4	—	2.4	1.2
These include:								
Cardiac valvular defects	0.8	—	—	—	100.0	—	—	—
Angina pectoris	0.3	—	—	—	100.0	—	—	—
Myocardial infarction	0.3	—	—	—	100.0	—	—	—
Myocardial fibrosis	2.0	—	—	—	100.0	—	—	—
Essential hypertension	3.5	—	—	0.1	97.2	—	—	2.8
Digestive diseases	11.1	5.3	2.3	—	59.6	28.3	11.8	—
These include:								
Acute gastritis	0.3	1.2	0.1	—	18.7	75.1	6.2	—
Enterocolitis	0.1	3.5	0.1	—	2.7	94.6	2.7	—
Chronic gastritis	4.2	—	0.1	—	97.2	—	2.8	—
Gastric and duodenal ulcers	3.2	—	0.6	—	84.2	—	15.8	—
Chronic hepatitis and cirrhosis	0.7	—	0.1	—	87.5	—	12.5	—
Cholelithiasis	0.3	—	0.2	—	60.0	—	40.0	—
Renal and urinary tract diseases	1.1	—	1.5	—	42.3	—	57.7	—
Thyroid diseases	0.5	—	0.4	—	55.6	—	44.4	—
Other internal diseases	2.5	5.4	0.1	0.1	64.3	28.5	3.6	3.6
Total	37.6	16.2	4.5	1.8	62.6	26.9	7.5	3.0

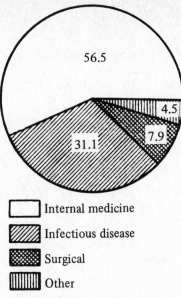

Internal medicine

Infectious disease

Surgical

Other

Figure 10

Distribution of hospitalizations of the adult population in various hospital departments according to the group of diseases chiefly cared for by internists (in percentages of the total)

to the surgical department. Forty percent of patients with cholelithiasis and 15.8% of those with gastric and duodenal ulcers are sent to the surgical department (Table 17).

The intensive age indexes of the hospitalization rate of the population are shown in Table 18 and Figure 11.

The hospitalization rate, closely following the age characteristics of the sickness rate, increases with age. For every 1,000 adolescents 37.4 are hospitalized. In the age group 40 to 49 this figure is almost doubled (71.4) and reaches its maximum at

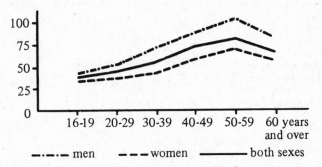

Figure 11

Average age indexes of hospitalization of the adult urban population for the group of diseases chiefly under the care of internists

Table 18

AVERAGE AGE INDEXES OF HOSPITALIZATION FOR THE GROUP OF

(number of cases of hospitalization per 1,000

Disease	16–19 years			20–29 years		
	men	women	both sexes	men	women	both sexes
Infectious hepatitis	1.9	1.3	1.6	1.3	0.9	1.1
Sore throat	2.4	2.4	2.4	2.5	2.5	2.5
Influenza	4.5	1.1	2.8	4.3	2.6	3.5
Colds	1.3	1.5	1.4	1.6	1.5	1.6
Helminthic infestations	0.7	1.2	0.9	1.0	1.2	1.1
Rheumatic fever	3.9	4.1	3.9	2.2	2.7	2.4
Metabolic diseases and allergic disorders	—	—	—	0.7	0.7	0.7
These include:						
Diabetes mellitus	—	—	—	0.3	—	0.2
Bronchial asthma	—	—	—	0.3	0.5	0.4
Respiratory diseases	6.5	5.9	6.3	7.2	3.8	5.5
These include:						
Acute bronchitis	0.1	—	0.1	0.2	0.2	0.2
Chronic bronchitis	—	—	—	0.5	0.1	0.3
Bronchopneumonia	4.8	3.1	3.9	4.5	2.3	3.4
Pulmonary fibrosis, emphysema	—	—	—	—	—	—
Circulatory diseases	1.6	1.4	1.5	1.8	1.7	1.6
These include:						
Cardiac valvular defects	0.3	0.2	0.2	0.7	0.8	0.7
Myocardial fibrosis from myocarditis	—	—	—	—	—	—
Angina pectoris	—	—	—	—	—	—
Myocardial infarction	—	—	—	—	—	—
Myocardial fibrosis from atherosclerosis	—	—	—	—	—	—
Essential hypertension	0.9	0.6	0.8	0.7	0.2	0.4
Digestive diseases	10.9	6.3	8.6	20.4	10.4	15.2
These include:						
Acute gastritis	1.1	1.4	1.3	1.7	2.0	1.9
Chronic gastritis	2.0	0.8	1.4	5.8	1.3	3.4
Enteritis and colitis	5.4	2.5	3.9	4.4	3.7	4.0
Chronic hepatitis, cirrhosis	—	—	—	0.7	0.4	0.6
Gastric and duodenal ulcers	1.6	0.2	0.9	5.5	0.6	2.9
Cholelithiasis	—	0.1	0.1	—	—	—
Renal and urinary tract diseases	1.8	1.3	1.4	1.1	2.5	2.3
Thyroid diseases	0.1	0.4	0.2	—	0.8	0.4
Other diseases	6.6	6.4	6.4	7.7	5.4	6.5
Total	42.2	33.3	37.4	51.7	36.6	44.4

DISEASES CHIEFLY UNDER THE CARE OF INTERNISTS FOR FIVE CITIES
population of the corresponding age and sex)

	Age groups										
30–39 years			40–49 years			50–59 years			60 years and over		
men	women	both sexes	men	women	both sexes	men	women	both sexes	men	women	both sexes
1.1	0.6	0.8	1.2	0.8	0.0	0.6	0.4	0.5	1.1	1.6	1.5
1.8	1.3	1.5	1.2	0.8	1.8	0.6	0.5	0.5	0.2	0.1	0.2
4.8	2.7	3.7	5.9	2.5	3.9	4.3	3.6	3.9	3.6	1.6	2.2
2.4	1.4	1.8	1.7	1.4	1.5	1.5	1.2	1.3	2.3	1.4	1.8
0.4	0.5	0.6	0.8	0.9	0.9	0.9	0.7	0.8	0.3	0.5	0.5
3.2	3.6	3.2	2.9	5.5	4.4	3.5	4.0	3.7	1.9	1.5	1.7
0.2	0.6	0.4	2.1	1.1	1.4	1.1	2.8	1,7	1.4	2.0	1.8
0.1	0.2	0.2	0.9	0.2	0.5	—	0.5	0.3	1.2	1.2	1.2
0.1	0.3	0.2	1.0	0.8	0.9	1.1	1.5	1.3	0.2	0.5	0.4
10.2	5.0	6.2	15.7	8.0	11.2	20.2	11.0	14.5	17.7	10.2	12.7
0.4	0.3	0.3	0.1	0.3	0.2	0.3	0.4	0.3		0.1	0.1
0.7	0.1	0.4	1.7	0.6	1.1	2.2	0.6	1.2	2.2	1.1	1.4
6.3	3.4	4.7	7.8	5.1	6.2	8.0	7.3	7.5	9.4	6.7	7.7
0.3	0.1	0.1	1.9	0.5	1.1	4.6	0.8	2.3	3.4	0.7	1.5
3.4	4.3	4.1	11.5	10.3	10.8	25.9	16.4	20.0	27.5	16.1	19.8
0.5	1.3	1.0	0.6	1.2	0.9	0.5	1.3	0.9	0.2	1.1	0.8
0.1	0.3	0.2	0.7	0.5	0.6	0.7	0.5	0.6	0.4	0.7	0.5
—	0.1	0.1	0.4	0.2	0.3	1.1	0.4	0.6	0.6	0.4	0.4
0.1	0.1	0.1	0.2	—	0.1	1.5	0.1	0.6	2.0	0.3	0.8
—	0.1	0.1	2.7	1.2	1.8	8.1	3.4	5.3	9.5	4.6	6.2
1.0	1.6	1.4	4.9	6.0	5.5	11.3	9.1	9.9	11.2	6.7	8.1
30.0	11.3	19.1	34.0	16.9	23.9	30.6	17,2	22.2	14.6	11.6	12.9
1.9	1.1	1.4	1.8	2.1	2.0	1.9	1.7	1.8	0.3	1.2	0.9
7.3	2.4	4.5	7.7	5.1	6.2	6.0	4.9	5.0	3.6	2.7	3.0
4.2	2.2	3.0	7.4	2.0	4.1	6.0	2.5	3.9	2.4	1.9	2.0
0.7	0.7	0.7	1.4	0.3	0.8	6.4	0.5	0.8	0.5	0.6	0.6
11.3	0.8	5.2	10.2	1.3	4.9	10.7	0.6	4.6	2.0	0.2	0.8
0.2	0.3	0.3	0.3	0.3	0.3	0.1	1.2	0.8	0.9	0.7	0.8
2.6	3.3	3.0	3.1	2.4	2.7	3.0	2.5	2.7	2.5	2.6	2.6
0.4	2.3	1.6	0.2	1.4	0.9	0.3	1.5	1.0	0.2	0.8	0.6
9.0	5.4	6.9	9.3	7.3	8.3	8.5	6.9	7.5	7.5	5.0	5.8
69.5	42.3	53.9	80.6	59.3	71.4	101.0	68.7	80.1	80.8	55.0	64.1

the age of 50 to 59 (80.1). At the age of 60 and over, the hospitalization rate drops to 64.1.

As indicated above, the data of sickness rate, attendance and hospitalization were subjected to the evaluation of experts. In the opinion of the experts, for the purpose of satisfying the patients' need (according to sickness rate) for hospital care 6.5 cases of additional hospitalization per 1,000 population over 16 (Table 19)

Table 19

NUMBER OF CASES OF HOSPITALIZATION PER 1,000 POPULATION OVER 16

Disease	Actual number	Added by experts	Total	Average duration of treatment in days
Infectious hepatitis	1.1	0.2	1.3	25.7
Sore throat	1.6	0.1	1.7	5.4
Influenza	3.5	0.5	4.0	7.6
Colds	1.6	—	1.6	7.5
Rheumatic fever	3.5	0.7	4.2	31.1
Metabolic diseases and allergic disorders	1.1	0.2	1.3	20.5
These include:				
Diabetes mellitus	0.3	0.1	0.4	20.9
Bronchial asthma	0.5	0.1	0.6	21.5
Respiratory diseases	9.0	0.9	9.9	15.7
These include:				
Acute bronchitis	0.2	—	0.2	6.7
Chronic bronchitis	0.6	—	0.6	13.2
Bronchopneumonia	5.2	0.5	5.7	14.1
Pulmonary fibrosis, emphysema	0.7	0.1	0.8	17.8
Circulatory diseases	8.4	1.5	9.9	23.4
These include:				
Cardiac valvular defects	0.8	—	0.8	21.5
Angina pectoris	0.3	—	0.3	20.0
Myocardial infarction	0.3	0.1	0.4	53.7
Myocardial fibrosis	2.0	0.1	2.1	26.0
Essential hypertension	3.6	1.2	4.8	21.3
Digestive diseases	18.7	1.8	20.5	11.4
These include:				
Acute gastritis	1.6	—	1.6	4.6
Chronic gastritis	4.3	0.5	4.8	12.3
Enteritis and colitis	3.7	0.4	4.1	6.0
Chronic hepatitis and cirrhosis	0.8	—	0.8	19.6
Gastric and duodenal ulcers	3.8	0.4	4.2	21.4
Cholelithiasis	0.5	0.2	0.7	18.0
Renal and urinary tract diseases	2.6	0.3	2.9	13.0
Thyroid diseases	0.9	0.1	1.0	17.8
Other internal diseases	8.1	0.2	8.3	—
Total for the group of diseases chiefly under the care of internists	60.1	6.5	66.6	—

were required. The highest number of cases of additional hospitalization was recommended for essential hypertension (1.2 per 1,000 population over 16), rheumatic fever (0.7), chronic gastritis (0.5), gastric and duodenal ulcers (0.4).

Standards of Therapeutic-Prophylactic Care of the Urban Population in the Field of Internal Medicine

The calculations of the norms of outpatient-polyclinic care of the adult population in the field of internal medicine are given in Table 20.

The number of outpatient therapeutic visits to internists with consideration of the corrections made by experts is 1,642.5 per 1,000 population over the age of 16, and in the calculation per 1,000 of the whole population, 1,269.7.

The frequency of the chronic cases detected through the comprehensive medical checkups requiring medical care among the population subject to medical checkups in the next few years is 59.8 per 1,000 population over 16 (per 1,000 of the whole population, 46.2).

In calculation of the need for medical visits associated with the chronic diseases detected in the population who will need medical checkups in the next few years, we used as a basis the average number of visits per disease calculated from the actual sickness rate with consideration of the corrections made by the experts.

The number of additional medical visits for chronic diseases detected among the population subject to medical checkups is 204.2 per 1,000 population over 16 or 157.8 per 1,000 of the whole population.

Therefore, the total number of medical visits for the established morbidity rate, according to the data of sickness rate and the results of medical checkups, is 1,846.7 per 1,000 population over 16 or 1,427.5 per 1,000 of the whole population.

In calculating the number of visits for the dispensary care of patients we considered the instructions of the public health agencies, the data in the literature, and the work experience of leading therapeutic-prophylactic institutions.

We provided complete coverage with dispensary care for cases of rheumatic fever, cardiac valvular defects, myocardial infarction, essential hypertension, diabetes mellitus, chronic suppurative disease of the lungs, chronic hepatitis and cirrhosis, gastric and duodenal ulcer and cholelithiasis.

Of the total number of cases of chronic gastritis and thyroid disease only persons with diseases whose clinical course requires regular treatment, in the experts' opinion, were assigned to dispensary care. Of the total number of patients with chronic gastritis 44.6% were assigned to dispensary care; of those with thyroid diseases, 36.8% (Table 21).

Dispensary care of patients with the chronic diseases listed requires 351.7 visits per 1,000 adult population or 271.9 per 1,000 of the whole population.

Provision has also been made for regular observations of certain groups of the

Table 20

STANDARDS OF OUTPATIENT-POLYCLINIC CARE OF THE URBAN

Nosologic entity	Average morbidity for five cities (by sickness rate)	Total number of visits of internists (actual number + that added by experts)	Number of visits of internists per disease (actual number + that added by experts)	Frequency of newly detected cases among the population groups subject to medical checkups
Infectious hepatitis	1.7	6.3	3.7	—
Sore throat	48.1	76.2	1.6	—
Influenza	78.8	191.3	2.4	—
Colds	135.4	363.9	2.7	—
Helminthic infestations	2.2	3.6	1.6	—
Rheumatic fever	11.4	47.3	4.1	3.4
Metabolic diseases and allergic disorders	4.8	12.5	2.6	0.2
These include:				
Diabetes mellitus	0.6	1.8	3.0	6.1
Bronchial asthma	1.4	5.0	3.6	0.1
Respiratory diseases	41.6	89.5	2.2	2.3
These include:				
Acute bronchitis	8.8	18.3	2.1	—
Chronic bronchitis	10.5	16.6	1.6	0.5
Bronchopneumonia	9.7	23.6	2.4	—
Pulmonary fibrosis, emphysema	3.9	9.3	2.4	1.4
Circulatory diseases	59.1	213.0	3.6	22.8
These include:				
Cardiac valvular defects	2.8	11.8	4.2	2.5
Myocardial fibrosis from myocarditis	5.6	16.9	3.0	0.1
Angina pectoris	1.0	2.8	2.8	0.5
Myocardial infarction	0.5	3.3	6.6	
Myocardial fibrosis from atherosclerosis	18.5	59.9	3.2	7.4
Essential hypertension	21.5	90.2	4.2	13.6
Circulatory diseases	74.0	201.1	2.7	15.2
These include:				
Acute gastritis	14.3	32.9	2.3	—
Chronic gastritis	28.5	78.5	2.7	8.9
Enteritis and colitis	9.7	13.9	1.4	—
Chronic hepatitis and cirrhosis	1.8	7.0	3.9	0.3
Gastric and duodenal ulcers	6.9	31.3	4.5	2.6
Cholelithiasis	0.6	3.0	3.7	0.2
Renal and urinary tract diseases	13.1	24.5	1.9	0.6
Thyroid diseases	5.1	17.4	3.0	6.4
Other internal diseases	10.3	12.2	1.5	0.2
Total	486.2	1,258.8	2.6	59.8
Medical consultation visits for other diseases	—	383.7	—	—
Total for 1,000 population over 16	—	1,642.5	—	59.8
Per 1,000 population of all ages	—	1,269.7	—	46.2

POPULATION IN THE FIELD OF INTERNAL MEDICINE (1966–1970)

| Number of additional therapeutic visits of internists for newly detected cases | Number of therapeutic visits of internists with corrective factor for newly detected cases | Number of visits in dispensary care of patients | Prophylactic checkups | | | | Total visits to internists |
			of workers of industrial enterprises	of adolescents	of the rest of the population	total	
—	6.3	—	—	—	—	—	—
—	76.2	—	—	—	—	—	—
—	191.3	—	—	—	—	—	—
—	363.9	—	—	—	—	—	—
—	3.6	—	—	—	—	—	—
13.9	61.2	—	—	—	—	—	—
0.7	13.2	—	—	—	—	—	—
0.3	2.1	—	—	—	—	—	—
0.4	5.4	—	—	—	—	—	—
5.3	94.8	—	—	—	—	—	—
—	18.3	—	—	—	—	—	—
0.8	17.4	—	—	—	—	—	—
—	23.6	—	—	—	—	—	—
3.4	12.7	—	—	—	—	—	—
115.9	328.9	—	—	—	—	—	—
10.1	21.9	—	—	—	—	—	—
0.3	17.2	—	—	—	—	—	—
1.4	4.8	—	—	—	—	—	—
—	3.3	—	—	—	—	—	—
23.7	83.6	—	—	—	—	—	—
57.1	147.3	—	—	—	—	—	—
47.1	248.2	—	—	—	—	—	—
—	32.9	—	—	—	—	—	—
24.0	102.5	—	—	—	—	—	—
—	13.9	—	—	—	—	—	—
1.2	8.2	—	—	—	—	—	—
11.7	43.0	—	—	—	—	—	—
0.7	3.7	—	—	—	—	—	—
1.8	26.3	—	—	—	—	—	—
19.2	36.6	—	—	—	—	—	—
0.3	12.5	—	—	—	—	—	—
204.2	1,463.0	—	—	—	—	—	—
—	—	—	—	—	—	—	—
204.2	1,846.7	351.7	169.0	84.6	312.0	565.5	2,764.0
157.8	1,427.5	271.9	122.6	61.4	226.1	410.1	2,109.5

Table 21

INTERNISTS' WORK LOAD FOR DISPENSARY CARE OF CHRONIC DISEASE PATIENTS (per 1,000 population over 16)

Disease	Patients needing dispensary care according to sickness rate data	Frequency of observations	No. of visits	Patients detected who need dispensary care in medical checkups of population groups needing periodic medical checkups	No. of visits	Total patients needing dispensary care	Total visits in connection with dispensary care of patients
Infectious hepatitis	1.7	3	5.1	—	—	1.7	5.1
Rheumatic fever	11.4	4	45.6	3.4	13.6	14.8	59.2
Diabetes mellitus	0.6	4	2.4	0.1	0.4	0.7	2.8
Suppurative disease of the lungs	0.9	2	1.8	0.2	0.4	1.1	2.2
Cardiac valvular defects	2.8	2	5.6	2.4	4.8	5.2	10.4
Angina pectoris	1.0	3	3.0	0.5	1.5	1.5	4.5
Myocardial infarction	0.5	12	6.0	—	—	0.5	6.0
Essential hypertension		21.5	—	86.6	46.6	36.1	133.2
This includes:							
Essential hypertension, stage I	7.7	2	15.4	5.5	11.0	13.2	26.4
Essential hypertension, stage II	11.8	4	47.2	7.7	30.8	19.5	78.0
Essential hypertension, stage III	2.0	12	24.0	0.4	4.8	2.4	28.8
Chronic gastritis	12.7	2	25.4	4.0	8.0	16.7	33.4
Hepatitis, cirrhosis	1.8	3	5.4	0.3	0.9	2.1	6.3
Gastric and duodenal ulcers	6.9	4	27.6	2.6	10.4	9.5	38.0
Cholelithiasis	0.8	3	2.4	0.2	0.6	1.0	3.0
Nephritis, nephosis	1.2	2	2.4	0.3	0.6	1.5	3.0
Thyroid disease	2.1	4	8.4	2.4	9.6	4.5	18.0
Total:							
Per 1,000 population over 16	72.8	—	254.9	30.0	97.4	102.8	351.9
Per 1,000 of the entire population	56.3	—	197.2	23.2	75.3	79.5	272.2

healthy population with the aim of timely detection of the initial stages of disease, at which time the therapeutic measures are most effective.

The work load in prophylactic checkups is determined with consideration of the directives of the USSR Ministry of Health on this subject as well as instructions on methods and instructions on the annual prophylactic checkups of various groups of the healthy population combined according to type of work or age.

The number of visits in connection with prophylactic checkups of workers with

Table 22

STANDARDS FOR HOSPITAL CARE OF THE ADULT URBAN POPULATION FOR 1966–1970

Disease	Number of cases hospitalized (per 1,000 population over 16)				Average duration of hospital treatment (in days)	Distribution according to hospital departments			
	actually hospitalized	added by the experts	for diseases detected among population groups undergoing routine checkups	Total		internal medicine	infectious disease	surgical	other
Infectious hepatitis	1.1	0.2	—	1.3	25.7	—	1.3	—	—
Sore throat	1.6	0.1	—	1.7	5.4	—	0.3	—	1.4
Influenza	3.5	0.5	—	4.0	7.6	—	4.0	—	—
Colds	1.6	—	—	1.6	7.5	—	1.6	—	0.3
Rheumatic fever	3.5	0.7	1.0	5.2	31.1	4.9	—	—	—
Metabolic diseases and allergic disorders	1.1	0.2	0.2	1.5	20.5	1.5	—	—	—
These include:									
Diabetes mellitus	0.3	0.1	0.1	0.5	20.9	0.5	—	—	—
Bronchial asthma	0.5	0.1	0.1	0.7	21.5	0.7	—	—	—
Respiratory diseases	9.0	0.9	0.4	10.3	15.7	10.3	—	—	—
These include:									
Acute bronchitis	0.2	—	—	0.2	—	0.2	—	—	—
Chronic bronchitis	0.6	—	—	0.6	13.2	0.6	—	—	—
Bronchopneumonia	5.2	0.5	—	5.7	14.1	5.7	—	—	—
Pulmonary fibrosis, emphysema	0.7	0.1	0.3	1.1	17.8	1.1	—	—	—
Circulatory diseases	8.4	1.5	4.8	14.7	23.4	14.5	—	0.2	—
These include:									
Cardiac valvular defects	0.8	—	0.7	1.5	21.5	1.5	—	—	—
Angina pectoris	0.3	—	0.1	0.4	20.0	0.4	—	—	—
Myocardial infarction	0.3	0.1	—	0.4	53.7	0.4	—	—	—
Myocardial fibrosis	2.0	0.1	0.6	2.7	26.0	2.7	—	—	—
Essential hypertension	3.6	1.2	2.3	7.1	21.3	7.1	—	—	—

Table 22 (continued)

Disease	Number of cases hospitalized (per 1,000 population over 16)				Average duration of hospital treatment (in days)	Distribution according to hospital departments			
	actually hospitalized	added by the experts	for diseases detected among population groups undergoing routine checkups	Total		internal medicine	infectious disease	surgical	other
Digestive diseases	18.7	1.8	4.0	24.5	11.4	17.0	5.1	2.4	—
These include:									
Acute gastritis	1.6	—	—	1.6	4.6	0.3	1.2	0.1	—
Chronic gastritis	4.3	0.5	1.3	6.1	12.3	6.0	—	0.1	—
Enteritis and colitis	3.7	0.4	—	4.1	6.0	0.1	3.9	0.1	—
Chronic hepatitis and cirrhosis	0.8	—	0.1	0.9	19.6	0.8	—	0.1	—
Peptic ulcer	3.8	0.4	1.4	5.6	21.4	5.0	—	0.6	—
Cholelithiasis	0.5	0.2	0.1	0.8	18.0	0.5	—	0.3	—
Genitourinary diseases	2.6	0.3	0.1	3.0	13.0	1.5	—	1.5	—
Thyroid diseases	0.9	0.1	1.0	2.0	17.8	1.6	—	0.4	—
Other internal diseases	8.1	0.2	0.1	3.1	18.1	2.9	—	0.1	0.1
Total for the group of diseases treated mainly by internists	60.1	6.5	11.6	78.2	—	54.2	17.6	4.6	1.8
Diseases of the internal type	—	—	—	—	—	10.6	0.9	—	—
Total per 1,000 population over 16	—	—	—	—	—	64.8	18.5	—	—
Per 1,000 of the total population	43.0	4.7	8.3	56.0	—	44.6	13.1	3.4	1.4
Number of beds per 1,000 population over 16	—	—	—	—	—	3.3	0.84	—	—
Number of beds per 1,000 of the total population	—	—	—	—	—	2.3	0.6	—	—

consideration of the number of examinations was 169.0 per 1,000 population over 16.

For the prophylactic checkups of adolescents of both sexes and dispensary examination of draftees 84.6 visits per 1,000 population over 16 are planned.

Prophylactic checkups of the rest of the population (312.0 per 1,000 population over 16) include checkups of boat transport workers, public dining room and public utility workers, workers in children's institutions as well as single checkups associated with the issuing of certificates to those entering schools, filling in sanatorium-health resort cards, etc.

Therefore the total number of visits for prophylactic checkups of the healthy population is 565.6 per 1,000 inhabitants over 16 or 410.1 per 1,000 of the whole population.

The population requirement of hospital care, as has already been pointed out, is also determined with consideration of the expansion of hospitalization for the various nosologic entities.

Calculations on the amount of hospital care are shown in Table 22. This table shows the distribution of patients in the various hospital departments and the average length of treatment for various diseases.

Hospital treatment for cardiovascular diseases was the longest: for myocardial infarction, 50 days; rheumatic fever, 38 days; essential hypertension, 23 days. Next were bronchial asthma, 20.5 days; gastric and duodenal ulcers, 19.5 days. Shortest hospital treatment was for helminthic infestations, 4.3 days; sore throat, colds, acute gastritis, enterocolitis and acute bronchitis, 5.4–7.8 days.

It should be noted that the figures for the average duration of treatment are to a considerable extent arbitrary and depend on the age distribution of those hospitalized, the timeliness of hospitalization, the individual characteristics of the course of the disease, as well as the number of beds available. Therefore, in calculating the number of internal medical and infectious disease beds per 1,000 population the average number of days the patient was in the respective departments was taken from data of records for the USSR for 1962 (internal medicine, 17.2 days; infectious disease, 13.5 days).

Standards of Therapeutic-Prophylactic Care of the Urban Population in the Field of Surgery

Incidence of Predominantly Surgical Diseases in the Urban Population

Table 23 shows the average figures for the prevalence of diseases in the population of five cities for which patients usually apply to surgeons (first group) and in the treatment of which physicians of other specialties also participate (second group).

These data show that the people of these cities usually suffer from various injuries that make up over half of the visits to surgeons; among them comparatively mild mechanical injuries without involvement of bones or joints are predominant.

In the second place after injuries are diseases of the bones, muscles, tendons, ganglia, joints, then phlegmons, abscesses, furuncles and carbuncles.

For the purpose of eliminating the influence of possible differences in the age and sex structure of the population on the total morbidity, the indexes were standardized by the direct method. The age and sex distribution of the urban population of the USSR according to the 1959 census was used as the standard. The standardization changed the actual total morbidity rate very little.

Between the sexes there are essential differences in the figures for the prevalence of various diseases. In men injuries are much more frequent than in women. Women suffer more often from acute and chronic appendicitis.

As is evident from Table 23, the incidence of acute and chronic appendicitis in men is 8.6; in women, 12.0 per 1,000 population of the respective sex. Hernias, phlegmons and abscesses are encountered more often in men. Women suffer more often from carcinoma and other malignant neoplasms.

The prevalence of many diseases is substantially different among the populations of different age groups (see Table 24 and Figures 1, 2, 3 and 4).

Table 23
AVERAGE FIGURES FOR THE PREVALENCE OF DISEASES AND INJURIES SEEN
CHIEFLY BY SURGEONS IN THE POPULATION OF FIVE CITIES
(number of cases of diseases or injuries per 1,000 city population according to sex)

Disease	Actual morbidity rate figures			Standardized morbidity rate figures		
	men	women	both sexes	men	women	both sexes
First group						
Mechanical injuries:						
with injury to internal organs	0.7	0.4	0.5	0.8	0.3	0.5
without injury to bones or joints	86.2	39.4	60.8	85.0	37.2	58.8
with injury to bones or joints	16.6	7.0	11.3	16.2	6.8	11.0
Burns	10.4	6.2	8.1	10.2	5.9	7.7
Frostbites	1.0	0.3	0.6	0.8	0.2	0.5
Other injuries	9.6	4.8	6.9	0.9	4.6	6.5
Carcinomas and other malignant tumors	2.9	3.7	3.3	2.8	3.7	3.4
Appendicitis:						
acute	6.0	7.9	7.1	5.8	7.4	6.7
chronic	2.6	4.1	3.4	2.5	3.6	3.1
Acute intestinal obstruction	0.2	0.2	0.2	0.2	0.2	0.2
Hernias	4.4	2.5	3.3	4.6	2.6	3.5
Bone diseases	5.6	4.3	4.9	5.3	3.8	4.5
Muscle and tendon diseases	27.3	22.5	24.6	27.0	20.9	23.5
Joint diseases	13.0	12.6	12.8	12.5	11.8	12.0
Phlegmons and abscesses	15.1	11.8	13.2	14.9	11.4	12.9
Second group						
Foreign body in the eye	13.9	4.1	8.4	13.7	3.4	7.8
Benign tumors	4.5	9.2	7.1	4.4	8.3	6.5
Peptic ulcers	9.7	1.5	5.1	9.3	1.3	4.8
Rectal diseases	1.8	1.3	1.5	1.7	1.3	1.4
Stones in kidneys and urinary tracts	2.2	1.9	2.0	2.1	1.8	1.9
Total	233.7	145.7	185.1	220.7	136.5	177.2

Mechanical injuries are noted in all age groups but more often in the age group capable of working most actively (from 20 to 50) (Figure 12).

In children burns are found most often under age 4; in adults, between 20 and 30.

Acute and chronic appendicitis are found in all age groups but most often between 14-19, 20-29 and 30-39 (Figure 13).

Of considerable interest are data showing which specialists are seen first by patients with diseases treatable mainly by surgeons (Table 25).

As is evident from Table 25, surgeons are most important in making the diagnosis in cases of injuries and acute appendicitis.

In 20% of cases injuries to internal organs are diagnosed by internists. These are

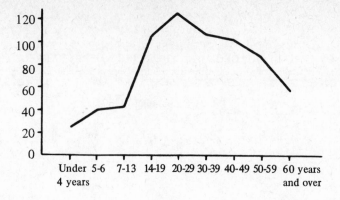

Figure 12

Average age indexes for the incidence of injuries (number of injuries per 1,000 population of the corresponding age)

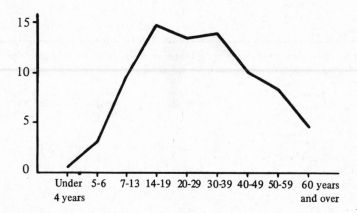

Figure 13

Average age indexes for the incidence of appendicitis in the population (number of cases per 1,000 population of the corresponding age)

largely injuries without breaks in the skin. When wounds are present the patients go to surgeons as a rule.

In the diagnosis of chronic appendicitis, internists (32.1%) and pediatricians (21.4%) participate, aside from the surgeons who diagnose 46.5% of the cases, because adults with abdominal pain not uncommonly go to internists, while children are referred to pediatricians; only after the diagnosis is clarified are they sent to surgeons for deciding on operation.

Surgeons (23.9%), internists (19.6%), oncologists (21.7%), and mostly obstetri-

Table 24

AVERAGE FIGURES FOR MORBIDITY RATE AND INJURIES IN THE POPULATION OF FIVE CITIES

(number of cases of diseases or injuries per 1,000 population of both sexes)

Disease	Age groups									total
	under 4 years	5–6 years	7–13 years	14–19 years	20–29 years	30–39 years	40–49 years	50–59 years	60 and over	
First group										
Mechanical injuries:										
with injury to internal organs	0.04	0.1	0.5	0.4	0.8	0.7	0.7	0.2	0.1	0.5
without injury to bones or joints	14.4	29.3	30.8	73.9	89.1	74.8	68.2	54.1	34.6	60.8
with injury to bones or joints	2.7	3.9	5.6	11.4	13.0	12.8	15.2	15.9	12.2	11.3
Burns	5.8	3.3	2.1	7.5	12.9	9.4	8.6	6.4	3.8	8.1
Frostbites	0.1		0.2	1.7	0.7	0.4	0.3	0.2	0.1	0.6
Other injuries	1.8	3.8	4.3	8.6	7.0	7.6	7.3	9.5	6.6	6.9
Carcinoma and other malignant tumors	—	0.1	—	0.1	0.4	1.8	5.8	10.7	17.1	3.3
Appendicitis:										
acute	0.3	2.3	6.8	10.8	9.1	9.2	6.6	4.4	3.0	7.1
chronic	0.1	0.7	2.6	3.8	4.2	4.5	3.3	3.7	1.4	3.4
Acute intestinal obstruction	0.2	0.3	—	0.1	—	0.1	0.4	0.3	1.3	0.2
Hernias	5.5	2.7	1.1	2.1	1.5	2.8	5.6	6.4	7.2	3.3
Bone diseases	1.1	2.2	1.9	3.3	4.0	5.4	8.4	8.0	4.5	4.9
Muscle and tendon diseases	1.4	0.6	3.3	10.8	25.6	35.0	47.8	41.2	22.3	24.6
Joint diseases	0.8	1.6	3.3	5.9	9.4	14.0	23.8	28.2	18.3	12.8
Phlegmons and abscesses	10.8	8.4	7.3	18.9	18.4	14.6	13.0	9.7	5.2	13.2
Second group										
Foreign body in the eye	0.4	0.8	1.9	6.8	14.3	12.5	10.0	6.2	2.9	8.4
Benign tumors	1.2	1.1	1.4	3.2	5.6	7.7	16.9	10.8	6.8	7.1
Peptic ulcers		0.1	0.1	1.4	5.1	9.8	9.7	8.1	2.4	5.1
Rectal diseases	0.8	0.6	0.3	0.2	1.4	2.2	2.5	3.0	1.3	1.5
Stones in kidneys and urinary tracts	0.3	0.1	0.3	0.5	1.7	2.5	4.0	4.3	2.3	2.0
Total	47.74	62.0	73.8	171.4	171.4	227.8	258.1	231.3	153.4	185.1

Table 25

PARTICIPATION OF PHYSICIANS OF DIFFERENT SPECIALTIES IN MAKING THE DIAGNOSIS OF DISEASE (in percentages of the total number of cases of each disease) IN THE GROUP OF DISEASES WHICH ARE LARGELY SURGICAL

Disease	Internists	Surgeons	Otorhinolaryngologists	Ophthalmologists	Phthisiologists	Neuropathologists	Psychiatrists	Dentists	Dermatovenereologists	Obstetricians and gynecologists	Pediatricians	Oncologists	Other specialists
First group													
Mechanical injuries:													
with injury to internal organs	20.0	80.0	—	—	—	—	—	—	—	—	—	—	—
without injury to bones or joints	1.3	95.2	0.6	1.0	—	0.6	—	0.1	—	0.2	1.0	—	1.3
with injury to bones or joints	4.4	88.5	0.9	—	—	1.6	—	—	—	—	2.4	—	0.9
Burns	4.5	71.8	2.0	15.4	—	—	—	—	3.2	—	2.5	—	0.6
Frostbites	25.0	75.0	—	—	—	—	—	—	—	—	—	—	—
Other injuries	8.4	77.6	2.8	4.7	—	1.9	—	—	—	—	2.8	—	1.8
Carcinoma and other malignant tumors	19.6	23.9	—	—	—	—	—	—	—	34.8	—	21.7	—
Appendicitis:													
acute	11.1	75.7	—	—	—	—	—	—	—	—	10.4	—	2.8
chronic	32.1	46.5	—	—	—	—	—	—	—	—	21.4	—	—
Acute intestinal obstruction	33.3	66.7	—	—	—	—	—	—	—	—	—	—	—
Hernias	7.0	80.6	—	—	—	—	—	—	—	2.7	9.7	—	—
Bone diseases	41.2	33.4	0.3	—	—	3.1	—	0.9	—	—	21.1	—	—
Muscle and tendon diseases	62.9	22.7	0.6	—	—	11.8	—	0.2	—	0.1	1.7	—	—
Joint diseases	36.8	46.5	—	—	—	10.0	—	0.5	—	0.4	5.6	—	—
Phlegmons and abscesses	2.4	77.1	0.4	1.2	—	—	—	0.8	10.9	1.2	6.0	—	0.2
Second group													
Foreign body in the eye	—	4.0	1.4	94.6	—	—	—	—	—	—	—	—	—
Benign tumors	3.8	51.7	2.1	—	—	1.7	—	—	3.4	31.4	1.7	4.2	—
Peptic ulcers	92.7	6.4	—	—	—	—	—	—	—	—	—	—	0.9
Rectal diseases	8.8	82.4	—	—	—	—	—	—	—	5.9	2.9	—	—
Stones in kidneys and urinary tracts	39.0	47.5	—	—	—	1.7	—	—	—	1.7	—	—	10.1

cian-gynecologists (34.8%) take part in diagnosing carcinoma and other malignant tumors.

Peptic ulcer is diagnosed largely by internists, and only 6.4% of the cases by surgeons; rectal diseases, on the other hand, are diagnosed by surgeons in 82.4% and by internists in only 8.8% of cases.

In making the diagnosis of bone, muscle, tendon and joint disease physicians of various specialties participate but mostly surgeons and internists.

Participation in making the diagnosis does not, however, fully define the work volume of physicians in various specialties in patient care. This volume may be judged on the basis of the distribution of all outpatient visits for the various diseases among physicians of the various specialties, about which we shall speak more below.

The data given on the morbidity rate according to the sickness rate data obtained even when surgical aid is fully available cannot give a complete idea of the prevalence of the various diseases. People usually go to the physician when they have a disorder of function of an organ or pain. However, there are diseases which in the initial stages give no subjective sensations. Therefore, comprehensive medical checkups aid in detecting many latent diseases and making the appropriate corrections in the rate

Table 26
FREQUENCY OF DETECTION OF CHRONIC DISEASE IN
COMPREHENSIVE MEDICAL CHECKUPS IN STUPINO
(per 1,000 population of the corresponding sex)

Disease	Both sexes	Men	Women
First group			
Mechanical injuries	0.3	0.4	0.2
Burns	—	—	—
Frostbites	—	—	—
Other injuries	0.1	—	0.2
Carcinoma and other malignant tumors	2.3	1.6	2.8
Appendicitis:			
acute	—	—	—
chronic	7.0	2.0	10.8
Acute intestinal obstruction	—		
Hernias	19.0	19.5	18.6
Bone diseases	1.5	2.3	0.9
Muscle and tendon diseases	5.5	7.0	4.3
Joint diseases	18.9	20.4	17.7
Second group			
Foreign body in the eye	—	—	—
Benign tumors	29.4	17.4	38.8
Peptic ulcers	6.6	11.6	2.8
Rectal diseases	0.5	0.7	0.3
Stones in kidneys and urinary tracts	0.7	0.2	1.1
Total	91.8	83.1	98.5

and distribution of the total morbidity of the population according to attendance at the therapeutic-prophylactic institutions, which is of great importance for purposes of planning standards. With the data on the so-called "exhaustive" morbidity available, it is possible to determine the actual need for therapeutic-prophylactic care by the population.

Data on the incidence of the cases newly detected by routine medical checkups are shown in Table 26.

From Table 26 it is evident that through medical checkups of the population quite often benign tumors (29.4 per 1,000 population), hernias (19.0), joint diseases (18.9), chronic appendicitis (7.0), peptic ulcers (6.6), diseases of muscles and tendons (5.5) and others, previously unknown from attendance at therapeutic-prophylactic institutions, are detected.

During the course of medical checkups made by experienced physicians some of the chronic diseases, for which patients' visits had been recorded and of which these physicians had been unaware, were not confirmed, and this was taken into account in determining the standards of therapeutic-prophylactic care in the field of surgery.

At the same time, the medical checkups offered the opportunity of determining the frequency of the chronic cases actually needing some form of medical care, which is very important to know for planning standards.

Urban Population Attendance at Outpatient-Polyclinic Institutions

The rate and distribution of the population morbidity essentially determine also the number of outpatient visits for therapy. However, visits to surgeons by patients with so-called related diseases for the purpose of obtaining consultations should be taken into account also. In addition, the work volume of surgeons in the prophylactic care of the population, as determined basically by the principles and directives of the USSR Ministry of Health, must be added.

In the evaluation by experts of the attendance data in various instances a clearly inadequate number of therapeutic visits for a number of diseases was found.

The average age indexes of the attendance for the existing morbidity rate (sickness rate) of the population are shown in Table 27 and Figure 14.

From Table 27 it is evident that per 1,000 urban population during the year the largest number of visits are for mechanical injuries without injury to bones or joints (85.4), muscle diseases (47.3), injuries with bone and joints included (44.5), joint diseases (31.7), etc. In one year 415.9 visits were made per 1,000 population for the diseases listed in the table.

The greatest number of visits by men to outpatient-polyclinic institutions were for phlegmons and abscesses, injuries, peptic ulcers, hernias, rectal diseases, bone, muscle and joint diseases; by women, for neoplasms and acute appendicitis.

Thus, the number of visits for acute appendicitis (essentially, postoperative) per

Table 27

AVERAGE AGE INDEXES OF ATTENDANCE OF THE URBAN POPULATION FOR THE GROUP OF DISEASES CARED FOR LARGELY BY SURGEONS (number of outpatient-polyclinic visits for therapeutic purposes per 1,000 population of the corresponding age and sex)

Disease	Distribution by age									Total		
	under 4 years	5–6 years	7–13 years	14–19 years	20–29 years	30–39 years	40–49 years	50–59 years	60 and over	men	women	both sexes
First group												
Mechanical injuries:												
with injury to internal organs	—	—	0.7	1.3	3.9	1.6	5.3	0.8	0.7	2.6	1.9	2.2
without injury to bones or joints	16.3	37.6	30.0	64.5	125.9	109.8	110.8	98.8	54.3	121.9	57.3	85.4
with injury to bones or joints	4.1	7.2	9.8	22.8	54.5	53.5	71.4	83.0	33.6	70.7	24.4	44.5
Burns	4.0	7.4	1.1	12.2	44.8	28.6	26.6	28.0	8.9	37.2	11.8	22.7
Frostbites	—	—	0.1	1.9	1.7	1.0	1.3	0.9	1.3	1.9	0.6	1.2
Other injuries	2.9	7.9	13.5	22.3	22.7	21.1	23.9	31.9	27.4	30.1	13.5	20.8
Carcinoma and other malignant tumors	—	0.2	—	0.4	0.6	6.2	29.2	41.3	49.2	12.0	13.6	12.8
Appendicitis:												
acute	0.3	2.6	10.7	20.8	29.6	22.6	17.6	14.4	3.4	16.7	17.9	17.4
chronic	0.5	1.3	5.5	9.0	11.8	16.0	11.5	11.6	3.6	8.1	10.9	9.7
Acute intestinal obstruction	0.2	0.3	—	0.1	—	0.1	0.6	0.1	3.0	0.5	0.3	0.4
Hernias	5.2	4.9	1.5	2.9	5.0	6.8	14.0	16.6	12.9	10.9	5.0	7.5
Bone diseases	5.1	7.4	6.4	6.2	10.8	20.4	39.1	17.3	15.1	22.2	12.2	16.4
Muscle and tendon diseases	2.9	0.4	5.6	15.4	45.8	63.9	102.0	77.0	38.2	54.0	42.0	47.3
Joint diseases	0.6	3.3	6.5	10.3	23.2	33.4	62.8	73.7	44.2	34.4	29.6	31.7
Phlegmons and abscesses	16.6	16.4	13.0	24.0	39.9	30.3	34.0	19.6	7.4	35.2	18.4	25.7
Second group												
Foreign body in the eye	0.2	0.7	2.3	5.3	20.8	17.4	14.6	8.9	2.9	21.5	3.2	11.1
Benign tumors	3.2	4.9	2.7	8.3	16.0	23.4	67.1	31.5	24.7	14.7	29.8	23.2
Peptic ulcers	—	—	0.2	4.9	28.3	51.8	46.0	41.9	13.9	52.6	6.7	26.7
Rectal diseases	0.8	0.5	0.3	—	2.5	4.5	7.9	9.6	6.0	4.7	3.2	3.9
Stones in kidneys and urinary tracts	0.8	—	0.3	0.6	5.2	7.4	9.1	9.0	8.0	5.5	5.1	5.3
Total	63.8	103.0	110.2	233.2	493.0	519.8	694.8	615.9	358.7	557.5	307.4	415.9

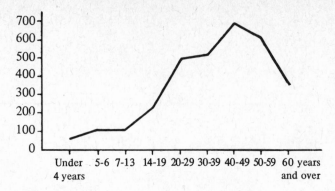

Figure 14

Average age indexes of outpatient attendance for therapeutic purposes by the urban population for the group of diseases cared for mainly by surgeons (number of therapeutic visits per 1,000 population of the corresponding age)

1,000 men was 16.7; per 1,000 women, 17.9; for acute intestinal obstruction these figures were, respectively, 0.5 and 0.3; for hernia, 10.0 and 5.0.

Particularly great differences in the attendance of men and women are seen for superficial injuries: for men, 121.9, and for women, 57.3; for injuries including bones 22.2 and 12.2; phlegmons and abscesses, 35.2 and 18.4; peptic ulcers, 52.6 and 6.7.

The attendance rate in the various age groups is in relationship with the morbidity (as judged by sickness rate).

As has been mentioned above, for the purpose of defining the work volume of the surgeon it is very important to determine the proportions of therapeutic visits for each disease group cared for by surgeons and physicians in other specialties.

The distribution of outpatient visits among physicians in various specialties in Stupino is shown in Table 28.

We took into account also all cases of prophylactic visits, among which were checkups of children, draftees, workers in industrial enterprises, workers in the public dining room system, visits for the purpose of obtaining health certificates, examinations made for sending the patient to the Medical Commission for Testing Disability and sanatorium-health resort treatment, and house calls made during dispensary care of patients and other visits.

The sum of the visits actually made and those added by experts most completely depicts the volume of medical aid needed by virtue of the existing morbidity as judged by sickness rate (Table 29).

Visits to surgeons for the group of diseases for which the patients are treated mainly by physicians in other specialties amount to 109 per 1,000 population. This group included visits to surgeons for hemorrhoids, varicose veins, and obliterative endarteritis, which are in the class, "Diseases of circulatory organs"; for cholelithiasis,

Table 28

DISTRIBUTION OF ACTUAL VISITS FOR TREATMENT MADE IN THE VARIOUS MEDICAL SPECIALTIES
(in percentages of the total)

Disease	surgery	internal medicine	otorhinolaryngology	opthalmology	phthisiology	neurology	psychiatry	dentistry	dermatovenereology	obstetrics and gynecology	pediatrics	oncology
First group												
Mechanical injuries:												
with injury to internal organs	15.6	21.9	1.2	1.1		62.5		0.07	0.03		2.0	
without injury to internal organs	87.6	3.9	1.1	0.1		4.1		0.8			0.5	
with injury to bones or joints	94.0	2.5	0.6			1.0			1.9		0.8	
Burns	79.1	3.1		14.5								
Frostbites	87.5	12.5										
Other injuries	75.0	6.0	2.0	2.4		5.1		5.1	2.4		1.0	1.0
Carcinoma and other malignant tumors	31.1	10.3	1.1		1.6					36.9	0.6	18.4
Appendicitis:												
acute	83.3	9.5				0.3				0.6	6.3	
chronic	53.2	29.9								2.6	14.3	
Acute intestinal obstruction	57.0	43.0										
Hernias	84.0	7.8								2.0	6.2	
Bone diseases	44.45	7.0	0.5		0.05	5.6		41.0			1.4	
Muscle and tendon diseases	20.9	60.1	0.3	0.1		16.4		0.2	0.5	0.3	1.2	
Joint diseases	37.6	41.8				16.5		0.2		0.6	3.3	
Phlegmons and abscesses	76.0	2.7	0.8	0.4				2.0	13.8	0.8	3.5	
Second group												
Foreign body in the eye	5.9	0.8		93.3								
Benign tumors	45.3	5.3	1.3	0.6		4.7			2.0	35.6	0.8	4.4
Peptic ulcers	14.2	85.8										
Rectal diseases	87.1	7.2								2.9	1.4	1.4
Stones in kidneys and urinary tracts	49.0	47.6				2.0				1.4		

Distribution of visits for treatment in the various medical specialties

Table 29
VISITS TO PHYSICIANS OF ALL SPECIALTIES OF OUTPATIENT-POLYCLINIC
INSTITUTIONS FOR TREATMENT PURPOSES FOR DISEASES CARED FOR
LARGELY BY SURGEONS

Disease	Average incidence (according to sickness rate per 1,000 population)	Number of visits for treatment			Average number of visits per disease
		actually made	added by the experts	total	
First group					
Mechanical injuries:					
with injury to internal organs	0.5	2.2	0.13	2.33	4.6
without injury to bones or joints	60.8	85.4	15.8	101.2	1.6
with injury to bones or joints	11.3	44.5	2.67	47.17	4.1
Burns	8.1	22.7	2.86	25.56	3.2
Frostbites	0.6	1.2		1.2	2.0
Other injuries	6.9	20.8	0.66	21.46	3.0
Carcinoma and other malignant tumors	3.3	12.8	0.89	13.69	4.1
Appendicitis:					
acute	7.1	17.4	0.45	17.85	2.5
chronic	3.4	9.7	0.04	9.74	2.9
Acute intestinal obstruction	0.2	0.4		0.4	2.0
Hernias	3.3	7.5	0.17	7.67	2.3
Bone diseases	4.9	16.4	3.43	19.83	4.0
Diseases of muscles, tendons and ganglia	24.6	47.3	29.9	77.2	3.1
Diseases of joints	12.8	31.7	4.77	36.47	2.8
Phlegmons and abscesses	13.2	25.7	3.3	29.0	2.2
Second group					
Foreign body in the eye	8.4	11.1	1.38	12.48	1.5
Benign tumors	7.1	23.2	3.3	26.5	3.7
Rectal diseases	1.5	3.9	0.18	4.08	2.6
Peptic ulcers	5.1	26.7	1.38	28.08	5.5
Stones in kidneys and urinary tracts	2.0	5.3	0.45	5.75	2.9
Total	185.1	415.9	71.76	487.66	

echninococcosis and liver abscess, and gastric polyposis, which are included in the class; "Digestive diseases"; for diseases of the renal pelvices, ureters, bladder and other diseases of the kidneys and urinary organs, which are in the class, "Diseases of the kidneys and urinary organs."

Patients with these diseases are cared for basically by internists and urologists.

The figures presented in Table 29 show that the average number of treatment visits per disease is greatest for injuries involving the internal organs (4.6), peptic ulcers (5.5), injuries involving the bones and joints (4.1), and carcinomas or other malignant tumors (4.1).

Hospitalization of the Urban Population for Diseases Cared for Largely by Surgeons

The average intensive indexes for hospitalization of the population for five cities are shown in Table 30 and Figure 15. Among the patients hospitalized for diseases cared for largely by surgeons, injuries (8.8 per 1,000 population) are in first place; acute appendicitis (5.2) in second place; diseases of bones, muscles and joints (2.6), third; further, benign tumors (1.7), hernias (1.4), etc.

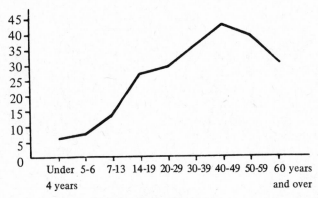

Figure 15

Average age indexes of hospitalization of urban population for the group of diseases chiefly under the care of surgeons (numbers of cases hospitalized per 1,000 population of the corresponding age)

Men are hospitalized more often for injuries (12.6) than women (5.6); on the other hand, more women are hospitalized for acute appendicitis (the number of women hospitalized is 5.9, men 4.2, per 1,000 population of the corresponding sex). Women are also hospitalized more often for tumor (benign and malignant); men, for peptic ulcers.

Table 31 gives an idea of the distribution of the patien's for the various departments of the hospitals.

From Table 31 it is seen that the great majority of patients with diseases cared for chiefly by surgeons are hospitalized in the surgical department. Patients with appendicitis, as a rule, are admitted to the surgical department, with the exception of a small number of children with acute appendicitis who are admitted for a certain period to the pediatric infectious disease department because of difficulties in the diagnosis.

On the basis of estimates by experts, corrective factors were introduced into the indexes of the population hospitalized, and thereby erors made by physicians as well

Table 30

AVERAGE INDEXES OF HOSPITALIZATION FOR FIVE CITIES (per 1,000 population)

Disease	Number of cases hospitalized														
	under 4 years			5–6 years			7–13 years			14–19 years			20–29 years		
	men	women	both sexes	men	women	both sexes	men	women	both sexes	men	women	both sexes	men	women	both sexes
First group															
Mechanical injuries:															
with injury to internal organs	—	—	—	0.1	0.1	0.1	0.5	0.16	0.3	0.6	0.1	0.3	0.4	0.16	0.3
without injury to bones or joints	0.5	0.3	0.4	1.9	1.3	1.7	3.6	2.0	2.9	5.0	2.4	3.7	7.1	2.7	4.6
with injury to bones or joints	0.9	0.6	0.8	1.5	0.6	1.1	2.0	0.5	1.3	5.7	1.3	3.5	5.0	1.8	3.4
Burns	0.9	1.1	1.0	0.5	0.2	0.4	0.6	0.16	0.4	0.9	0.26	0.6	1.5	0.7	1.0
Frostbites	—	—	—	—	—	—	—	—	—	0.4	0.2	0.2	—	—	—
Other injuries	0.1	0.2	0.2	0.2	0.16	0.2	0.7	0.4	0.5	2.0	0.7	1.4	1.4	0.8	1.0
Carcinoma and other malignant tumors	—	—	—	—	—	—	—	—	—	—	0.1	—	0.5	0.3	0.4
Appendicitis:															
acute	0.2	0.04	0.1	0.7	1.0	0.8	3.8	5.4	4.6	7.0	11.1	8.9	5.2	7.9	6.6
chronic	—	—	—	0.1	0.8	0.4	0.3	1.4	0.9	1.1	1.8	1.4	1.2	2.9	2.1
Acute intestinal obstruction	—	0.25	0.1	—	0.1	0.1	0.7	0.14	0.4	0.2	0.08	0.1	—	—	—
Hernias	0.9	0.3	0.6	1.9	0.1	1.0	0.4	0.05	0.2	3.0	—	1.5	1.4	0.3	0.8
Bone diseases	—	0.25	0.1	0.2	0.08	0.1	0.1	0.4	0.2	0.7	0.47	0.6	0.6	0.3	0.4
Diseases of muscles and tendons	—	—	—	—	—	—	0.4	0.16	0.3	0.3	0.38	0.3	1.0	0.25	0.6
Joint diseases	0.1	1.9	1.0	0.1	0.2	0.1	—	—	—	0.9	0.48	0.7	1.6	0.9	1.4
Phlegmons and abscesses	1.3	1.6	1.4	0.9	0.7	0.8	1.2	1.0	1.1	2.2	1.4	1.8	1.6	1.6	1.6
Second group															
Foreign body in the eye	—	—	—	0.1	—	0.1	0.2	—	0.1	—	—	—	0.2	—	0.1
Benign tumors	0.5	0.1	0.3	—	—	—	0.1	0.06	0.1	0.9	0.4	0.6	0.3	1.6	1.0
Peptic ulcers	—	—	—	0.1	0.02	0.1	0.3	0.17	0.3	1.6	0.24	0.9	5.5	0.6	2.9
Rectal diseases	0.4	0.2	0.3	0.1	0.5	0.3	0.1	0.2	0.1	0.2	0.06	0.2	0.4	0.3	0.4
Stones in kidneys and urinary tracts	0.1	0.1	0.1	0.1	0.06	0.1	0.1	0.2	0.2	0.2	0.3	0.3	0.6	0.44	0.5
Total	5.9	6.94	6.4	8.5	5.92	7.4	15.1	12.4	13.9	32.9	21.77	27.0	35.5	23.55	29.1

Table 30 (continued)

Disease	30–39 years men	women	both sexes	40–49 years men	women	both sexes	50–59 years men	women	both sexes	60 years and over men	women	both sexes	total men	women	both sexes
First group															
Mechanical injuries:															
with injury to internal organs	0.6	0.3	0.4	0.6	0.3	0.4	0.6	0.16	0.3	0.2	0.3	0.2	0.4	0.23	0.3
without injury to bones or joints	7.4	2.6	4.7	7.1	2.9	4.6	4.1	3.1	3.4	4.8	2.1	3.0	5.2	2.3	3.6
with injury to bones or joints	5.7	1.8	3.5	6.3	2.2	3.9	5.9	2.9	4.0	3.7	4.5	4.2	4.3	1.84	3.0
Burns	0.9	0.36	0.6	1.9	0.8	1.2	0.2	1.1	0.8	0.9	0.7	0.8	1.1	0.6	0.8
Frostbites	0.2	0.03	0.1	—	—	—	0.1	—	0.04	—	—	—	0.1	0.01	0.1
Other injuries	1.4	0.6	0.9	1.9	0.6	1.1	1.8	1.0	1.3	0.5	0.7	0.7	1.3	0.6	0.9
Carcinoma and other malignant tumors	1.2	1.4	1.3	2.5	4.1	3.6	7.2	4.3	5.3	8.3	6.8	7.3	1.4	1.84	1.6
Appendicitis:															
acute	5.9	8.7	7.5	4.8	5.0	4.9	2.6	3.8	3.3	1.3	2.5	2.2	4.2	5.9	5.2
chronic	1.8	2.5	2.2	1.3	2.1	1.8	1.0	1.0	1.0	0.3	0.5	0.5	0.9	1.8	1.4
Acute intestinal obstruction	0.2	0.05	0.1	0.2	0.2	0.2	0.1	0.2	0.1	1.4	1.0	0.9	0.2	0.2	0.1
Hernias	1.4	0.9	1.1	2.7	2.3	2.5	3.4	1.8	2.4	3.5	2.5	2.7	1.9	0.9	1.4
Bone diseases	1.5	0.8	1.0	0.7	0.6	0.6	1.3	0.45	0.8	0.7	0.15	0.3	0.7	0.4	0.5
Diseases of muscles and tendons	1.1	0.5	0.8	1.2	0.7	0.9	1.5	0.9	1.1	0.8	0.1	0.3	0.7	0.36	0.6
Joint diseases	2.2	1.4	1.8	4.9	1.8	3.1	3.0	2.5	2.7	3.8	1.4	2.2	1.9	1.1	1.5
Phlegmons and abscesses	1.0	0.6	0.8	1.0	0.8	0.9	1.4	0.7	1.0	1.6	0.3	0.7	1.3	1.0	1.2
Second group															
Foreign body in the eye	0.4	—	0.1	0.2	—	0.1	0.1	—	0.1	—	—	—	0.2	—	0.1
Benign tumors	0.7	3.1	2.1	1.6	7.0	4.9	1.5	4.4	3.3	2.6	0.9	1.5	0.8	2.4	1.7
Peptic ulcers	11.3	0.8	5.2	10.2	1.3	4.9	10.7	0.6	4.6	2.0	0.2	0.8	5.4	0.6	2.7
Rectal diseases	0.5	0.2	0.3	1.5	0.4	0.8	1.2	0.3	0.7	0.4	0.4	0.4	0.5	0.3	0.4
Stones in kidneys and urinary tracts	2.4	0.7	1.4	3.0	1.6	2.2	3.0	2.3	2.7	2.0	0.5	1.1	1.3	0.8	1.0
Total	47.8	27.34	35.9	53.6	34.7	42.6	50.7	31.51	38.94	38.8	25.55	29.8	33.8	23.18	28.1

Table 31

DISTRIBUTION OF PATIENTS HOSPITALIZED (in percent) ACCORDING TO HOSPITAL DEPARTMENTS

Disease	Hospital departments								
	surgical	internal medicine	otorhino-laryngo-logical	ophthalmo-logical	neurological	gyneco-logical	pediatric	infectious disease (for adults)	other de-part-ments
First group									
Mechanical injuries:									
with injury to internal organs	80.0	20.0	—	—	—	—	—	—	—
without involving bones or joints	96.3c	—	—	—	—	3.7	—	—	—
with injury to bones or joints	93.4	4.8	—	—	1.8	—	—	—	—
Burns	70.7	—	15.3	7.0	—	—	7.0	—	—
Frostbites	100.0	—	—	—	—	—	—	—	—
Other injuries	61.5	—	—	38.5	—	—	—	—	—
Carcinoma and other malignant tumors	46.4	10.8	—	—	—	42.8	—	—	—
Appendicitis:									
acute	99.2	—	—	—	—	—	—	0.8	—
chronic	100.0	—	—	—	—	—	—	—	—
Acute intestinal obstruction	100.0	—	—	—	—	—	—	—	—
Hernias	95.5	—	—	—	—	—	4.5	—	—
Bone diseases	100.0	—	—	—	—	—	—	—	—
Muscle and tendon diseases	40.0	20.0	—	—	20.0	—	20.0	—	—
Joint diseases	35.5	35.5	—	—	18.4	5.3	5.3	—	—
Phlegmons and abscesses	77.8	—	—	—	—	11.1	11.1	—	—
Second group									
Foreign body in the eye	—	—	—	100.0	—	—	—	—	—
Benign tumors	39.1	—	2.3	—	10.3	46.0	—	2.3	—
Peptic ulcers	15.6	84.4	—	—	—	—	—	—	—
Rectal diseases	80.0	—	—	—	—	—	20.0	—	—
Stones in kidneys and urinary tracts	100.0	—	—	—	—	—	—	—	—

as refusals by hospitals to admit the patients because of bed shortages are eliminated from the calculations of the need for hospital care.

For the purpose of determining the standards of the population's hospital care requirement it is essential to take into account also the patients who did not seek medical aid but were detected through routine medical checkups and do need hospitalization.

The experts determined that in the group of patients with diseases newly detected through the medical checkups the following need hospitalization (per 1,000 population of both sexes):

patients with chronic appendicitis	6.4
patients with hernias	13.5
patients with joint diseases	0.7
patients with benign tumors	3.5
patients with rectal diseases	0.4
patients with kidney stones	0.1

For the purpose of planning standards it is also important to know the patients' average stay in bed.

The average duration of treatment (in days) in the hospitals of the cities of Dneprodzerzhinsk, Rubezhnoe and Stupino for the various nosologic entities is represented by the following figures:

First group

Mechanical injuries:	
with injury to internal organs	7.3
without injury to bones or joints	9.2
with injury to bones or joints	15.2
Burns	13.6
Frostbites	8.5
Other injuries	11.2
Carcinoma and other malignant tumors	19.9
Appendicitis:	
acute	9.4
chronic	8.1
Acute intestinal obstruction	8.2
Hernias	10.7
Bone diseases	15.9
Muscle and tendon diseases	10.3
Joint diseases	24.9
Phlegmons and abscesses	8.5

Second group

Foreign body in the eye	38.0
Benign tumors	11.6
Peptic ulcers	19.6
Rectal diseases	8.6
Stones in kidneys and urinary tracts	8.2

Standards of Therapeutic-Prophylactic Care of the Urban Population in the Field of Surgery

Having at our disposal the data for total morbidity (sickness rate), hospitalization and attendance at outpatient-polyclinic institutions as well as the data of comprehensive medical checkups and the corrective factors introduced by experienced medical experts from different specialties, we have a sufficiently solid basis for determining the standards for the requirement of hospital and outpatient-polyclinic care for the next few years, particularly since we have gained an idea not only about all the acute and chronic diseases from the sickness rate data but also on the chronic cases for which medical care is needed but for which the patients do not spontaneously apply to the physician. For such diseases the volume of additional medical care needs to be determined; however, it should be kept in mind that it will not be equal to the outpatient and hospital care actually existing for the diseases being analyzed. These conditions should be taken into account for the calculations of the standards of the population's medical care requirement.

Standards for Therapeutic-Prophylactic Care of the Urban Population for the Next Few Years (1966–1970)

In calculating the population's requirement of medical care in the next few years we used as a premise the fact that all the patients need it to the degree determined by the sickness rate with consideration of corrective factors introduced by the experts.

We also took into consideration the fact that in the next few years the conditions needed for making annual comprehensive medical checkups in which all the chronic cases might be detected will no longer obtain. Therefore, in the group of all the chronic cases needing medical care detected by comprehensive medical checkups only those found in population groups given prophylactic checkups (workers, children, adolescents) were used for purposes of introducing corrective factors into the attendance and hospitalization rates.

The number of all visits actually made for treatment purposes in the group of diseases cared for largely by surgeons amounts to 415.9 per 1,000 population of both sexes. To them the experts added 71.76 visits. Therefore, the total number of visits necessary will be 487.66. Of this number 294.6 (60.4%) of the visits will be to surgeons, and the rest, 193.06, to physicians in all the other specialties. The number of additional medical visits for the newly detected cases in various population groups subject to examination is 30.9 per 1,000 population. In addition, 109 visits to surgeons for treatment purposes will be in the group of patients cared for essentially by physicians in other specialties. Therefore, all the visits to surgeons for treatment purposes amount to 434.5 per 1,000 inhabitants per year.

In the majority of the cities of the Soviet Union patients with carcinoma and other malignant tumors and persons with premalignant states, among which are benign tumors with a tendency toward degeneration, some cases of peptic ulcers (callous ulcers, those with a tendency to degeneration, a stomach operated on for ulcer, etc.), cases of chronic appendicitis, sequelae of injuries (indolent ulcers, osteomyelitis, etc.), are now under the dispensary care of surgeons.

On the basis of figures on the morbidity, hospitalization and the participation of physicians in other specialties in patient care, as determined from the data in the city of Stupino, it is possible to determine the number of visits made to surgeons by way of dispensary care of chronic patients.

All patients with carcinoma and other malignant as well as benign tumors should be observed by physicians in various specialties both in the postoperative and pre-operative periods. Some of the visits for dispensary care of the patients (31.1% for

Table 32

PREVALENCE OF DISEASES TAKEN CARE OF MAINLY BY SURGEONS AMONG THE URBAN POPULATION ACCORDING TO SICKNESS RATE DATA AND MATERIAL OF ROUTINE COMPLETE MEDICAL CHECKUPS
(per 1,000 population of both sexes)

Disease	Average intensive morbidity indexes for 5 cities (according to sickness rate)	Incidence of previously unknown surgical cases requiring medical care detected through routine medical checkups
First group		
Mechanical injuries:		
with injury to internal organs	0.5	
without injury to bones or joints	60.8	
with injury to bones or joints	11.3	
Burns	8.1	
Frostbites	0.6	
Other injuries	6.9	
Carcinoma and other malignant tumors	3.3	2.2
Appendicitis:		
acute	7.1	
chronic	3.4	0.3
Acute intestinal obstruction	0.2	
Hernias	3.3	3.7
Bone diseases	4.9	0.5
Diseases of muscles and tendons	24.6	4.0
Joint diseases	12.8	9.2
Phlegmons and abscesses	13.2	
Second group		
Foreign body in the eye	8.4	
Benign tumors	7.1	20.1
Peptic ulcers	5.1	6.7
Rectal diseases	1.5	0.2
Stones in kidneys and urinary tracts	2.0	0.7
Total	185.1	47.6

carcinoma and other malignant tumors and 45.3% for benign tumors) will be by surgeons; others will be distributed among physicians of different specialties (obstetrician-gynecologists, oncologists, internists, etc.).

With house calls or routine checkups of patients every month for those with carcinoma or other malignant tumors and with four visits a year by patients with benign tumors, the number of surgeons' visits for carcinoma and other malignant tumors will amount to 12.3, for benign tumors, 12.8.

Patients with peptic ulcers are observed largely by internists, but those who require or have undergone operation are observed by surgeons. Of all the patients hospitalized with this condition 15.6% were treated in the surgical department.

Including routine checks of patients once a month, the number of surgeons' visits will amount to 9.6 per 1,000 population.

Surgeons should periodically check all patients with hernias not less than twice a year, during the postoperative period four times a year. The number of surgeons' visits in connection with this condition will be 9 per 1,000 population.

Considering the frequency of checkups of patients with chronic appendicitis to be four times, the rate of visitation of the patients by the surgeons will be 13.6 per 1,000 urban population.

Surgeons are responsible for 87.1% of the visits in the care of patients with rectal disease. Based on this and including monthly checkups, the number of visits for these conditions will be 15.6 per 1,000 inhabitants per year.

Surgeons will take care of 49% of all visits to patients with stones in the kidneys and urinary tracts. It should be taken into consideration that postoperative patients require frequent checkups. According to our data, 50% of patients with stones in kidneys and urinary tracts are treated in the surgical department of the hospital.

Including four checkups of patients not operated on by surgeons and no less often than once a month in the postoperative period, the number of visits per year will be 8 per 1,000 urban population.

For dispensary care of patients with diseases of the bones, muscles and joints as well as with the sequelae of trauma, we used the fraction of the most seriously ill patients who had been hospitalized in the surgical department largely for operative therapy (patients with osteomyelitis, indolent ulcers, scars after burns, nonuniting fractures, contractures of joints, etc.). With a checkup each month the number of surgeons' visits for these diseases will be 30 per 1,000 population.

For acute appendicitis in the postoperative period the surgeons will have to make an average of four checks on the patient, which will amount to 20.8 visits per 1,000 population.

For acute intestinal obstruction 50.6% of patients are sent to a surgical hospital for operation. In the postoperative period these patients need a monthly checkup by the surgeon. The number of house calls will be 1.2 per 1,000 population. All patients operated on in the surgical department for phlegmons and abscesses should be checked by surgeons no less than twice, which will amount to 1.6 visits per 1,000 population.

To this group we should add visits by way of dispensary care for the group of diseases in which the patients are cared for largely by physicians in other specialties, principally by internists. These are diseases of the thyroids for which the patients were hospitalized in the surgical department, hemorrhoids, varicose veins, endarteritis obliterans, cholelithiasis, diseases of the renal pelvices, other diseases of the liver, bile ducts and digestive organs, diseases of kidneys and urinary tracts, other diseases of the endocrine system, and chronic suppurative lung diseases. With a checkup per month, the number of visits for these conditions will be 42 per 1,000 population per year. To them should be added visits by patients who are not seriously affected with these conditions, detected through medical checkups, and who, according to the decision of the experts, need hospitalization and dispensary observation (7.7 per 1,000 population). With four checkups of the patients the number of visits for these patients will come to 30.8 per 1,000 inhabitants per year.

The total number of surgeons' visits by way of dispensary care will be 207.3 per 1,000 urban population per year.

As has been pointed out, dispensary care provides not only patient care but also regular observation of a certain group of the healthy population for timely detection of disease in the early stage.

To determine the volume of prophylactic care of the population by the surgeons, we took into account the directives, letters on methods and instructions of the Ministry of Health of the USSR existing on this matter.

In accordance with the directive of the Ministry of Health of the USSR No. 136 dated September 7, 1957, workers in various branches of industry engaged in enterprises under hazardous working conditions, in hot shops, as well as at work connected with the danger of injury, etc., are subject to regular medical checkups. Surgeons are to participate in these checkups along with other specialists. The total number of prophylactic visits to surgeons by workers in the various enterprises will be 10.7 per 1,000 population.

According to directive No. 321 of the Ministry of Health of the USSR, *Concerning the Status and Measure for Further Improvement of Outpatient-Polyclinic Care of the Urban Population,* 7-year-old children should have a dispensary examination before starting school. The number starting school yearly is 19.7 per 1,000 urban population.

Therefore, the number of prophylactic visits to surgeons for preschool children will be 19.7 per 1,000 population, the same as for other specialists. School age children (from 7 to 15) are all subject to annual prophylactic checkups by surgeons, which will be 134.1 per 1,000 population.

Adolescents must also be given a regular medical checkup by physicians of the various specialties. This has been provided for by a directive of the Ministry of Health of the USSR, No 354, dated 30 July 1963, *Concerning Measures for the Further*

Table 33

NORMS FOR HOSPITALIZATION OF THE POPULATION IN THE SURGICAL DEPARTMENT FOR 1966–1970

Disease	No. of cases of disease per 1,000 population	No. of cases hospitalized			Average duration of treatment	Distribution of hospitalized patients among the departments of the hospitals per 1,000 population							
		actual	according to experts' data	total		surgical	internal medicine	ENT	ophthalmological	neurological	infectious diseases	obstetric-gynecological	pediatric
First group													
Mechanical injuries:													
with injury to internal organs	0.5	0.3	—	0.3	7.3	0.24	0.06	—	—	—	—	—	—
without injury to bones or joints	60.8	3.6	0.08	3.68	9.2	3.55	—	—	—	—	—	0.13	—
with injury to bones or joints	11.3	3.0	0.04	3.04	15.2	2.85	0.14	0.12	0.05	0.05	—	—	0.05
Burns	8.1	0.8	—	0.8	13.6	0.58	—	—	0.05	—	—	—	—
Frostbites	0.6	0.1	—	0.1	8.5	0.1	—	—	—	—	—	—	—
Other injuries	6.9	0.9	—	0.9	11.2	0.6	—	—	—	—	—	—	—
Carcinoma and other malignant tumors	3.3	1.6	0.09	1.69	19.9	0.79	0.18	—	0.3	—	—	0.72	—
Appendicitis:													
acute	7.1	5.2	0.08	5.28	9.4	5.24	—	—	—	—	0.04	—	—
chronic	3.4	1.4	—	1.4	8.1	1.4	—	—	—	—	—	—	—
Acute intestinal obstruction	0.2	0.1	0.04	0.14	8.2	0.14	—	—	—	—	—	—	—
Hernias	3.3	1.4	—	1.4	10.7	1.34	—	—	—	—	—	—	0.06
Bone diseases	4.9	0.5	0.27	0.77	15.9	0.77	—	—	—	—	—	—	—
Diseases of muscles and tendons	24.6	0.6	0.04	0.64	10.3	0.16	0.16	—	—	0.16	—	—	0.16
Joint diseases	12.8	1.5	—	1.5	24.9	0.55	0.54	—	—	0.27	—	0.07	0.07
Phlegmons and abscesses	13.2	1.2	0.04	1.24	8.5	0.98	—	—	—	—	—	0.13	0.13
Second group													
Foreign body in the eye	8.4	0.1	—	0.1	38.0	—	—	—	0.1	—	—	—	—
Benign tumors	7.1	1.7	—	1.7	11.6	0.66	—	0.04	—	0.17	0.04	0.79	—
Peptic ulcers	5.1	2.7	—	2.7	19.6	0.42	2.28	—	—	—	—	—	0.08
Rectal diseases	1.5	0.4	—	0.4	8.6	0.32	—	—	—	—	—	—	—
Stones in kidneys and urinary tracts	2.0	1.0	—	1.0	8.2	1.0	—	—	—	—	—	—	—
Total	185.1	28.1	0.68	28.78		21.69	3.36	0.16	0.45	0.65	0.08	1.84	0.55

Improvement of Medical-Sanitary Care of Adolescents. According to data of the 1959 census, for every 1,000 city dwellers there are 69 adolescents from 15 to 18 years old. Therefore, the number of visits to the surgeon for dispensary care will also come to 69 per 1,000 population.

In addition, surgeons participate in prophylactic medical checkups of those being given drivers' licenses as well as certain categories of construction workers. The number of these is 38.6 per 1,000 urban population.

Therefore, the total number of prophylactic visits to surgeons will be 272.1 per 1,000 urban population.

Sufficiently complete outpatient-polyclinic care can be assured in the field of surgery in this way, if the number of all visits by the urban population to surgeons will come to no less than 913.9 per 1,000 population during the year (including 434.5 visits for treatment and 479.4 for prophylactic purposes).

The need for hospital care by the population is determined largely by the morbidity according to the sickness rate data of the population in outpatient-polyclinic institutions. Making routine complete medical checkups assists in detecting an additional number of persons needing hospital treatment for previously unknown surgical diseases, i.e., diseases not known from visits to outpatient-polyclinic departments. This made it possible to determine more correctly the population hospitalization requirement. The number of cases of patients hospitalized, on the average, for five cities is 28.1 per 1,000 population. To that the experts added 0.68. Therefore, the total hospitalization rate is 28.78. However, not all patients with these diseases need hospitalization in the surgical department. Some of them (25.9%) are hospitalized in other departments. The frequency of hospitalization in the surgical department is 21.68 per 1,000 population.

In addition, patients with the group of diseases usually cared for by other specialists are hospitalized in the surgical department; these amount to 3.5 per 1,000 population. Among these conditions are hemorrhoids, varicose veins and other vein diseases (0.9 per 1,000 population), diseases of the thyroid (0.3), endarteritis obliterans (0.14), cholelithiasis (0.12), diseases of the renal pelvices (0.3), other diseases of the kidneys and urinary tracts (0.84), other endocrine diseases (0.1), and chronic suppurative diseases of the lungs (0.2).

Therefore, the annual hospitalization rate will be 24.8 per 1,000 population if the average length of hospital stay is 13.3 days, and of bed operation, 330 days per year.

We deem it possible to use these figures for calculating beds for future years (1966-1970) for similar cities and, with the introduction of the necessary corrective factors, for care of the rural population in the same volume as in a given city (Table 33).

Standards of Therapeutic-Prophylactic Care
of the Urban Population in the Field of
Pediatrics

The data of the total morbidity (according to sickness rate at the therapeutic-prophylactic and pediatric institutions), the attendance and hospitalization obtained with fully available, obligatory and qualified care in the cities of Stupino, Chelyabinsk, Kopeisk, Dneprodzerzhinsk and Rubezhnoe were used as the basis for determining the standards of therapeutic-prophylactic care of the children. The total number of children studied in these cities was 82,814.

In addition, we made a complete medical checkup of the child population of the experimental districts of Stupino (2,849 persons), which permitted us to supplement the data on the incidence of chronic disease among the children and to determine the related additional attendance and hospitalization. So that the data on morbidity might be more reliable statistically and better suited to planning, we made calculations of the standards of therapeutic-prophylactic care of the children on the basis of the average figures for the five cities mentioned above. At the same time, we used a number of corrective factors worked out chiefly on the basis of the data for Stupino.

Total Morbidity of City Children (according to sickness rate data)

It is well known that in view of the comparatively high degree to which the population is provided with medical care and the quite satisfactory status of the initial records, the sickness rate data permit us correctly and quite completely to judge the morbidity of the population for the most manifest forms of pathology and acute diseases.

With respect to children, the sickness rate data approach the "exhaustive morbidi-

106

ty" [true morbidity] because certain groups, particularly infants, nursery school, kindergarten and schoolchildren, are under regular medical observation (S. Yu. Levina: "Zabolevaemost' detei rannego vozrasta" (Morbidity in Infants), *Sovetskoe Zdravookhranenie,* 1963, No. 3; P.G. Dzhamgarova, in the book: *Dispanserizatsiya gorodskogo naseleniya (Dispensary Care of the Urban Population),* edited by S. Ya. Freidlin. Leningrad, 1964; F. D. Turova: *Detskaya bol'nitsa s poliklinikoi (Children's Hospital with Polyclinic).* Moscow, 1964; and others). This contributes to maximum detection of the majority of types of pathology.

In Table 34 we present the intensive indexes of morbidity in children in all classes of disease (except for diseases of the mouth and teeth) in each of the cities and their average figures.

Table 34

INTENSIVE INDEXES OF THE TOTAL MORBIDITY (by the sickness rate) OF CHILDREN OF ALL AGES (per 1,000 children)

Class of disease	Stupino	Kopeisk	Chelya-binsk	Dnepro-dzer-zhinsk	Rubezhnoe	Average figures for 5 cities
Infectious diseases	337.5	235.9	525.4	270.6	310.1	318.0
Parasitic diseases	40.1	36.3	21.7	30.6	17.8	31.4
Injuries	56.1	44.0	61.4	31.5	9.0	45.3
Poisoning	1.6	1.7	2.75	2.5	0.6	1.9
Vitamin deficiency diseases	3.6	17.8	4.6	2.3	5.8	11.6
Rheumatic fever	10.3	6.3	6.75	2.5	1.1	6.0
Metabolic diseases and allergic disorders	10.1	19.4	7.4	9.2	3.3	13.9
Neoplasms	4.2	0.6	0.85	0.5	1.4	1.0
Endocrine diseases	0.9	0.4	0.3	0.2	0.3	0.4
Hemopoietic diseases	3.4	1.3	0.7	0.7	—	1.2
Mental disorders	1.6	1.0	2.2	—	—	1.2
Nervous diseases	11.2	4.3	6.9	3.5	2.0	5.2
Eye diseases	31.2	24.0	39.7	33.1	19.7	28.4
ENT diseases	394.8	275.8	317.6	335.9	428.4	310.9
Respiratory diseases	85.5	135.9	107.1	113.2	122.2	122.8
Circulatory diseases	11.7	12.7	9.3	13.5	15.0	12.1
Digestive diseases	70.6	77.7	37.3	59.5	60.0	65.3
Diseases of bones, muscles, and joints	21.8	3.5	2.7	4.4	1.3	4.6
Skin diseases	35.5	39.7	63.8	36.2	16.2	42.7
Diseases of kidneys and urinary organs	6.4	4.1	2.95	5.4	8.1	4.4
Congenital defects	1.9	1.8	0.7	0.2	0.3	1.3
Diseases of the newborn	1.9	1.4	1.6	1.7	—	1.4
Other diseases	57.4	4.7	8.4	71.8	52.8	18.2
Total diseases (not including oral and dental diseases)	1,200.4	950.3	1,232.1	1,029.0	1,075.4	1,049.2

In comparing the morbidity indexes of children in various cities it is evident that the greatest attendance is noted for the following four classes of disease: ENT (25.7– 40.1% of the total number of cases), mainly because of common colds, infectious diseases, respiratory diseases and digestive diseases.

In the various cities the attendance for these classes of disease ranged from 75% (for Stupino) to 85.7% (Rubezhnoe) of the total for children, determining thereby the total morbidity.

Certain differences in the total morbidity for the children of different cities may be explained chiefly by outbreaks of influenza and certain children's diseases, as well as in connection with the different numbers of mass prophylactic checkups of preschool and schoolchildren.

The high figures for the total morbidity of children in Chelyabinsk (1,232.1) are explained by the influenza epidemic during the year being studied (1959). As far as Stupino is concerned, the relatively high morbidity figures (1,200.4) are most likely connected with the fact that the most favorable conditions were created there for medical care of children (general, medical and nursing staff, etc.) and this accounted for the greater frequency of admissions for the mild forms of disease (colds, etc.). Despite certain differences in the rate and distribution of the morbidity in children in the different cities, certain rules and regulations may be noted, which make it possible to utilize the average data for these cities as statistically more reliable for final calculations and analysis.

Analysis of the morbidity figures for children according to sex made it possible to demonstrate only some of the differences in injuries (more in boys) as well as in rheumatic fever, chronic tonsillitis, sore throats, nervous and metabolic diseases (somewhat more in girls). For the remaining classes and the total morbidity the figures show only slight variations.

The standardization made did not introduce any substantial changes in the morbidity figures, which gives us reason to believe that the age and sex distribution for children in these cities is typical for the entire child population of the cities of the USSR.

According to the average morbidity figures for the children of five cities, infectious diseases (318) and ENT diseases (310.9 per 1,000 children) were in first and second places with regard to prevalence. In third and fourth places were, respectively, respiratory diseases (122.8) and digestive diseases (65.3). Injuries (45.3), skin diseases (42.7), parasitic diseases (31.4), and eye diseases (28.4) were much less often encountered. The prevalence of other diseases in children was very low.

Among the nosologic entities included in the class of ENT diseases the commonest were common colds (233.7), influenza (89.2), sore throat (79.6), measles (32.5), "minor infectious diseases"—chicken pox and rubella (25.5), pertussis (17.7), acute dysentery (13.9), and mumps (13.4).

Bronchopneumonia (73.7) and acute bronchitis (30.4) were the most frequent in the class of respiratory diseases; in the group of chronic nonspecific respiratory diseases the sickness rate was 15.9 per 1,000 children (not counting bronchial asthma). Among the digestive diseases acute gastrointestinal diseases were encountered most often: simple and toxic dyspepsia (21.6), enteritis and colitis (16.2), acute gastritis (4.7). Infectious hepatitis (5.9) and acute appendicitis (4.4 per 1,000 child population) were quite widespread.

The morbidity for these four classes of disease was 77.9% of the entire morbidity for the child population of five cities.

Therefore, the average figure for total morbidity according to sickness rate that we used for the children of the five cities was 1,049.2 (not including oral and dental diseases). This figure is quite close to a number of figures given in the literature, despite differences in the methods of introducing corrective factors into the morbidity rates. N. N. Govor ("Zabolevaemost' naseleniya Minska v 1955 i 1956 gg." (Morbidity of the Minsk Population in 1955 and 1956), *Sovetskoe Zdravookhranenie*, 1958, No. 7), who studied the morbidity according to sickness rate of the Minsk population for 1955 and 1956, points out that the total child morbidity was 1,129.8 per 1,000 children under 15.

According to the findings of A.A. Akhmedov, "Sdvigi v zabolevaemosti naseleniya g. Nukhi (Azerbaidzhanskaya SSR) za period s 1939 po 1959 g." (Changes in the Morbidity of the Nukha Population (Azerbaidzhan SSR) during the Period from 1939 through 1959), *Sovetskoe Zdravookhranenie*, 1964, No. 6, in the city of Nukha in 1959 the total child morbidity was 1,057.6.

A detailed study of the morbidity for 1958 made by the Scientific Methods Bureau of Sanitary Statistics of the Ministry of Health of the USSR (Brushlinskaya, Levina and others) in a number of cities of the RSFSR showed that the child morbidity was 1,223.

We believe that the last figure is somewhat too high, because the authors did not alphabetize the stubs used for statistical purposes and thereby did not exclude the possibility of duplication of admissions.

Comparison of the morbidity figures for the various climato-geographic regions of the country shows that with adequate provision of medical care the effect of different natural factors on the morbidity figures is equalized to a considerable degree by various social measures (medical care, nutrition, housing and others), which assure the rise in material and cultural levels of the population.

Proceeding with the analysis of the morbidity figures for children at various periods in their lives, it should be noted that we use as a basis the idea that they are conditioned by anatomico-physiological characteristics, by the reactivity of the body, by environmental conditions, as well as by the nature of the medical care of the children.

According to our data, the highest figures for total morbidity in Stupino are noted in children from one to two years old (2,495.6); the lowest, from 13 to 15

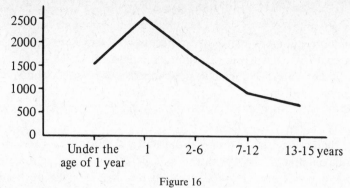

Figure 16

Age indexes for the total morbidity (according to sickness rate) of children in Stupino, not including oral diseases and dental diseases (number of cases per 1,000 children of the corresponding age)

(669.3). Below the age of one the morbidity was 1,515.3 per 1,000 children of this age (see Figure 16).

The lower morbidity figures in children during the first year of life can be explained most probably by the rising material and cultural levels of the population and government concern for mothers and children.

The data of Stupino show that the morbidity in children during the first year of life is much lower, both with regard to the total level and by comparison with the morbidity of children during the second year, which apparently should be considered another confirmation of a relatively new tendency in age morbidity changes in recent years, in contrast to the bulk of data in the literature (R. B. Kogan: "Sdvigi v zabolevaemosti detei Moskvy (po dannym vyborochnykh issledovanii 1951–1953 i 1956 gg.)" (Changes in the Morbidity of Moscow Children (according to data of selective studies for 1951–1953 and 1956)), *Sovetskoe Zdravookhrananie*, 1958, No. 7; N. N. Govor: "Zabolevaemost' naseleniya Minska v 1955 i 1956 gg." *Sovetskoe Zdravookhranenie*, 1958, No. 7; V. A. Mozglyakova and V. E. Ganina: "Nekotorye rezul'taty izucheniya zabolevaemosti gorodskogo naseleniya USSR v 1958–1959 gg." (Some Results of Study of the Morbidity of the Urban Population of the USSR in 1958–1959), *Zdravookhranenie*, 1963, No. 1; and others).

According to the data of S. Yu. Levina's study ("Zabolevaemost' detei rannego vozrastra," *Sovetskoe Zdravookhranenie*, 1963, No. 3), in 1958 for 65 cities of the RSFSR the morbidity of children in the second year of life (2,071.5) is also somewhat higher than for children under the age of one (2,056.3).

A. A. Perelygina ("Sostoyanie zdorov'ya i zabolevaemost' detei pervykh dvukh let zhizni, po dannym nepreryvnogo nablyudeniya v detskikh konsul'tatsiyakh" (State of Health and Morbidity of Children in the First Two Years of Life, According to the Data of Continuous Observation in Pediatric Consultoria), *Vosprosy Okhrany Materinstva i Detstva*, 1962, No. 10) presents the following figures

Table 35

AGE INDEXES FOR CHILD MORBIDITY IN STUPINO FOR CERTAIN
CLASSES OF DISEASE AND SPECIFIC, MOST FREQUENT DISEASES
(per 1,000 children of the corresponding age of both sexes)

Class of disease and specific diseases	Age groups				
	under one year	from one year to two years	2–6 years	7–12 years	13–15 years
Infectious diseases	230.9	603.8	531.4	273.7	173.7
These include:					
influenza	72.2	176.1	143.2	83.5	63.8
sore throat	23.3	153.0	142.6	101.2	89.2
ENT diseases	699.3	1,025.4	580.7	236.9	165.7
These include:					
colds	561.1	855.3	402.3	109.6	44.6
Respiratory diseases	95.6	213.9	151.7	52.6	23.1
These include:					
bronchopneumonia	74.6	117.4	69.7	18.4	5.6
Digestive diseases	172.5	155.2	65.8	56.3	40.6
Injuries	11.6	56.7	48.8	51.5	90.0
Skin diseases	56.0	94.3	46.9	23.6	18.3
Eye diseases	25.7	83.9	48.8	21.7	12.0
Other diseases	177.1	262.4	208.5	186.6	145.9
Total (not including oral and dental diseases)	1,515.3	2,495.6	1,682.6	902.9	669.3

for child morbidity in Rostov-on-Don for 1959–1960, according to the data of continuous observation: under the age of one, 1,658; in the second year of life, 2,008 cases per 1,000 children of the corresponding age.

From Table 35 it is evident that common colds and infectious diseases, respiratory and digestive diseases are most frequent in the pathology of children in all age groups. These diseases are the cause of 70.1% of all admissions for disease in children under the age of one; 73.2% in the second year; 68.4% from two to six years; 54.4% from 7 to 12, and 42.2% from 13 to 15 years.

Simultaneously with the reduction in the proportion of these diseases in older children there is a rise in the importance of such diseases as injuries, parasitic disease, rheumatic fever, etc.

The rise in morbidity during the second year of life is accounted for chiefly by the increase in the number of colds (from 561.1 to 855.3), respiratory diseases (from 95.6 to 213.9, chiefly from an increase in bronchopneumonia), and infectious diseases (from 230.9 to 603.8) (see Table 35).

The increase in the incidence of these diseases in children in the second year of life is explained by the closer contact with the environmental conditions and with other children, because under the age of one children usually live under artificially improved conditions.

In contrast to this group of the most common diseases, the incidence of digestive diseases begins to drop as early as the second year of life (from 172.5 to 115.2).

Beginning with the third year of life there is a considerable drop in the incidence of colds and respiratory (particularly bronchopneumonia) and infectious diseases.

The rate and distribution of the morbidity in school age children (7–15) are appreciably different from those in preschool children. In first and second places during school age (7–12 and 13–15) are infectious diseases (273.7 and 173.7, respectively) and ENT diseases (236.9 and 165.7).

In third place from 7 to 12 years of age are digestive diseases (56.3); at 13–15, traumata (90). The variations in the age indexes of child morbidity are determined by the prevalence primarily of colds (from 855.3 at the age of one to two to 44.6 from 13 to 15), infectious diseases (from 603.8 in the second year of life to 173.7 from age 13 to 15) as well as bronchopneumonia (from 117.4 at the age of one to two to 5.6 from 13 to 15).

Aside from these conditions, variations in the age indexes are noted also for other classes of disease. Thus, the incidence of injuries reaches a considerable degree as early as the second year of life (56.7 per 1,000 children). It remains at approximately the same level until high school age, when traumatism becomes more than $1\frac{1}{2}$ times as frequent.

Attendance at Outpatient-Polyclinic Institutions by City Children

The attendance of children at outpatient-polyclinic institutions for treatment purposes is directly related to the distribution and rate of morbidity. The variation in the total attendance is most often connected with conditions of different degrees of prevalence in different cities (influenza, colds, children's diseases). The visits to pediatricians and physicians in other specialties for other diseases are relatively stable.

The experts' evaluation of the attendance was made on the basis of final diagnoses, which was facilitated by preliminary alphabetization and collection of statistical record cards copied from various types of initial records for each child.

In making the evaluation we were guided by the nature of the disease, its severity, and its duration in accordance with the child's age and with current principles of treatment of children for various diseases. We made changes in the number of repeat visits when the latter showed a discrepancy from current clinical experience and the nature of the disease. At the same time, the analysis permitted us to make adjustments in the distribution of the visits for the corresponding medical specialties.

The number of house calls and polyclinic visits was estimated in accordance with the principle of predominant treatment of sick children at home, permitting repeat treatment visits to the polyclinic for acute diseases during recovery and, for chronic diseases, when not in an acute period. For colds and sore throats from colds we planned a minimum of two visits, one of which was a house call. For follicular and lacunar tonsillitis, mumps and chicken pox, an average of three visits was planned, two of which were house calls. For the treatment of pneumonia an average of four to five house calls was planned. In view of the data for the most common diseases this number of visits stems from the duration of the disease as well as from previous studies (Turova, Nazarova, Abramova, Gashimova and others) and from the experience of the leading therapeutic-prophylactic institutions.

In Table 36 the total child attendance at therapeutic-prophylactic institutions of Stupino and average figures for five cities are shown.

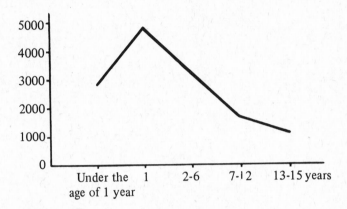

Figure 17

Age indexes of attendance of children for treatment in Stupino (number of visits per 1,000 children of the corresponding age)

Simultaneously, the table shows the corrections in the attendance figures made by experts in different specialties.

From Table 36 it is evident that the bulk of treatment visits both for Stupino and as average figures for the 5 cities it is 2. For the subsequent workup of standards of diseases, and respiratory and digestive diseases.

The average number of treatment visits per child under age 15 per year (not including oral and dental diseases) for the city of Stupino is 2.2; according to the average figures for these cities it is 2. For the subsequent workup of standards of outpatient-polyclinic care of children we are using the average actual figures for these cities supplemented by the corrective factors of the experts.

In analyzing the characteristics of the child attendance for treatment according to age (see Figure 17), we may also note the direct relationship between this and the morbidity rate and distribution.

Table 36

CHILD ATTENDANCE AT OUTPATIENT-POLYCLINIC INSTITUTIONS FOR TREATMENT (per 1,000 children of all ages)

Class of disease	Stupino			Average figures for five cities			Additions by the experts		Average attendance figures with additions by the experts	
	morbidity	attendance	average number of visits per disease	morbidity	attendance	average number of visits per disease	per 1,000 children	per disease	per 1,000 children	per disease
Infectious diseases	337.5	626.8	1.9	318.0	571.2	1.8	170.0	0.5	741.2	2.3
Parasitic diseases	40.1	66.9	1.7	31.4	49.1	1.6	16.3	0.5	65.4	2.1
Injuries	56.2	79.8	1.4	45.3	51.5	1.1	18.8	0.4	70.3	1.5
Rheumatic fever	10.3	25.7	2.5	6.0	11.0	1.8	5.6	0.9	16.6	2.7
Nervous diseases	11.2	38.3	3.4	5.2	15.7	3.0	10.1	1.9	25.8	4.9
Eye diseases	31.2	50.8	1.6	28.4	47.5	1.7	18.9	0.7	66.4	2.4
ENT diseases	394.9	720.2	1.8	310.9	719.2	2.3	233.8	0.7	953.0	3.0
Respiratory diseases	85.5	191.6	2.2	122.8	207.7	1.7	51.3	0.4	258.9	2.1
Circulatory diseases	11.7	24.8	2.1	12.1	25.0	2.1	4.0	0.3	29.0	2.4
Digestive diseases	70.7	124.9	1.8	65.3	105.1	1.6	18.0	0.3	123.1	1.9
Diseases of bones, muscles and joints	21.8	32.9	1.5	4.6	14.7	3.2	4.3	0.9	19.0	4.1
Skin diseases	35.6	49.9	1.4	42.7	47.2	1.1	20.9	0.5	68.1	1.6
Diseases of kidneys and urinary organs	6.4	11.4	1.8	4.4	12.5	2.8	2.9	0.7	15.4	3.5
Other classes of disease	87.3	140.3	1.6	52.1	124.9	2.4	37.9	0.7	162.8	3.1
Total (not including oral and dental diseases)	1,200.4	2,184.3	1.8	1,049.2	2,002.2	1.9	612.8	0.6	2,615.0	2.5

The highest attendance figures were noted for children between the ages of one and two (4.8), which corresponds to the highest morbidity indexes that we established among children in the given age group. Beginning with the ages of two to six (3.1), the average number of treatment visits per child per year decreases steadily, reaching the minimum figures at the ages of 13–15 (1.1 visit per year per child of the corresponding age) (Figure 17).

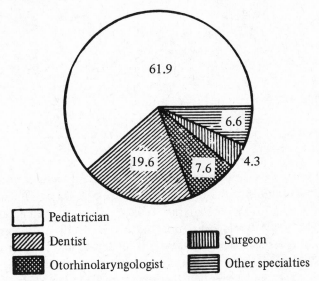

Figure 18

The distribution of treatment visits by children among physicians of the various specialties (in percentage of the total)

Figure 18 and Table 37 show the distribution of treatment visits among physicians of the various specialties in the town of Stupino. The data include also visits to physicians of the various specialties added by the experts when estimating the visitation rate.

From Figure 18 it is evident that pediatricians are responsible for the greatest amount (61.9%) of treatment to children. The high proportion of therapeutic visits in the field of stomatology (19.6%) is, to a considerable degree, connected with preliminary familiarization with the dental status of children through mass prophylactic checkups by dentists of the child population of Stupino.

Next, according to amount of treatment care, are otorhinolaryngology (7.6%), surgery (4.3%), ophthalmology (2%), dermatology (1.5%). The degree of participation by physicians of other specialties is slight (less than 1%).

Considering that in a number of cases stomatological care is determined separately from the other types of medical care, we are also presenting data on the distribution of treatment visits not including oral and dental diseases (see Table 37).

Table 37
DISTRIBUTION OF TREATMENT VISITS AMONG PHYSICIANS IN VARIOUS
SPECIALTIES ACCORDING TO THE DATA OF STUPINO
(in percentages of the total)

| | Totals | Including the following specialties | | | | | | | | | | |
		pediatrics	surgery	otorhino-laryngology	ophthalmology	tuberculosis	neuropathology	psychiatry	stomatology	dermato-venereology	gynecology	logopedics
Total treatment visits (not including oral and dental diseases)	100.0	76.6	5.4	9.5	2.4	0.6	1.2	0.2	0.4	1.9	0.2	1.6

In consideration of the adjustments made by the experts, pediatricians are responsible for the bulk of treatment visits for such classed of disease as infectious diseases
(93.2%), respiratory (97.5%), circulatory (86.6%) diseases, rheumatic fever (90.5),
hemopoietic (97.3%), vitamin deficiency and neonatal (100%) diseases. For such
very common diseases as colds (together with influenza) and sore throats, pediatricians made 98.3 and 93.3% of all treatment visits, respectively.

An analysis of the data shows that the general pediatrician (district pediatrician)
participates to various degrees in the treatment of all diseases in children and is the
main figure in children's health even where there is adequate provision of specialized
care. This is largely connected with the polyclinic system of child treatment, according
to which all patients with acute disease are treated at home. As a rule, the district
pediatrician makes the initial house call to the sick child. The sick child sees the specialist as early as the second visit, at the pediatrician's recommendation, for specialized treatment as well as for consultation or for maintenance on dispensary
supervision.

Through a differential account of all treatment visits to the polyclinic and house
calls in the field of pediatrics we determined that 61.6% are polyclinic visits and
38.4% house calls.

By working out the figures obtained for visits to pediatricians at the polyclinic and
for their house calls for different classes of disease, with consideration of the corrections made by the experts, we obtained the figures shown in Table 38.

For sore throat 48.8% of the patients came to the polyclinic and 51.2% were house
calls; for influenza, 51.4 and 48.6%, respectively; for colds 55.4 and 44.6%; for
chronic tonsillitis, 66.5 and 33.5%; for conjunctivitis, 72 and 28%, etc.

It should be noted that the relatively high number of treatment visits to the poly-

Table 38
RATIO OF POLYCLINIC VISITS TO HOUSE CALLS
IN THE FIELD OF PEDIATRICS

Disease	Proportion of visits (in percentages of their total)	
	polyclinic	house call
Infectious diseases	52.2	47.8
Parasitic diseases	95.4	4.6
Injuries	90.9	9.1
Poisoning	64.7	35.3
Vitamin deficiency diseases	96.4	3.6
Rheumatic fever	78.5	21.5
Metabolic diseases and allergic disorders	77.2	22.8
Neoplasms	100.0	—
Endocrine diseases	100.0	—
Hemopoietic diseases	100.0	
Mental disorders	100.0	
Nervous diseases	81.3	19.7
Eye diseases	76.8	23.2
ENT diseases	58.6	41.4
Respiratory diseases	60.8	39.2
Circulatory diseases	88.6	11.4
Oral and dental diseases	75.9	24.1
Digestive diseases	72.0	28.0
Diseases of bones, muscles and joints	86.1	13.9
Skin diseases	82.8	17.2
Diseases of kidneys and urinary organs	79.7	20.3
Diseases of male genital organs	71.4	28.6
Diseases of female genital organs	100.0	—
Congenital defects	92.8	7.2
Diseases of the newborn	76.9	23.1
Diseases not included in the nomenclature and not designated correctly	74.4	25.6
Total	61.6	38.4

clinic is accounted for to a considerable degree by repeat visits during convalescence, which were added by the experts.

While the attendance for treatment is determined chiefly by the rate and nature of child morbidity, the attendance for prophylactic care depends primarily on the instructions of public health agencies and work experience of pediatric therapeutic-prophylactic institutions. The amount of prophylactic care depends to a large degree on the provision of the pediatric polyclinics, preschool institutions and schools with medical personnel, on the number of preschool children's institutions as well as on the cultural level of the population.

Proceeding with an analysis of the attendance for prophylactic purposes, it should be noted that the amount of prophylactic care is connected, to a considerable degree, with the age of the children. Regular visits by children under the age of three, checkups of preschool children, dispensary care of children six to seven years old starting school, prophylactic checkups of schoolchildren as well as other prophylactic visits, among which are those connected with registration in nurseries, kindergartens, schools, admission to sanatoria, etc., should be considered prophylactic visits.

In determining the amount of prophylactic care it is essential to consider dispensary care of the children according to their state of health, regardless of age, including observations of children with chronic disease (rheumatic fever, chronic pneumonia, bronchial asthma, chronic tonsillitis and some others), convalescents from acute diseases (epidemic hepatitis, dysentery, bronchopneumonia), as well as children with frequent diseases of the upper respiratory tract who are physically weakened and have serious functional abnormalities in the cardiovascular and nervous systems, eyes and locomotor apparatus (F. D. Turova: "K voprosu ob obsluzhivanii re-) konvalestsentov posle zaboleniya pnevmoniei" (The Problem of Convalescent Care after Pneumonia), *Pediatriya*. 1960, 3; *Dispanserizatsiya gorodskogo naseleniya*, edited by S. Ya. Freidlin. Leningrad, 1964; E. S. Mikhailova: "K voprosu o dispanserizatsii bol'nkh grippom i katarom verkhnikh dykhatel'nykh putei" (The Problem of Dispensary Care of Patients with Influenza and Colds), *Sovetskoe Zdravookhranenie*, 1963, 6; V. P. Vager: "Nablyudenie za bol'nymi v period vyzdorovleniya" (Observation of Patients during the Recovery Period), *Sovetskoe Zdravookhranenie*, 1958, 12; L. G. Lekarev: "Programma KPSS i voprosy dispanserizatsii" (The CPSU Program and Problems of Dispensary Care), *Sovetskoe Zdravookhranenie*, 1962, 3).

In all these types of prophylactic care, from time to time, apart from the general pediatrician, physicians in a number of the more limited specialties participate.

Table 39 shows data on prophylactic checkups of children in Stupino for 1961. From the table it is evident that the bulk of prophylactic visits by children was taken care of by pediatricians (81 % of all prophylactic visits), and only 19 % by the specialists in the more limited fields, chiefly ophthalmologists (5.7%), dentists (4.3%), otorhinolaryngologists (2.9%), dermatologists (2.8%) and surgeons (2.7%). Physicians in the other specialties took care of 0.6% of the prophylactic visits. The average number of prophylactic visits per child under the age of 15 was 2.6, of which 2.1 visits were to pediatricians and 0.5 to specialists in the other fields.

The number of prophylactic visits to children under the age of one year was, on the average, 4.8. Through the work of a number of authors (K. A. Gashimova: *K metodike vyyavleniya norm potrebnosti v poliklinicheskoi pomoshchi detyam (Methods of Showing the Norms for Polyclinic Care Requirements by Childrne)*, Candidate Thesis. Moscow, 1935; R. I. Arkad'yeva: "Opyt dispansernogo nablyudeniya detei rannego i doshkol'nogo vozrasta v rabote detskoi polikliniki" (Experience

Table 39
FIGURES FOR THE PROPHYLACTIC CARE OF CHILDREN IN STUPINO (1961)

Type of prophylactic care	Total prophy-lactic visits	Including the following specialties						
		pedi-atrics	oph-thal-mol-ogy	stoma-tology	oto-in laryn-gology	derma-tology	surgery	other special-ties
Physicians' visits to children under the age of one year (per 1,000 children of the given group)	4,878.9	4,804.2	9.3	2.4	7.0	—	32.6	23.4
Checkups of preschool and school age children (with dispensary care of those starting school) (per 1,000 children of all ages)	2,703.4	2,558.9	42.2	25.3	22.4	20.0	14.9	19.9
Checkups of schoolchildren (per 1,000 children of this group)	1,826.6	1,134.4	209.4	161.8	106.5	106.0	98.6	9.8
Other prophylactic visits (per 1,000 children of all ages)	282.2	269.4	3.7	2.6	2.0	1.9	1.9	0.6
Total per 1,000 children	2,587.9	2,096.2	147.3	111.0	75.4	73.7	69.8	14.5
in %	100.0	81.0	5.7	4.3	2.9	2.8	2.7	0.6

in the Dispensary Observation of Infants and Preschool Children in the Work of the Pediatric Polyclinic) in the book: *"Ambulatorno-Poliklinicheskoe Obsluzhivanie Naseleniya.* Moscow, 1959; F. D. Turova: *"Detskaya bol'nitsa s poliklinikoi"* *(Children's Hospital and Polyclinic)*, Moscow, 1964; N. S. Nazarova and E. V. Abramova: "O normakh potrebnosti v poliklinicheskoi i statsionarnoi pomoshchi detskogo naseleniya g. Moskvy" (Norms for the Requirement of Polyclinic and Hospital Care by the Child Population of Moscow), *Sbornik Nauchnykh Rabot Instituta Organizatsii Zdravookhraneniya i Istorii Meditsiny imeni N. A. Semashko.* Moscow, 1957; and others), the number of prophylactic visits proposed for the first year of life was 8 to 14. Through Ministry of Health of the USSR Directive No. 321 dated July 20, 1960, 13 prophylactic visits were established for children under the age of one year.

In Czechoslovakia, in the first year of life each child is seen by a pediatrician 12.4 times on the average (Z. Štych, *Československé Zdravotnictvi*, Praha, 1962, and others). On the basis of studies which they made, N. S. Nazarova and E. V. Abramova point out that even in the best polyclinics children under the age of one were seen on an average 7–8 times for prophylactic purposes.

According to the data for Stupino, physicians attended preschool and school age children for prophylactic purposes an average of 2.7 times; of these the pediatrician accounted for 2.6. Specialists (oculist, dentist, otorhinolaryngologist, dermatologist and surgeon) examined the children of this age for prophylactic purposes generally once before the children were registered in school. The number of visits obtained is clearly inadequate, because children under the age of three are subject to dispensary care. This applies chiefly to children in the second year of life (M. S. Meller: "Zabolevaemost' detei rannego vozrasta" (Infant Morbidity), in the book: *Sostoyanie Zdorov'ya Nasleneiya Moskvy.* Moscow, 1946; F. D. Turova: "Poliklinicheskoe obsluzhivanie detei vtorogo goda zhizni" (Polyclinic Care of Children in the Second Year of Life), *Pediatriya,* 1957, No. 8; and others).

School age children, according to the data which we obtained, were checked for prophylactic purposes an average of 1.8 times; of these, 1.1 by the pediatrician (school physician). To a considerable degree this corresponds to the official instructions of public health agencies.

As a result of the analysis made, it is evident that the amount of prophylactic care of children in Stupino is inadequate. Therefore, in subsequent calculations of the number of prophylactic visits needed we shall consider the instructions of the public health agencies, data in the literature, and the work experience of the leading pediatric therapeutic-prophylactic institutions.

Hospitalization of City Children

The intensive indexes of hospitalization of the child urban population are shown in Table 40.

It is known that the hospitalization rate depends, on the one hand, on the morbidity rate and distribution and, on the other, on the quality of outpatient-polyclinic care and the capacity of the hospitals in various cities.

The highest figure for children hospitalized is noted in Rubezhnoe (217), although the morbidity figures there were comparatively low (1,075.4).

The relatively low figure for hospitalization in Stupino (119.4) is largely due to the fact that the incidence of bronchopneumonia in children there is the lowest (39.3) of all the cities compared (in Kopeisk, 75.3; in Chelyabinsk, 68.4; in Dneprodzerzhinsk, 78.9; and in Rubezhnoe, 46.9 per 1,000 children). Though it is adequately provided with beds for somatic diseases in children (1.3 per 1,000 population), it should be taken into account that Stupino is, at the same time, the district center, and its hospital provides admission for a large number of children from the rural environs.

A characteristic of hospitalization of children common to all the cities is the fact that it is largely made up of cases included in the four classes of most prevalent diseases—infectious, respiratory, digestive, and ENT (Table 41).

The hospitalization rate for the four classes of diseases noted was 82.7% for Stupino, 79% for Kopeisk, 75% for Chelyabinsk, 75.5% for Dneprodzerzhinsk, and 86.8% of the total of all children hospitalized in these cities for Rubezhnoe.

On the average, per 1,000 children of the five cities, there were 157.2 cases hospitalized (Table 42).

Table 40
INTENSIVE INDEXES FOR HOSPITALIZATION OF CHILDREN
(Number of cases hospitalized per 1,000 children under 15)

Class of disease	Stupino	Kopeisk	Chelyabinsk	Dnepro-dzerzhinsk	Rubezhnoe
Infectious diseases	40.5	41.4	42.3	24.2	51.3
Parasitic diseases	4.8	15.3	12.8	14.7	13.4
Injuries	4.4	5.9	5.3	2.8	2.9
Poisoning	0.3	1.3	1.5	0.7	0.2
Vitamin deficiency diseases	0.2	0.3	0.1	0.3	0.2
Rheumatic fever	4.7	3.4	4.4	1.4	0.4
Metabolic diseases and allergic disorders	0.1	0.9	0.6	0.2	0.1
Neoplasms	0.1	0.1	0.05	—	0.1
Endocrine diseases	0.1	0.05	0.05	—	—
Hemopoietic diseases	0.5	0.4	0.7	0.3	—
Mental disorders	0.2	0.05	—	—	—
Nervous diseases	0.6	0.5	0.7	0.9	0.9
Eye diseases	0.3	0.8	1.3	0.2	
ENT diseases	12.8	20.8	11.4	16.1	25.8
Respiratory diseases	15.6	44.5	27.7	40.9	76.6
Circulatory diseases	0.5	1.2	1.0	1.0	1.8
Digestive diseases	29.8	25.5	17.7	18.9	34.6
Diseases of bones, muscles and joints	1.1	0.9	0.7	0.2	0.2
Skin diseases	0.6	1.3	1.0	1.7	1.4
Diseases of kidneys and urinary organs	0.8	1.5	1.1	1.4	4.4
Other diseases	1.4	1.3	1.7	6.7	2.7
Total cases (not including oral and dental diseases)	119.4	167.4	132.1	132.6	217.0

Table 41
DISTRIBUTION OF HOSPITALIZATION OF CHILDREN
(in % of the total)

Class of disease	Stupino	Kopeisk	Chelyabinsk	Dnepro-dzerzhinsk	Rubezhnoe
Infectious diseases	33.9	24.7	32.0	18.3	23.6
Respiratory diseases	13.1	26.6	21.0	39.8	35.3
Digestive diseases	25.0	15.3	13.4	14.2	16.0
ENT diseases	10.7	12.4	8.6	12.2	11.9
Other diseases	17.3	21.0	25.0	24.5	13.2
Total	100.0	100.0	100.0	100.0	100.0

The largest number hospitalized are noted for infectious diseases (41.1), respiratory (40.8), digestive (24.4), ENT (18.1), and parasitic diseases (13.7).

We did not find any differences between the number of boys and girls hospitalized. Thus, according to the averages for three cities (Stupino, Kopeisk, Chelyabinsk),

Table 42

AVERAGE FIGURES FOR HOSPITALIZATION OF THE CHILD POPULATION
OF FIVE CITIES

Class of disease	Per 1,000 children of all ages				
	No. of cases actually hospitalized	additions by the experts	total figures for hospitalization (including the experts' additions)	Actually hospitalized per 100 admissions	Average length of stay in bed (in days)
Infectious diseases	41.1	1.4	42.5	12.9	13.2
Parasitic diseases	13.7	—	13.7	43.7	14.5
Injuries	5.2	0.2	5.4	11.4	9.1
Poisoning	1.1	—	1.1	58.1	20.5
Vitamin deficiency diseases	0.2	—	0.2	2.0	12.0
Rheumatic fever	3.3	—	3.3	55.4	32.7
Metabolic diseases and allergic disorders	0.6	—	0.6	4.6	24.0
Neoplasms	0.1	—	0.1	8.8	1.0
Endocrine diseases	0.05	—	0.05	12.1	30.0
Hemopoietic diseases	0.4	—	0.4	36.0	14.7
Mental disorders	0.04	—	0.04	3.2	13.0
Nervous diseases	0.7	—	0.7	13.0	21.0
Eye diseases	0.8	—	0.8	2.7	12.5
ENT diseases	18.1	2.0	20.1	5.8	11.0
Respiratory diseases	40.8	0.8	41.6	33.2	15.4
Circulatory diseases	1.1	—	1.1	9.3	9.0
Digestive diseases	24.4	0.3	24.7	37.3	18.1
Diseases of bones, muscles and joints	0.8	—	0.8	16.5	11.3
Skin diseases	1.1	—	1.2	2.9	18.3
Diseases of kidneys and urinary organs	1.6	—	1.6	35.2	41.2
Other diseases	1.9	0.3	2.2	7.5	11.7
Total cases (not including oral and dental diseases)	157.2	5.0	162.2	15.0	15.4

the hospitalization rate for boys was 154.7 and for girls, 153.5. According to the data of five cities these figures were, respectively, 158.4 and 156.1.

The average figures for hospitalization presented for the three and the five cities are very close and can serve as a criterion for evaluating the hospitalization rate in cities that are adequately provided with hospital beds.

The average figures for hospitalization obtained for the five cities were supplemented using the corrective factors introduced by the experts on the basis of children hospitalized in Stupino. We considered that the changes made by the experts are typical of cities adequately (in accordance with existing standards) supplied with beds.

In the expert evaluation of the hospitalization data we were guided by the nature of the illness, its severity and duration in accordance with the age of the child and the current principles of indications for hospitalization of children with various diseases.

Specifically, we planned additional hospitalzation in cases of severe, acute, and chronic diseases or those with a doubtful prognosis (acute cholecystitis, chronic tonsillitis with frequent exacerbations, all forms of cerebral concussion, pneumonia and dysentery in infants, and others). Thereby we appropriately reduced the number of house calls for treatment purposes. In a number of cases we noted the unreasonableness of hospitalization for relatively mild and brief diseases (colds, ascariasis, worms, and some others).

Thus, the average figure for hospitalization rate that we derived for five cities with consideration of additions made by the experts was 162.2 per 1,000 children of all ages (under 15).

The average length of stay in bed was 15.4 days, the longest hospital treatment being for diseases of the kidneys and urinary organs (41.2), rheumatic fever (32.7), endocrine diseases (30), metabolic diseases and allergic disorders (24), nervous diseases (21), poisoning (20.5), skin diseases (18.3), digestive (18.1) and respiratory (15.4 days) diseases.

The hospitalization of children in the different age groups has its own specific characteristics, as is distinctly seen in Figure 19.

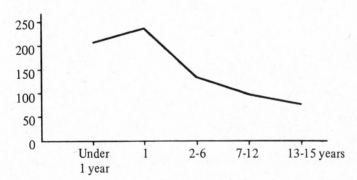

Figure 19

Age indexes for hospitalization of children in Stupino (the number of cases hospitalized per 1,000 children of the corresponding age)

The highest hospitalization figures were noted in children in the second year of life (231.7); the lowest, at the ages of 13–15 (76.6). The characteristics of the age indexes of hospitalization for the most common nosologic entities are shown in Table 43.

From Table 43 it is evident that the main causes of hospitalization in the first year of life are bronchopneumonia (51.3), dyspepsia (44.3), colds and influenza (together, 37.3) and dysentery (30.3); in the second year of life, also peneumonia (56.6), dysen-

Table 43

AGE INDEXES FOR HOSPITALIZATION OF CHILDREN IN STUPINO
FOR THE VARIOUS NOSOLOGIC ENTITIES
(per 1,000 children of the corresponding age)

Disease	Age groups				
	under 1 year	1–2 years	2–6 years	7–12 years	13–15 years
Acute dysentery	30.3	44.0	9.1	1.8	1.6
Scarlet fever	2.3	18.9	48.8	24.3	2.4
Sore throat	—	4.2	0.7	2.2	—
Influenza	14.0	4.2	1.9	1.8	—
Colds	23.3	14.7	1.9	0.4	—
Rheumatic fever			2.0	7.0	6.4
Bronchopneumonia	51.3	56.6	17.6	2.9	—
Injuries	—	2.1	2.0	6.3	5.6
Simple and toxic dyspepsia	44.3	—	—	—	—
Enteritis and colitis	9.3	29.4	2.6	1.5	2.4
Acute and chronic appendicitis	—	—	—	7.0	9.6
Infectious hepatitis	2.3	0.7	20.2	15.4	6.4
Other diseases	30.1	56.9	28.1	26.6	42.2
Total	207.2	231.7	134.9	97.2	76.6

tery (44), enterocolitis (29.4), influenza and colds (18.9) and, in addition, scarlet fever (18.9).

At the age of two to six scarlet fever (48.8) is the first place in hospitalization rate; infectious hepatitis (20.2), in second place; pneumonia (17.6), in third place; and, finally, dysentery (9.1), in fourth place. The hospitalization rate for the other diseases is much lower.

The main reasons for hospitalization at early school age (7–12) are also scarlet fever (24.3) and infectious hepatitis (15.4), but, in addition, rheumatic fever (7), appendicitis (7) and trauma (6.3).

At later school age (13–15), with the lowest hospitalization rate, the main causes are appendicitis (9.6), infectious hepatitis and rheumatic fever (6.4 each) and trauma (5.6).

The hospitalization rate for the other nosologic entities not included in Table 43 is low.

Table 44

AGE INDEXES OF THE AVERAGE HOSPITALIZATION TIME
(in days)

Disease	under 1 year	1–2 years	2–6 years	7–12 years	13–15 years
All diseases	12.6	13.1	15.5	17.2	15.2
Including bronchopneumonia	15.1	15.5	14.0	18.9	—

The age characteristics of length of hospital treatment are conditioned, on the one' hand, by the amount of time which has elapsed between onset of disease and hospitalization and, on the other, by the severity and duration of the pathological process. In addition, therapeutic-diagnostic possibilities of therapeutic institutions, conditioned by the achievements of medical science and technology, have an influence on the duration of hospital treatment.

Of great interest are data on the distribution of children hospitalized according to hospital departments (see Figure 20).

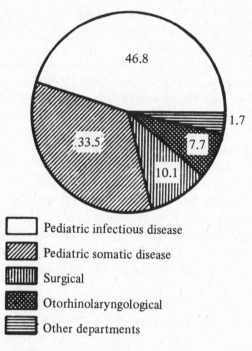

☐ Pediatric infectious disease

▨ Pediatric somatic disease

▥ Surgical

▩ Otorhinolaryngological

☰ Other departments

Figure 20
Distribution of hospitalized children according to hospital departments (in percentage of the total)

As is evident from Figure 20, the bulk of children are hospitalized in the pediatric infectious disease department (46.8%) and pediatric somatic disease department (33.7%). Eighty and a half percent of the children hospitalized are placed in these basic departments of the children's hospital. The number of children hospitalized in the surgical department (10.1%), chiefly for appendicitis, trauma and hernias, is quite considerable. Hospitalization in the ENT department (7.7%) is due mainly to chronic tonsillitis.

According to the data which we obtained, hospitalization in other departments is insignificant: 0.4% in the ophthalmological department; 0.1%, tuberculosis; 0.1%, nervous disease; 0.2%, dental; 0.7%, dermatological; and 0.2%, gynecological.

The data given on the distribution of children hospitalized according to hospital departments may be used for determining the proportions among the separate types of specialized hospital care for the child population.

The State of Health of Stupino Children According to the Data of Complete Medical Checkups

A complete medical examination is necessary for clarifying morbidity data, because prophylactic checkups of children by physicians in different specialties cover by no means all children's groups, particularly preschool age, in the everyday practice of therapeutic-prophylactic institutions.

Actually, as a result of a complete medical checkup of children with the participation of all the main specialists (pediatrician, orthopedic surgeon, otorhinolaryngologist, ophthalmologist, neuropathologist, psychiatrist, dermatologist and logopedist), we obtained information on quite a large number of such indistinct or occult diseases and pathological states as chronic tonsillitis, refractive errors, postural abnormalities, and others.

In making the examination we ascribed particular importance to a careful history. Physical examination data were compared with past diseases shown in the statistical record card, which was attached to the medical examination card. Anthropometry was carried out according to the generally accepted standard method.

Aside from the main and associated diagnosis, data on physical development and blood pressure, a record of all past infectious and various nonspecific diseases was made on the record card. In recording the disease we noted its stage, degree, form and location.

Children suspected of rheumatic fever were given functional tests and electrocardiograms, and were seen in consultation by the rheumatologist. On all children not in specific groups we performed tuberculin tests, and when tuberculosis was suspected they were seen in consultation by the phthisiologist. Children with abdominal pain were investigated for helminths and giardia. In various children blood, urine, stool, and gastric juice were taken for analysis, and they were given an X-ray examination.

Chest fluorography was performed on all children from the age of 12 onward. In all doubtful cases we were assisted by workers of the Roentgeno-Radiological Institute. Some children were sent for consultation to the Moscow scientific research institutes and hospitalized. In the most complicated cases the child was sent for consultation to the Pediatric Institute of the Ministry of Health of the RSFSR. During the examinations the physicians made recommendations for diets and treatment. After the examination we, in cooperation with the corresponding specialists, outlined the plan and volume of treatment-health and organizational measures for each child needing them for the calendar year.

In all, we examined about 4,000 children in the experimental districts, but in the workup the data on only 2,849 children, in which all the other members of the family had undergone examinations, were included. This was done so as not to distort the age and sex distribution of the morbidity of the entire population under study, because our investigation was part of the comprehensive work. Considering the relatively small number of children examined, we are giving the results of examinations based on the entire child population without dividing it into separate age groups. See the text below for details on age characteristics of certain diseases.

In Table 45 data are given on unrecorded cases and some pathological states in the sickness rate data and for those detected from making a medical examination.

From Table 45 it is evident that the composition of "newly detected" diseases, in medical examinations, and pathological conditions is substantially different from the distribution of morbidity reflected in sickness rate data.

The examinations showed up mainly chronic cases in the phases of remission and compensation, incipient or indistinctly expressed forms of chronic disease as well as borderline states, and functional disorders that cannot be considered a disease in the current concept of the word. The prevalence of refractive errors, 205, and chronic tonsillitis, 77.6 (including its compensated form), was particularly great. Abnormalities such as speech disorders (along with stammering, 50.5), postural disorders (35.8) and retarded physical development (29.8) were detected somewhat less often.

As a result of the examination, in addition to the sickness rate data, such diseases as first to second degree rickets (181.8 per 1,000 children under the age of one), nervous diseases (19.3), rheumatic fever (1.6), enuresis (9.8), concomitant strabismus (9.8), residua of poliomyelitis (8.1), chronic nonspecific diseases of the respiratory organs (along with bronchial asthma, 7.7), and inactive forms of tuberculosis (6.7 per 1,000 children under 15) were detected. Other diseases and abnormalities were detected in quite small numbers (Table 45).

The figures for the prevalence of various diseases and pathological states detected on examination showed essential differences in the various age groups of children.

According to our data, the prevalence of chronic tonsillitis in children in Stupino was 91.2 per 1,000 children of all ages; of these, 13.6 sought medical care, and 77.6 were detected through medical examination.

The greatest prevalence of chronic tonsillitis according to the medical examination data was noted in children from 7 to 12 years old (100.5), 13–15 years of age (86.6) and 2 to 6 years old (56.3 per 1,000 children of the corresponding age).

According to the data we obtained, the number of cases of rheumatic fever in Stupino children was 21.8 per 1,000 children of all ages, of which 10.3 came to see physicians during the year.

Chronic nonspecific respiratory diseases (chronic bronchitis, chronic suppurative respiratory diseases, bronchial asthma) were noted in 23.8 per 1,000 children under

Table 45

FREQUENCY OF NEWLY DETECTED CASES AND PATHOLOGICAL STATES
ACCORDING TO THE DATA OF MEDICAL EXAMINATIONS
(No. of cases per 1,000 children under 15)

Name of disease	No. of cases	Name of disease	No. of cases
Tuberculosis (all forms)	6.7	Other diseases of the ear, nose, throat, larynx and sinuses	8.1
Helminthic infestation	2.1		
Giardiasis	3.2	Chronic nonspecific respiratory diseases	7.0
Rickets, first and second degrees	13.3 (181.8)*		
Rheumatic fever	11.6	Functional cardiovascular disorders	31.3
Diabetes mellitus	0.4	Chronic appendicitis	4.6
Hypotrophy, second degree	1.4 (54.5)*	Uncomplicated hernias	4.9
Bronchial asthma	0.7	Other gastric and intestinal diseases	1.1
Other metabolic diseases and allergic disorders	2.1	Chronic hepatitis and other hepatic and biliary tract diseases	1.4
Benign tumors	3.2	Bone and joint diseases	2.8
Endocrine diseases	2.8	Skin diseases	1.4
Anemia	0.7	Diseases of the renal pelvices	0.7
Hemorrhagic diatheses	0.7	Cryptorchidism	2.5
Psychopathy	1.8	Female genital diseases	0.4
Oligophrenia	1.8	Congenital cardiac defects	1.8
Other mental disorders	0.7	Other congenital defects	1.8
Epilepsy	4.6	Scoliosis, first and second degrees	21.8
Neuroses	5.3	Pes planus	14.0
Stammering	19.3	Residua of poliomyelitis	8.1
Enuresis	9.8	Weakening and lagging in physical development (over one year old)	29.8
Other nervous diseases	14.0		
Conjunctivitis	0.4	Speech disorders (not including simple dyslalia)	31.2
Other eye diseases	1.8		
Malignant progressive myopia	2.1	Inaccurately designated diseases	1.4
Concomitant strabismus	9.8		
Errors of refraction and accommodation	205.0		
Chronic suppurative otitis media	2.8		
Adenoids	2.8		
Chronic tonsillitis	77.6		

* Per 1,000 children under one year of age.

15, according to our data, of which 16.1 came for medical care during the year, and 7.7 were detected on medical examination.

Determination of the need for medical care by the child population is closely connected with the study of a number of the basic indexes of their state of health.

Considering this, we included a study of physical development in the investigation program, in addition to the study of morbidity. In all, we made an anthropometric examination of about 3,000 children. Their standing height, weight and chest perimeter were measured.

The average figures for the anthropometric features calculated for Stupino children characterize their good level of physical development and are close to data obtained in recent years in a number of cities of the Soviet Union, particularly in Moscow (1957–1958) (G. P. Golovanova and V. Ya. Leont'ev, *Metodicheskoe posobie po otsenke fizicheskogo razvitiya detei doshkol'nogo i shkol'nogo vozrasta (Methodical Textbook on Evaluation of the Physical Development of Children of Preschool and School Age)*, edited by Professor A. G. Tseitlin. Moscow, 1960).

At the same time, groups of children were detected who lagged considerably in physical development (29.8 per 1,000 children) and who needed additional therapeutic-health measures.

Children with the chronic diseases and pathological states indicated in Table 45 need the most varied forms and degrees of medical care. Some diseases require only periodic recommendations by physicians (pes planus, scoliosis and others); in others surgical procedures are needed (chronic appendicitis, hernia, some types of benign tumors, cryptorchidism, etc.); in still others, dispensary observation and sanatorium-health resort care (rheumatic fever, chronic diseases of respiratory organs and others).

The level of "newly detected" indistinct chronic diseases and pathological states in children on medical examination is determined, in our opinion, to a great degree by inadequate coverage of some groups of children by prophylactic examinations of physicians in certain specialties, as well as at times inadequate attention by physicians, parents and teachers to the initial slight symptoms of the developing abnormality (frequent nasopharyngeal diseases, inattentiveness, disorders of sleep, appetite, visual acuity, hearing, speech, posture, etc.).

Further improvement of medical care of children and the growth of the sanitary-hygienic culture of the population should, in the final analysis, lead to sufficiently complete detection of these initial forms of diseases, which will create additional work for the therapeutic-prophylactic institutions.

Standards for Outpatient Therapeutic-Prophylactic Care of City Children

The data for the total morbidity, attendance and hospitalization of the child population obtained in cities relatively well provided with medical care and sufficiently complete records can serve as the basis for creating standards of therapeutic-prophylactic care.

The results of the expert evaluation of attendance and hospitalization data as well as the findings of complete medical examinations made in Stupino substantially supplement and render more accurate the estimate of the child population requirement of various types of therapeutic-prophylactic care.

Calculations of the standards of outpatient-polyclinic care of children in the field of pediatrics for therapeutic-consultative purposes are given in Table 46.

Table 46

STANDARDS OF OUTPATIENT-POLYCLINIC CARE OF CITY CHILDREN IN THE FIELD OF PEDIATRICS FOR 1966–1970

Disease	Average intensive morbidity figures (according to sickness rate) per 1,000 children for 5 cities	Average of all visits for treatment per 1,000 children			Average number of visits for treatment per disease	Incidence of diseases requiring medical care newly detected in medical examinations	Number of additional visits for treatment for the newly detected diseases	Total figures for previously unknown and newly detected cases	No. of outpatient visits for treatment to physicians of all specialties per 1,000 children	No. of visits for treatment to pediatricians per 1,000 children	Number of prophylactic visits to pediatricians per 1,000 children
		actually made	added by the experts	total		per 1,000 children	per 1,000 children				
Infectious diseases	318.0	571.2	170.0	741.2	2.3	6.7	15.4	324.7	756.6	705.2	—
Parasitic diseases	31.4	49.1	16.3	65.4	2.1	5.3	11.1	36.7	76.5	68.6	—
Injuries	45.3	51.5	18.8	70.3	1.5	—	—	45.3	70.3	8.4	—
Rheumatic fever	6.0	11.0	5.6	16.6	2.7	11.9	32.1	17.9	48.7	44.1	—
Nervous diseases	5.2	15.7	10.1	25.8	4.9	44.2	216.6	49.4	242.4	58.4	—
Eye diseases	28.4	47.5	18.9	66.4	2.4	12.6	30.2	41.0	96.6	14.9	—
ENT diseases	310.9	719.2	233.8	953.0	3.0	91.3	273.9	402.2	1,226.9	918.4	—
Respiratory diseases	122.8	207.6	51.3	258.9	2.1	6.7	14.1	129.5	273.0	266.2	—
Circulatory diseases	12.1	25.0	4.0	29.0	2.4	5.6	13.4	17.7	42.4	36.5	—
Digestive diseases	65.3	105.1	18.0	123.1	1.9	11.6	22.0	76.9	145.1	126.8	—
Diseases of bones, muscles and joints	4.6	14.7	4.3	19.0	4.1	2.8	11.5	7.4	30.5	12.9	—
Skin diseases	42.7	47.2	20.9	68.1	1.6	1.4	2.2	44.1	70.3	26.2	—
Diseases of kidneys and urinary organs	4.4	12.5	2.9	15.4	3.5	0.7	2.5	5.1	17.9	14.4	—
Other diseases	52.1	124.9	37.9	162.8	2.9	54.4	157.8	106.5	320.6	196.8	—
Total (not including oral and dental diseases)	1,049.2	2,002.2	612.8	2,615.0	2.5	255.2	802.8	1,304.4	3,417.8	2,497.8	—
Errors of refraction and accommodation	5.1	6.5	9.8	16.3	3.2	72.7	232.6	77.8	248.9	—	—
Total	1,054.3	2,008.7	622.6	2,631.3	—	327.5	1,035.4*	1,382.2	3,666.7	2,497.8	2,068
Number of outpatient visits to pediatricians by children per 1,000 of the whole population										747.1	618.5

* This number included visits connected with dispensary care of children.

The number of outpatient visits actually made for treatment purposes in all specialties was 2,008.7; with consideration of the corrections made by the experts, 2631.3 visits per 1,000 children.

The average number of visits for treatment to physicians of all specialties per disease (with consideration of the additions made by the experts) amounted to 2.5 for all diseases; for refractive errors, 3.2

The frequency of chronic cases needing treatment "newly detected" by medical examination amounted to 327.5 per 1,000 children, of which 72.7 were for refractive errors. The need for treatment visits over and above the number for prophylactic care of the children at the current level of medical care was determined by each specialist separately for each child by the expertise method during and after making the medical examination.

In calculating the need for treatment and dispensary visits (which in most cases may be considered equivalent) connected with "newly detected" chronic cases, we used as a basis the established average number of treatment visits per disease which had been compiled during the calculation of the actual sickness rate with consideration of corrective factors introduced by the experts.

The number of additional treatment visits for "newly detected" chronic cases determined this way was 802.8; including the visits connected with refractive errors the number was 1,035.4 per 1,000 children.

Therefore, the optimum number of visits for treatment in all specialties at the established morbidity, according to sickness rate data (1,054.3) and the results of complete medical examinations (327.5), was 3,666.7 per 1,000 children.

In considering the distribution of the established level of visits for treatment in the medical specialties we determined that the bulk of the visits for treatment (2,497.8) should be taken care of by pediatricians.

In calculating the number of prophylactic visits needed we took into account the directions of the public health agencies, data in the literature, and the work experience of the leading children's therapeutic-prophylactic institutions.

In the group of prophylactic visits we included examinations of healthy children in accordance with their ages as well as the visits associated with dispensary care of the children who had various chronic diseases that were not in an acute phase.

Data on the age and sex distribution of the urban population of the USSR were used for calculations of the prophylactic visits of healthy children in certain age groups.

According to Directive No. 321 of the Ministry of Health of the USSR dated July 20, 1960, children under one year old are to be examined by a pediatrician for prophylactic purposes 13 times a year (once a month and twice in the first month of life); children in the second year, four times (once every quarter); children in the third year, twice (half-yearly); and preschool children, once a year.

According to the "Instructions on the Work of the School Physician" approved by the Ministry of Health of the USSR on July 10, 1954, the school pediatrician should make a thorough medical examination of schoolchildren once a year.

On the basis of these principles, we determined the number of prophylactic visits to pediatricians by the children, which came to 2,068 per 1,000 children from birth to 15 years old; of these 871 were by children under one year, 264 by children in the second year, 132 by children in the third year, and 801 by preschool and school-children.

Therefore, the total number of visits to pediatricians which we consider optimal per 1,000 children under 15 should be 4,565.8 (1,365.6 per 1,000 of the entire population); of these 2,497.8 should be for treatment and 2,068 prophylactic (per 1,000 of the whole population the number of visits to the pediatrician for treatment should be 747.1; for prophylactic purposes, 618.5).

Standards for Hospital Care of Children

In determining standards for the hospital care requirement of children, we used as a basis the average data on the actual hospitalization in the five cities adequately supplied with beds, with consideration of the additions made by the experts to the sickness rate data and the results of complete medical examinations of children in Stupino, using the actual figures for the average length of hospital treatment (Table 47).

From the calculations given it is evident that at the established morbidity, according to the sickness rate data as supplemented by the data of complete medical exa-minations (1,304.4 per 1,000 children under the age of 15), the optimum index for the need for hospital treatment in all specialties was 242.6 (72.6 per 1,000 of the whole population), of which 157.2 were cases actually hospitalized, 5 were added by the experts according to the sickness rate data, and 80.4 were additions in connection with diseases found on examination. It should be noted that the majority of additional cases hospitalized in connection with the findings of medical examinations were for the chronic cases in the following groups: ENT diseases, 38.3 (mainly chronic tonsillitis), nervous diseases, 11.6 (congenital CNS diseases, epilepsy, severe forms of logoneuroses, and others), diseases of the digestive organs (mainly in connection with chronic appendicitis and hernias), 9.5. In this calendar year the indications for hospi-talization were determined by the appropriate specialists directly during medical examination.

Of the total number of all persons to be hospitalized, 84.2 per 1,000 children or 25.2 per 1,000 of the whole population were to be hospitalized in the pediatric somatic disease department; 59 and 17.6, respectively, in the pediatric infectious disease department.

It should be noted that the average length of hospital treatment is one of the essen-tial indexes for making up the plan of development of the hospital system.

Table 47

STANDARDS FOR HOSPITAL CARE OF CITY CHILDREN
FOR THE NEXT FEW YEARS (1966–1970)

Disease	No. of cases according to sickness rate and medical examination data (per 1,000 children)	No. of cases hospitalized (per 1,000 children				this includes	
		actual	added by the experts	for diseases detected by examination	total	in the department of stomatic diseases	in the pediatric infectious- disease department
Infectious diseases	324.7	41.1	1.4	—	42.5	3.1	37.9
Parasitic diseases	36.7	13.7	—	4.6	18.3	14.2	3.1
Injuries	45.3	5.2	0.2	—	5.4	0.4	—
Rheumatic fever	17.9	3.3	—	1.8	5.1	5.1	—
Nervous diseases	49.4	0.7	—	11.6	12.3	0.3	—
Eye diseases	41.0	0.8	—	1.1	1.9	—	—
ENT diseases	402.2	18.1	2.0	38.3	58.4	6.1	0.2
Respiratory diseases	129.5	40.8	0.8	2.1	43.7	42.3	1.4
Circulatory diseases	17.7	1.1	—	9.4	1.5	1.2	—
Digestive diseases	76.9	24.4	0.3	9.5	34.2	5.7	15.5
Diseases of bones, muscles and joints	7.4	0.3	—	1.4	1.7	0.5	—
Skin diseases	44.1	1.2	—	—	1.2	0.3	—
Diseases of kidneys and urinary organs	5.1	1.6	—	0.4	2.0	2.0	—
Other diseases	106.5	4.9	0.3	9.2	14.4	3.0	0.9
Total (not including oral and dental diseases)	1,304.4	157.2	5.0	80.4	242.6	84.2	59.0
No. of cases of children hospitalized per 1,000 of the entire population						25.2	17.6
Average length of hospital treatment in days						16.4	15.5

Comparison of the figures for the average length of hospital treatment obtained in various years and different cities shows that with improvement of medical care of children and a change in the distribution of their morbidity toward a reduction in the proportion of serious and long-lasting diseases (tuberculosis, severe forms of scarlet fever and a number of others) as well as in the number of complications (in the form of otitis, nephrosonephritis, etc.) and cases of intramural hospital disease, a regular reduction is noted in the average number of days spent in the hospital.

The average length of treatment in the pediatric somatic disease department, according to our data, was 16.4 days; in the pediatric infectious disease department, 15.5.

Standards of Therapeutic-Prophylactic Care of the Urban Population in the Field of Stomatology*

For the purpose of determining the standards of dental care in 1961, dentists made mass examinations of the urban population, a study of its sickness rate in the field of dentistry for a complete calendar year, as well as an experimental study of various organizational forms of outpatient dental care, furnishing dental clinics with new technical equipment, efficiency work, and improvement in methods of treating patients. The population was examined in Leningrad, Minsk, Petrozavodsk, Stupino (Moscow Region), and Tashkent. In all, over 48,000 persons were examined.

Data on the incidence of caries in the population of various cities, according to examination data, are given in Table 48.

The data of dental checkups presented in Table 48 give us an idea of the incidence of dental caries in various age groups of the population, but do not show the amount of dental treatment needed. For planning development of dental care the KPU/KP index, which is defined as the average number of teeth with caries which have been filled or extracted for caries per person examined, is very important. The KPU/KP index for various age and sex groups of the population of different cities is given in Table 49.

Table 49 shows that the average KPU/KP figures per person examined, that is, the incidence of dental caries in the population, show a quite definite pattern in various cities.

The average number of teeth affected by caries in women checked in all cities is much greater than in men. The KPU/KP index shows quite a definite tendency to rise with age. Thus, while in schoolchildren (7–12 years) there are from two to

* This section is brief, because the publication of a separate book on this subject is planned.

Table 48

THE INCIDENCE OF DENTAL CARIES IN THE POPULATION OF DIFFERENT CITIES EXAMINED

Age in years	Proportion of persons with caries in % of the number examined				
	Tashkent	Minsk	Stupino	Petrozavodsk	Leningrad
1–2	5.9	2.7	5.2	5.8	19.0
3–6	37.7	47.0	63.9	63.9	76.0
7–12	60.2	79.1	89.5	85.0	94.9
13–15	53.6	77.8	84.5	93.1	96.0
16–19	56.5	74.6	80.9	92.8	93.3
20–29	77.3	81.6	86.2	96.7	96.1
30–39	89.9	91.6	92.6	98.1	98.5
40–49	95.1	95.0	97.2	99.3	99.3
50–59	99.1	98.5	99.1	99.6	99.6
60 and over	97.8	99.6	98.6	99.3	100.0
Total for the entire population	70.1	80.6	87.2	92.5	96.2
This includes:					
men	58.9	72.0	84.9	89.2	94.1
women	75.8	84.2	89.9	94.2	97.1

Table 49

KPU/KP INDEX IN VARIOUS CITIES

Age in years	City				
	Tashkent	Minsk	Stupino	Petrozavodsk	Leningrad
1–2	0.3	0.1	0.2	0.2	0.9
3–6	1.4	1.7	3.1	2.8	3.8
7–12	2.1	3.0	3.9	3.9	4.9
13–15	1.6	2.9	3.0	4.8	6.3
16–19	2.3	3.2	3.8	5.2	6.2
20–29	4.3	4.3	4.5	6.2	7.9
30–39	8.3	6.9	6.8	8.7	10.4
40–49	12.0	10.6	10.6	11.4	13.2
50–59	18.3	16.6	16.3	15.5	18.8
60 and over	22.1	24.1	24.6	22.6	23.5
Total	5.9	7.8	7.8	8.1	10.5
This includes:					
men	3.1	6.0	6.6	6.7	8.6
women	7.2	9.1	8.8	8.8	11.3

five carious teeth per child, subsequently the incidence rises, and in the age group over 60 there are 22–24 carious teeth per person examined.

The figures given in Table 49 give us an idea of the total population requirement of treatment for dental caries and its complications. More detailed information on the nature of this need and the degree to which it is satisfied by the existing system of therapeutic-prophylactic institutions may be obtained through an analysis of the various components of the KPU/KP index (Table 50).

Table 50

AVERAGE NUMBER OF TEETH FILLED AND REQUIRING EXTRACTION FOR CARIES PER PERSON EXAMINED NEEDING TREATMENT IN DIFFERENT CITIES

	City				
	Tashkent	Minsk	Stupino	Petrozavodsk	Leningrad
No. of teeth needing treatment	1.1	0.8	1.2	2.3	1.7
No. of teeth filled	0.6	1.7	0.9	1.3	3.1
No. of teeth extracted	3.5	4.8	5.1	3.9	5.3
No. of teeth needing extraction	0.7	0.5	0.6	0.6	0.5
Average KPU/KP index	5.9	7.8	7.8	8.1	10.5

The data given in Table 50 show that at the time of examination the population of these cities was not adequately or uniformly provided with dental care. Thus, while there were 7.8 teeth affected with caries as an average per inhabitant, of these only 0.9 had been filled, while 1.2 needed treatment. The number of teeth needing extraction was half that of the number needing treatment, an average of 0.6 per person. Noteworthy is the great loss of teeth from previous extractions, expecially in the older age groups.

On the average for the Tashkent population, 35% of the teeth needing treatment for caries had been filled; in Stupino, 42%; Petrozavodsk, 36%; Minsk, 60%; and Leningrad, 64%.

The figures for the prevalence of periodontosis among the different sex groups of the population examined are shown in Table 51.

According to our data, periodontosis is most prevalent in Tashkent, where it affects up to 7% of the entire population checked. The incidence of periodontosis in men is higher in all groups than in women.

The data obtained confirm the fact that periodontosis is most prevalent among the population older than 30 (particularly after 50).

In all, of the 1,141 persons in Stupino in which clinically manifest periodontosis was found, 1,118 (98%) had a greater or lesser number of carious teeth; in Leningrad, 98.7%; in Minsk, 96.2%; in Tashkent, 92%.

Table 51
INCIDENCE OF PERIODONTOSIS IN THE POPULATION
(No. of persons with clinical signs of periodontosis in % of the total number examined)

Age group	City			
	Tashkent	Minsk	Stupino	Leningrad
16–19 years	4.5	—	0.3	0.3
20–29 "	5.5	0.8	0.5	2.6
30–39 "	9.7	2.3	3.9	6.4
40–49 "	19.8	5.8	10.9	12.9
50–59 "	21.3	10.6	19.7	19.9
60 and over	19.3	9.9	22.2	17.8
For the entire city population examined	7.0	3.1	5.8	6.9
Standardized indexes	8.8	2.9	5.5	6.3

As a result of the examination made, some additional data were obtained which were not indexes of the population morbidity, but rather characterized the additional need for dental care and application of dentures and the degree to which it was fulfilled. We present some of them.

The number of persons needing removal of dental calculus in Stupino was, on the average, 24.8% of those examined; in Minsk, 34.6%; in Tashkent, 10.6%; in Leningrad, 9.1%. In all cities this figure in men was $1\frac{1}{2}$–2 times higher than in women.

The number of persons who had lost all their teeth at the age of 60 or over in Stupino was 27.1% of the men and 24.6% of the women; in Minsk, 23.3 and 27.1%, respectively; in Leningrad, 16.5 and 17.4%; in Petrozavodsk, 23.9 and 29.6%.

Conducting mass examinations of the population in various regions of the country permitted us to obtain very important information for the purpose of judging the need for dental care and planning its development in the Soviet Union.

For the purpose of determining standards, the incidence of dental and oral disease in the population according to sickness rate at the therapeutic-prophylactic institutions for a full calendar year is very important.

Because of the inadequate provision of dental care and inadequate attention to the condition of the teeth and mouth by part of the population, the sickness rate data usually cannot give a complete idea of the "true" or, as often said, "exhaustive" morbidity of the population. However, these data are needed for determining the frequency of outpatient visits for various forms of dental and oral disease, because the amount of outpatient dental care for the year and the number of dentists needed for this work can be judged on the basis of such data.

The sickness rate data are also necessary for the purpose of establishing the frequency and dynamics of exacerbations of the carious process during the year and for determining the amount of hospitalization for dental and oral diseases.

Considering the fact that the population morbidity is usually studied according to sickness rate data at the medical institutions, as well as the fact that study of the morbidity according to sickness rate data is technically much easier than study of morbidity by mass population surveys, we decided to compare the data of these two sources on the incidence of dental and oral disease in the same population of four territorial districts of Stupino.

It should be pointed out that prior to the collection of the sickness rate data the dental department of the Stupino City Hospital had its staff reinforced; the population of the four experimental districts examined from January 1, through December 31, 1961, had the opportunity of obtaining the necessary aid in full volume in the dental field. Therefore, the data given below permit us to judge the sickness rate and attendance at the institutions by the population under the conditions of fully available and obligatory dental care.

From Table 52 it is evident that with comparatively adequate availability of dental care per 1,000 inhabitants during the year there were 345.01 admissions, of which 306.43 (88.81%) were for dental caries and its complications, 11.09 (3.21%) for periodontosis, 7.66 (2.24%) for diseases of the oral mucosa and 19.3 (5.74%), for other dental and oral diseases.

Table 52

MORBIDITY OF THE POPULATION IN THE EXPERIMENTAL DISTRICTS OF STUPINO, ACCORDING TO SICKNESS RATE DATA IN 1961

Diagnosis	No. of admissions per 1,000 population	Proportion, in % of total
Dental caries and its immediate complications	306.43	88.81
Periodontosis	11.09	3.21
Diseases of the oral mucosa (gingivitis, stomatitis)	7.66	2.24
Other dental and oral diseases	19.83	5.74
Total	345.01	100.00

Of considerable interest are data which characterize the age indexes of the population sickness rate for the various nosologic entities (Table 53).

It is significant that the complicated forms of caries are more than twice as common as uncomplicated forms. From Table 54 it is evident also how important periodontosis becomes in elderly persons.

Tables 55 and 56 extend our ideas of the quality of dental care of the population in the experimental districts of Stupino.

From Table 55 it is seen that according to examination data 78.6% of the population of the experimental districts needs dental care, whereas actually only 34.8% of this population came for treatment during the year.

Table 53
INTENSIVE AGE INDEXES OF THE POPULATION SICKNESS RATE FOR THE VARIOUS NOSOLOGIC ENTITIES
(No. of cases of admissions during the year per 1,000 population of the corresponding age group)

Age	Dental caries and its immediate complications	Periodontosis	Diseases of the oral mucosa	Other oral and dental diseases	Total diseases
Under one year	—	—	37.30	2.33	39.63
1–2 years	29.35	—	100.63	6.29	136.27
3–6 years	369.14	—	31.25	16.17	416.66
7–12 years	421.27	—	6.25	4.05	431.57
13–15 years	325.09	0.80	—	7.17	333.06
16–19 years	220.33	1.71	2.56	9.40	234.00
20–29 years	269.04	2.72	2.99	19.59	294.34
30–39 years	360.91	7.99	2.88	31.28	403.06
40–49 years	331.75	23.79	2.85	31.71	390.10
50–59 years	291.28	34.67	2.89	27.93	356.77
60 years and over	150.07	31.81	0.69	9.68	192.25

Table 54
THE DISTRIBUTION OF THE SICKNESS RATE IN DIFFERENT AGE GROUPS OF THE POPULATION FOR DENTAL AND ORAL DISEASES
(in % of the total number of admissions for each age group)

Age	Caries	Pulpitis	Perio-dontitis	Perio-dontosis	Stoma-titis	Phleg-mon, osteo-myelitis, periosti-tis, and abscess	Second-ary caries	Other	Total, in %
Entire population	26.8	22.6	33.4	3.2	2.2	1.7	2.0	6.1	100
Under one year	—	—	—	—	94.1	—	—	5.9	100
1–2 years	4.6	4.6	7.6	—	73.8	4.6	—	4.8	100
3–6 years	32.5	22.7	28.4	—	7.4	2.0	2.7	4.3	100
7–12 years	31.0	19.5	42.2	—	1.4	1.3	2.7	1.9	100
13–15 years	29.9	27.7	34.4	0.2	—	2.8	2.6	2.4	100
16–19 years	25.9	25.5	38.3	0.7	1.0	1.4	2.9	4.3	100
20–29 years	28.3	27.0	32.3	0.9	1.0	1.9	1.9	6.7	100
30–39 years	27.5	23.9	34.2	1.9	0.7	1.3	2.3	9.2	100
40–49 years	23.9	23.0	34.9	6.0	0.7	2.0	1.1	8.4	100
50–59 years	21.9	19.4	36.9	9.7	0.8	2.1	1.2	8.1	100
60 years and over	14.3	12.5	47.8	16.5	0.8	1.7	1.4	5.5	100

Table 55

NEED OF DENTAL CARE AND SICKNESS RATE OF THE POPULATION
DURING THE CALENDAR YEAR

Age	% actually seeking dental care	% needing dental care (according to examination data)	% affected by caries (according to examination data)
Total	34.8	78.6	87.22
Under one year	4.4	1.1	—
1–2 years	13.6	6.4	5.25
3–6 years	41.6	60.1	63.88
7–12 years	43.4	80.7	89.53
13–15 years	33.3	76.2	84.55
16–19 years	23.3	72.4	80.87
20–29 years	29.4	73.9	86.24
30–39 years	40.3	86.0	92.63
40–49 years	39.0	91.3	97.22
50–59 years	35.6	89.0	99.17
60 years and over	19.2	77.2	98.63

For what has been presented the conclusion may be drawn that even the sickness rate figure for oral and dental disease that we obtained (345.01 per 1,000 population), which is more than $1\frac{1}{2}$ times the best analogous figures (Kiev), does not depict the true picture of the population morbidity; for this reason, given the existing level of dental care, the amount of dental equipment available, the organizational forms, and the level of sanitary culture of the population, we cannot be limited to a study of the sickness rate for determining sufficiently reliable standards for the requirement of dental care, but we must resort to mass population surveys.

The degree to which outpatient-polyclinic care in the field of dentistry is needed depends on the sickness rate (morbidity), the repetition factor (the number of visits per new admission with experimental corrections), and the visits connected with dispensary care of the patients with certain forms of disease.

In Table 56 we give the calculations for determining the standards of outpatient-polyclinic care, but the standards of dental care show that they are essentially different in the various age groups.

The increase in the dental care requirement in the older age groups is due to the age indexes, the incidence of periodontosis, and mucosal diseases.

Characteristic of these age groups is a marked increase in the need for dental surgery because of third–fourth degree periodontosis (20–30% requirement) and complicated forms of caries that cannot be treated. Noteworthy also is the fact that with reduction in the need for visits for treatment of dental caries and its complications, which begins as early as the 7–12-year-old group, the need for visits for dental extraction begins to rise steadily.

Table 56

STANDARDS FOR OUTPATIENT-POLYCLINIC CARE OF THE URBAN POPULATION IN THE FIELD OF STOMATOLOGY IN 1966–1970

Visits for	No. of visits per disease	Per 1,000 population										
		No. of visits by inhabitants aged:										Total visits
		0–2 years	3–6 years	7–12 years	13–15 years	16–19 years	20–29 years	30–39 years	40–49 years	50–59 years	60 years and over	
1. Dental caries and its complications												
This includes:												
in connection with dental extraction	1.0	—	16.79	54.94	19.34	24.95	70.38	79.33	89.86	88.86	106.65	550.39
in connection with treatment of uncomplicated caries	0.88	7.25	133.6	197.98	56.70	64.51	185.20	148.76	91.56	44.05	21.38	950.99
in connection with treatment of complicated caries	1.8	—	37.25	71.45	25.47	31.71	74.31	54.11	32.79	16.52	12.05	355.66
Total from caries		7.25	187.65	324.37	101.51	121.17	329.89	282.20	213.50	149.43	140.08	1,857.04
2. Periodontosis:												
first–second degree	10.0	—	—	—	—	1.6	8.24	43.48	79.03	81.10	71.33	284.78
third–fourth degree	0.3	—	—	—	—	0.08	0.77	1.87	1.86	1.86	1.48	6.06
3. Diseases of the oral mucosa	3.0	0.89	0.23	—	0.89	0.18	6.18	19.24	31.64	31.89	23.90	115.04
Total visits for diseases		8.14	187.87	324.37	102.40	122.95	344.39	345.69	326.04	264.28	236.78	2,262.9
4. Prophylactic care	One visit per healthy person	32.3	27.6	12.8	7.6	11.8	28.4	13.2	3.6	0.6	0.8	138.7
Total visits connected with morbidity and prophylactic care		40.44	215.47	337.17	110.0	134.75	372.79	358.89	329.64	264.88	237.59	2,400.9

The amount of prophylactic care (fourth division in Table 56) is determined on the basis of the need for prophylactic examinations of the "healthy population," in which no carious teeth were detected on examination (the KPU index), i. e., 12.8% or 128 persons per 1,000 population, not counting children in the first year of life. This means that during the first year of life observation by the pediatrician of the correct cutting of teeth is adequate, and consultation with the dentist is required only exceptionally.

Beginning with the second year of life and in all other age groups, one prophylactic visit per year is the accepted number for those in whom no caries is detected on examination.

The number of actual visits per inhabitant of the experimental districts of Stupino was 1.9.

With the rate and distribution of the morbidity in the Stupino population obtained (according to examination data) and with the number of visits mentioned, the number of visits per inhabitant per year in connection with disease for the various age groups will be the following:

0–2 years	0.2		20–29 years	1.7
3–6 "	2.4		30–39 "	1.9
7–12 "	2.7	} 2.1	40–49 "	2.5
13–15 "	2.1		50–59 "	3.6
16–19 "	2.0		60 years and over	4.4

The average per inhabitant is 2.26, or, in round numbers, 2.3.

The standards for the number of visits needed for each of the age groups were compiled through an experimentally developed, substantial reorganization of dental care and with good technical equipment.

Standards of Therapeutic-Prophylactic Care of the Urban Population in the Field of Orthodontics

Specialized dental care, including orthodontics, is an important division of out-patient-polyclinic care of the population. Orthodontics, particularly the application of dentures, assures the prevention of deformities of the jaws and alveolar processes as a result of premature extraction of teeth in childhood, while in adults it prevents deformities of the rows of teeth and the overloading of individual teeth.

At the present time, development of the system of dental institutions is being planned without consideration of the need for dentures by the population. To date, the basic planning standards have not been determined for this mass type of medical care.

We determined the standards of orthodontic care for the population on the basis of data characterizing the involvement of the masticatory apparatus in 48,260 persons in the cities of Minsk, Leningrad, Stupino, Tashkent, and Petrozavodsk.

Mass dental examinations of the population, according to a specially worked out program, were organized for the purpose of obtaining these data.

On a card showing the arrangement of the teeth a note was made for every tooth on the degree of atrophy of the socket, and the teeth and roots needing extraction were noted. In the examination and in filling out the card, the suitability of the dentures and their longevities were noted as an obligatory matter.

A column was also introduced in the orthodontic section indicating the need of the patient for dentures of various designs with simultaneous mention of the number of dentures needed. As a result it became possible to determine the number of visits needed, which depends on the type of design of the denture as well as the amount of work time and material needed for making the dentures.

For each age and sex group we included in the program of development of the

143

material the compilation of figures characterizing the need for various kinds of dentures, the degree to which they were provided with dentures (pàrtial and complete), the amount of denture application needed and already accomplished, and the need for prophylactic observation only. These indexes were determined per 1,000 population. In addition, the development program provided for obtaining data on the average longevities of various kinds of dentures.

Included in the examination of those needing dentures were those with relative and absolute indications for application of dentures according to N. I. Agapov: loss of 25% or more masticatory efficiency. In addition, among those needing dentures were those with indications of a cosmetic nature as well as persons in whom the Popov phenomenon had been diagnosed on examination.

A determination was also made of the need for additional dentures or change in the design of the existing dentures. In determining the indications for dentures, consideration was given to the functional condition of the rows of teeth and the residual capacity of their supporting apparatus.

The time of cutting of the teeth and the developmental characteristics of the jaws were taken into account in examining the age groups from 3–6 to 13–15.

During the course of the investigation we studied and worked out sickness rate data for orthodontic care with the aim of obtaining figures characterizing the doctor's work.

The data of mass dental examinations were subjected to evaluation by the experts and worked up according to a special program at a computer center.

Study of the data of the mass dental checkups of the population showed that the degree to which it needed orthodontic care was very great in all cities and averaged 55.7% of the number examined with very slight variations ($\pm$ 4.6%).

The population requirement of orthodontic care is conditioned by the persons who have slight anatomical deviations in the rows of teeth, which then need only prophylactic observation, and of persons who have indications for application of dentures.

The data of different cities reflecting the distribution of those with slight anatomical deviations of the rows of teeth without any indication for application of dentures are shown in Table 57.

From Table 57 one can see the increase in the proportion of those with anatomical deviations in the rows of teeth with age. This figure in all cities rises up to the age of 16–19, is maintained at about the same level from 20–29, and then gradually falls to practically zero at the age of 60.

The higher figures in the younger age groups for Stupino and Petrozavodsk are explained by the poor organization of dental care of the child population of these cities and the unsatisfactory treatment of complicated forms of caries. The average number of teeth lost per person examined in this group in the various cities is from 1.7 to 2.3.

Table 57
THE NUMBER OF PERSONS WITH DEFECTS IN THE ROWS OF TEETH NEEDING
ONLY PROPHYLACTIC OBSERVATION (per 1,000 of the population examined)

Age	Minsk	Tashkent	Stupino	Leningrad	Petrozavodsk
3–6 years	0.0	89.8	14.6	0.0	0.0
7–12 "	7.2	23.5	38.9	11.6	141.6
13–15 "	22.7	43.6	179.3	53.4	406.8
16–19 "	93.6	193.6	269.1	200.0	302.5
20–29 "	145.7	177.6	114.9	186.9	114.2
30–39 "	136.9	117.5	246.8	136.5	141.5
40–49 "	71.7	68.4	100.8	51.7	83.9
50–59 "	36.3	35.8	43.7	33.4	80.9
60 years and over	4.2	—	7.2	13.9	32.4
For the entire population (standardized index)	72.5	84.1	130.3	89.0	135.7

Table 58
AGE INDEXES OF THE NEED FOR ORTHODONTIC TREATMENT
(per 1,000 population examined)

Age	Minsk	Tashkent	Stupino	Leningrad	Petrozavodsk
3–6 years	25.5	47.6	51.2	80.7	96.3
7–12 "	75.8	96.2	127.1	78.8	166.6
13–15 "	93.6	54.2	120.0	232.5	206.8
16–19 "	138.8	139.6	149.0	281.8	205.1
20–29 "	323.8	389.0	333.1	491.3	290.1
30–39 "	583.7	667.8	586.0	738.3	520.5
40–49 "	799.8	804.2	807.9	825.8	654.6
50–59 "	929.2	885.6	922.9	924.2	802.8
60 years and over	965.7	903.2	986.2	902.0	928.5
For the entire population (standardized index)	438.7	459.7	452.3	514.7	413.5

Among the urban population examined, those with derangements of the rows of teeth requiring treatment by an orthodontist are very common. Data characterizing the need of the population examined for application of dentures are shown in Table 58.

The data given here depict the pattern of the increasing need for dentures in the population with age, common to all the cities investigated.

For purposes of eliminating possible differences in the degree to which the population examined in different cities was provided with orthodontic care, as well as for the most accurate representation of the pathology of the masticatory apparatus in this population group, we included those who were fully provided and who needed more dentures, as well as those who did not have dentures.

Noteworthy is the absence of essential differences in the figures for this requirement in the different cities, which permits us to suspect the existence of certain age-dependent patterns for the occurrence of pathology in the rows of teeth needing orthodontic treatment. The fact that the figures for Leningrad are higher is explained by the fact that the highest prevalence of dental caries is noted in the population of this city.

Standardization of the age indexes of the need for application of dentures made by the direct method (as a standard the composition of the urban population of the USSR, according to data of the All-Union Census of 1959, was used) permitted us to determine that the general need of the population of these cities for this type of medical care is approximately the same.

Of considerable interest is the clear-cut relationship that we showed between denture requirement and sex. Table 59 shows data characterizing this relationship.

Table 59
STANDARDIZED INDEXES OF THE NEED FOR ORTHODONTIC
TREATMENT IN PERSONS OF DIFFERENT SEX
(per 1,000 population)

Sex	Minsk	Tashkent	Stupino	Leningrad	Petro-zavodsk
Women	505.4	525.4	500.2	577.3	452.2
Men	353.3	383.9	388.5	458.5	360.4

From Table 59 it is evident that in all these cities women need dentures more than men do. This may be explained by the fact that dental caries in women pursue a more active course. At the same time, the absence of significant differences in the requirement for application of dentures between the women and the men of different cities is noteworthy. As has been pointed out above, the relatively higher figures in persons of both sexes in Leningrad are also slightly greater (10%) than the averages.

The age and sex characteristics of involvement of the masticatory apparatus of the population investigated are supplemented by the data characterizing the increase in the average number of teeth lost with age. Workup of the examination data permitted us to determine that in the various cities the average number of teeth lost per person examined was from 4.8 to 5.6.

A detailed workup of these data permitted us to determine also the clear-cut pattern of more active loss of teeth in aging women.

The nature of destruction of the masticatory apparatus in connection with age is shown by the data on persons examined who had lost all their teeth. Thus, at the age 30–39 the number who were edentulous was 1.1 per 1,000; at 40–49, 10.2; 50–59, 5.7; and in the group over 60, 248.1.

We supplemented the mass dental examinations, with the aim of determining the level and nature of pathology of the masticatory apparatus in the population examined, with a special study for determining the average longevities of dentures of various designs, with consideration of how suitable they were, as determined by the dentist during the examination. The data obtained on the average longevities of dentures of different designs considerably facilitate the calculations in planning orthodontic care of the population. Thus, the average longevity of the partial removable plastic dentures is five years; of full removable dentures and bridges, 10 years.

In determining the standards of the number of visits to orthodontic institutions needed for therapeutic and prophylactic purposes, one should have an exact idea not only of the number needing this type of medical care, but also of the amount and nature of care needed. The need for a special workup of the data of the dental examinations is due to the fact that orthodontic care has its own characteristic features, namely, that even with absolutely the same degree of derangement of the row of teeth different numbers of visits may be needed according to the type of denture design.

For example, the number of visits for making a bridge is from three to four; for a partial plastic denture, seven to eight. A workup of the data of mass dental examinations by means of determining the figures for the need for dentures of different designs per 1,000 population, examined together with the most accurate approach to determining the number of visits needed, also permits the determination of the amount of work needed by the orthodontist and dental technician and the requisite quantity of denture material.

It is also necessary to consider the fact that the person examined may need at the same time different kinds of dentures, for the preparation of which a greater number of visits will be required.

Table 60 shows data depicting the need for different kinds of dentures by the population examined.

Table 60
FIGURES FOR THE REQUIREMENT OF DIFFERENT KINDS OF
DENTURES (per 1,000 population examined)

Type of denture	Minsk	Tashkent	Stupino	Leningrad	Petro-zavodsk
Permanent dentures	329.3	311.4	294.6	378.4	264.9
Removable dentures	156.2	166.3	198.3	179.6	183.4

From Table 60 it is evident that the requirement for dentures of different kinds is about the same in all cities, after eliminating differences in the age composition of the population. Noteworthy are the insignificant differences in the requirement for removable dentures.

Table 61

THE DEGREE TO WHICH ORTHODONTIC CARE WAS NEEDED ON THE DAY OF EXAMINATION (the number of visits needed per 1,000 urban population)

Visits for	Number of visits per admission	Per 1,000 population										Total visits
		Number of visits of the inhabitants aged										
		0–2 years	3–6 years	7–12 years	13–15 years	16–19 years	20–29 years	30–39 years	40–49 years	50–59 years	60 years and over	
1. Production of bridges	3.2	—	—	—	—	34.89	170.23	206.68	161.04	107.16	46.88	726.88
2. Production of partial removable dentures	8.0	—	28.64	35.02	10.75	16.93	33.78	132.82	228.50	272.93	285.81	1,045.18
3. Production of full removable dentures	7.0	—	—	—	—	—	—	0.22	1.15	7.55	50.78	59.70
4. Examinations and appointments for treatment	1.0	—	4.77	11.67	3.58	9.50	49.81	70.23	66.11	56.29	51.08	323.04
5. Periodic prophylactic checkups	1.0	—	0.38	4.88	3.86	15.54	38.39	25.44	8.89	4.24	1.00	102.62
Total	—	—	33.79	51.57	18.19	76.86	292.21	435.39	465.69	448.17	435.55	2,257.42
In addition for:												
6. Full removable dentures	2.0	—	—	—	—	—	—	—	—	—	—	38.24
7. Replacement of bridges	3.2	—	—	—	—	—	—	—	—	—	—	51.23
8. Replacement of partial removable dentures	8.0	—	—	—	—	—	—	—	—	—	—	61.20
9. Replacement of full removable dentures	7.0	—	—	—	—	—	—	—	—	—	—	9.45
Total	—	—	—	—	—	—	—	—	—	—	—	2,417.54

The relationship between abnormalities of the masticatory apparatus and age and sex, which we noted above, is also maintained when we evaluate data showing the need for different kinds of dentures. For example, women need removable dentures in 215.5–239.8 cases per 1,000 examined; men, in 105.5–141.5 cases.

The work expenditures of dental technicians depend a great deal also on the number of artificial teeth in the dentures needed. We determined that 1,000 persons need 1,086.6 to 1,409.4 teeth in permanent dentures and 2,336.8–3,041.4 teeth in removable ones.

Further workup of the examination data permitted us to determine the degree to which the population is actually provided with orthodontic care and to distinguish the groups fully supplied with dentures on the day of the examination. This made it possible to refine the calculations determining the requirement standards.

We determined the figures for the number of visits, which permitted us to calculate the necessary number of visits per 1,000 population for complete satisfaction of the need for orthodontic care (Table 61).

The data given in Table 61 depict the full volume of therapeutic-prophylactic care of the urban population needed in the field of orthodontics. The great need for this type of medical care in the age groups over 30 attracts attention. However, it would be incorrect to propose these indexes as standards, because the population that has received orthodontic care will no longer need this type of care for several years, with the exception of a small group of persons with a newly occurring need for application of dentures and replacement of those which have become unsuitable.

Therefore, it becomes obvious that calculation of the standards of therapeutic-prophylactic care of the population in the field of orthodontics should be conducted with consideration of a number of factors. Thereby calculations must be made so as to assure an annual uniform load on the orthodontists. The main factors are the potentials of the staffs, the annual amount of care needed, the average longevities of different kinds of dentures, the annual increase in the need for orthodontic care, and the prediction of changes in the age-sex distribution.

Based on the number of prosthetic dentists in 1965, the standards for orthodontic care in the field of stomatology must be calculated so as to satisfy them for 10 years.

First of all, the amount of orthodontic care to be given annually must be determined. This includes visits for replacement of dentures which have become unsuitable and the repair of dentures. Every year it is necessary to give therapeutic-prophylactic care to children and adolescents, that is, to groups which even at present need stomatological dispensary care.

Therefore, the amount of care needed annually in orthodontics per 1,000 population will come to 263.67 visits: for the care of the child population, 103.55 visits per year, and of the adult population, 160.12 visits per year. Of the remaining 2,153.87 visits it is planned to satisfy 10% of the need per year, that is, 215.38 visits per year per 1,000 inhabitants (Table 62).

Table 62
STANDARDS OF ORTHODONTIC CARE OF THE
URBAN POPULATION PER 1,000 POPULATION FOR A YEAR

Visits for	No. of visits per year
Making bridges	72.68
Making partial removable dentures	171.48
Making full removable dentures	5.97
Replacement of bridges	51.23
Replacement of partial removable dentures	61.20
Replacement of full removable dentures	9.45
Examination and appointments for treatment	50.32
Consultations and regular examinations	18.47
Repair of removable dentures	38.24
Number of visits for the year	479.0

For the purpose of providing care for the visits to orthodontic institutions in the volume indicated (479 visits per 1,000 population per year) with the work of the orthodontist as it is at present, 1.3–1.4 orthodontists will be needed per 10,000 population.

Standards of Therapeutic-Prophylactic Care of the Urban Population in the Field of Obstetrics and Gynecology

The list of gynecological diseases and abnormalities and diseases related to pregnancy, delivery, and the postnatal period given in Table 63 was made up essentially in accordance with the official disease nomenclature accepted in the USSR. However, we excluded abortions (induced and spontaneous), which cannot be considered disease in the true sense of the word, from the class of diseases of pregnancy, pathology of labor and the postnatal period.

Data on the sickness rate of women for abortions and deliveries are included on a separate line.

The amount of outpatient-polyclinic and hospital care given by obstetrician-gynecologists to women admitted for abortions was taken into account in our analysis of the attendance and hospitalization data on women and, finally, in the calculation of the population requirement of the type of specialized medical care under study. On the other hand, we considered it necessary to give the figures for the prevalence of neoplasms of the female genitals, which are cared for usually by obstetrician-gynecologists, but which in the existing nomenclature are put in the class of "Neoplasms."

In addition, the following were included in the group "Other diseases of the female genitals," given in our list, aside from diseases included in it according to the official nomenclature: diseases of the external genitals and vagina (with the exception of seropurulent and trichomonal vaginitis).

We found it necessary to list the morbidity figures for diseases characteristic of the female sex only in the calculations not only for women but also for the entire population (both sexes), in order to determine the standards for the whole population requirement of various types of specialized medical care.

151

Table 63

AVERAGE INTENSIVE INDEXES OF THE INCIDENCE OF GYNECOLOGICAL DISEASE,
DISEASES OF PREGNANCY, PATHOLOGY OF LABOR AND THE POSTNATAL PERIOD
ACCORDING TO SICKNESS RATE DATA FOR THE POPULATION OF FIVE CITIES

| Disease and condition | No. of admissions per year per 1,000 population | | |
| | Average intensive indexes | | Standardized indexes |
	women	both sexes	women
I. Gynecological diseases	84.8	46.6	79.5
1. Vaginitis	15.1	8.4	13.9
2. Uterine diseases	28.9	15.9	27.7
These include: polyposis of the cervix	2.7	1.5	2.6
cervicitis (acute and chronic)	8.6	4.8	8.4
cervical erosions	7.8	4.2	7.6
endometritis, metroendometritis and other inflammatory processes of the uterus	6.5	3.7	6.3
abnormalities of position of the genital organs	3.3	1.7	2.8
3. Diseases of the ovaries and tubes	24.4	13.3	22.5
These include: oophoritis and salpingitis	11.7	6.5	13.9
ovarian cysts	3.3	1.8	2.9
4. Other gynecological diseases	16.4	9.0	15.4
These include: parametritis	1.3	0.7	1.2
menstrual disorders	5.0	2.8	4.5
II. Diseases of pregnancy, pathology of labor and the postnatal period	14.9	8.2	14.0
1. Diseases of pregnancy	8.6	5.3	8.7
These include: toxemias of pregnancy	3.3	1.8	3.0
2. Pathology of labor	2.6	1.4	2.6
These include: ruptures of birth passages	1.4	0.7	1.4
3. Diseases of the postnatal period	2.7	1.5	2.7
These include: mastitis	2.5	1.4	2.4
III. Neoplasms of the female genitals	5.9	3.1	5.3
These include: malignant	1.2	0.6	1.1
benign	4.7	2.5	4.2
Total for the group of diseases and pathological states cared for chiefly by obstetrician-gynecologists	105.6	57.9	98.8
In addition:			
IV. Term deliveries	36.9	20.0	
V. Abortions	61.2	33.2	

From Table 63 it is evident that per 1,000 women there are 84.8 admissions for diseases included in the class of gynecological diseases.

The analogous figures, given in published studies of recent years, based on a detailed analysis of the total morbidity of the population in different cities, vary: in Kalinin (N.A. Frolova: "Zabolevaemost' naseleniya g. Kalinina, po dannym obrashchaemosti v 1958 g." (Population Morbidity in Kalinin according to Sickness

Rate Data for 1958), *Sovetskoe Zdravookhranenie,* 1963, No. 10), 45.7 per year per 1,000 women; in Ivanovo (*Materialy po zabolevaemosti naseleniya g. Ivanova* (*Data on Population Morbidity in Ivano*), edited by A.M. Merkov. Moscow, 1939), 52; in Leningrad (N. I. Turoverova: "Obshchaya zabolevaemost' (obrashchaemost') po boleznyam zhenskikh polovykh organov" (Total Morbidity (Sickness Rate) for Gynecological Diseases), *Zdravookhranenie Rossiiskoi Federatsii,* 1964, No. 1), 65.7; in Orel (E. I. Albats: "Materialy po obshchei zabolevamosti (obrashchaemosti) naseleniya Orla" (Data on the Total Morbidity (Sickness Rate) of the Orel Population), *Zdravookhranenie Rossiiskoi Federatsii,* 1964, No. 9), 114.1.

First place in the distribution of the morbidity for this class of disease is taken by the group of uterine diseases (34.1%), the bulk of which (66.1%) is made up of diseases of the cervix; in second place is the group of diseases of the ovaries and tubes (28.8%), among which adnexitis (48%) is predominant; in third place are other diseases of the female genitals (19.3%).

In the group of "Other diseases" the most common (30.5%) are various menstrual disorders.

If we undertake a more detailed grouping of diseases, the most prevalent will be diseases of the cervix (cervicitis and erosion), 19.1 per 1,000 women; then, seropurulent and trichomonal vaginitis, 15.1 per 1,000; and, finally, adnexitis, 11.7 per 1,000. Turoverova gives similar intensive and extensive indexes in her article.

Other authors (L. A. Averbukh, N. A. Petrova, and R. A. Mel'nikova) also point to the predominance of diseases of the cervix, vaginitis, and adnexitis in the morbidity distribution of gynecological diseases.

The sickness rate of women for diseases in the class of diseases of pregnancy, pathology of labor, and the postnatal period is 14.9 per 1,000 women per year.

According to the data of other authors, the corresponding intensive indexes are approximately the same.

Most common in the morbidity structure for this class of disease is the group of diseases of pregnancy (64.4%), of which one-third is due to toxemias (34.4%).

The group of postnatal diseases comprises 18.2% and consists almost wholly of postnatal mastitis.

There is a definite connection between morbidity rate and the age of the women. The age indexes of morbidity for diseases of the female genitals are given in Table 64 and Figure 21.

While in the 14–19-year age group the morbidity rate is 13 per 1,000 women of this age, at the 20–29-year-old level the morbidity rises almost 10 times and comes to 120.3 per thousand, and at the age of 30–39 it reaches its highest level (167.8 per 1,000). Afterward, there is a drop in the level.

The marked rise in morbidity is due to the onset of sexual life, childbearing, and particularly the increase in the number of abortions, the number of which is 124.9 per 1,000 women at the ages of 20–29 and 177.6 per 1,000 from 30 to 39.

Table 64

AVERAGE AGE INDEXES OF MORBIDITY FOR DISEASES OF THE FEMALE GENITALS, OF PREGNANCY, PATHOLOGICAL LABOR AND THE POSTNATAL PERIOD, AND ALSO OF BIRTHS AND ABORTIONS (according to sickness data for five cities)

No. of admissions per year per 1,000 population (women, both sexes together)

Disease and condition	0–4 years women	0–4 years both sexes	5–6 years women	5–6 years both sexes	7–13 years women	7–13 years both sexes	14–19 years women	14–19 years both sexes	20–29 years women	20–29 years both sexes	30–39 years women	30–39 years both sexes	40–49 years women	40–49 years both sexes	50–59 years women	50–59 years both sexes	60 years and over women	60 years and over both sexes
1. Vaginitis (including trichonomal)	—	—	—	—	0.4	0.2	2.1	1.1	16.1	8.8	22.8	12.8	26.7	16.0	24.9	15.0	8.3	5.9
2. Uterine diseases	—	—	—	—	0.2	0.1	3.1	1.5	42.0	22.1	60.5	34.0	53.4	31.0	18.7	11.5	4.3	2.8
These include: diseases of the cervix	—	—	—	—	0.2	0.1	1.8	0.8	29.9	15.7	39.4	22.1	34.8	19.9	12.2	7.4	3.0	1.9
endometritis, metroendometritis and other inflammatory processes of the uterus	—	—	—	—	—	—	—	—	9.0	4.8	16.6	9.3	11.6	6.8	2.6	1.6	—	—
abnormalities of position of the genital organs	—	—	—	—	—	—	—	—	3.1	1.6	4.5	2.6	7.0	4.3	3.9	2.5	1.3	0.9
3. Diseases of the ovaries and tubes	—	—	—	—	0.2	0.1	3.0	1.4	38.4	20.1	55.6	31.7	34.6	20.7	9.3	5.7	1.9	1.3
These include: oophoritis and salpingitis	—	—	—	—	—	—	3.0	1.4	25.6	13.5	32.0	18.1	21.4	13.0	6.2	3.7	—	—
ovarian cysts	—	—	—	—	—	—	—	—	4.5	2.3	9.2	2.3	—	—	—	—	—	—
4. Other gynecological diseases	0.9	0.4	1.1	0.5	0.8	0.4	4.8	2.3	23.7	12.5	29.2	16.6	26.4	16.6	15.2	9.3	5.1	3.4
These include: parametritis	—	—	—	—	—	—	—	—	1.3	0.6	2.3	1.3	3.0	1.9	2.3	1.3	—	—
menstrual disorders	—	—	—	—	0.5	0.2	2.1	1.6	8.9	4.8	7.7	4.4	8.3	5.2	2.2	1.3	—	—
Total for the class of gynecological diseases	0.9	0.4	1.1	0.5	1.6	0.8	13.0	6.3	120.2	63.5	167.8	95.1	141.1	84.3	68.1	41.5	19.6	13.4
5. Diseases of pregnancy	—	—	—	—	—	—	4.1	2.0	26.2	13.7	17.9	10.1	2.9	1.7	0.2	0.1	—	—
6. Pathology of labor	—	—	—	—	—	—	2.0	0.9	9.1	4.9	3.7	2.0	0.8	0.5	0.3	0.2	—	—
7. Diseases of postnatal period	—	—	—	—	—	—	2.2	1.1	6.9	3.7	5.8	3.4	1.0	0.6	0.4	0.3	—	—
Total for the class of diseases of pregnancy, pathology of labor and the postnatal period	—	—	—	—	—	—	8.3	4.0	42.2	22.3	27.4	15.5	4.7	2.8	0.9	0.6	—	—
8. Malignant neoplasms of the female genitals	—	—	—	—	—	—	—	—	—	—	0.9	0.5	3.5	2.1	2.7	1.6	2.1	1.4
9. Benign neoplasms of the female genitals	—	—	—	—	—	—	—	—	1.7	0.8	3.7	2.1	18.4	10.9	7.4	4.6	1.2	0.8
Total for the group of diseases and pathological conditions chiefly cared for by the obstetrician-gynecologist	0.9	0.4	1.1	0.5	1.6	0.8	21.3	10.3	164.2	86.6	199.8	113.2	167.7	100.2	79.1	48.3	22.9	15.6
In addition:																		
10. Term deliveries	—	—	—	—	—	—	31.8	15.5	109.9	55.9	70.7	39.7	5.8	3.5	0.8	0.5	—	—
11. Abortions	—	—	—	—	—	—	18.9	9.2	124.9	63.6	177.6	99.6	36.1	21.4	1.9	1.2	0.7	0.5

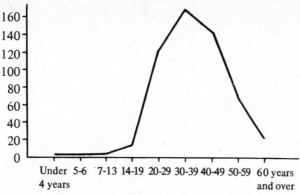

Figure 21

Average age indexes of population morbidity for gynecological diseases for five cities (number of admissions per year per 1,000 women of the corresponding age)

The age characteristics of the sickness rate for the group of gynecological diseases are also proper to the group of pathology of pregnancy, labor and the postnatal period (Figure 22). The difference here is only that the morbidity rate is highest at ages 20–29 (42.2); at 40–49 it drops sharply to 4.7 per 1,000 women.

It is perfectly natural that the dynamics of the sickness rate for diseases of pregnancy, pathology of labor, and the postnatal period repeats the tendency of the age indexes for the number of women in labor.

The highest birth rate is from 20–29 years of age (109.9 of term deliveries per 1,000 women of this age).

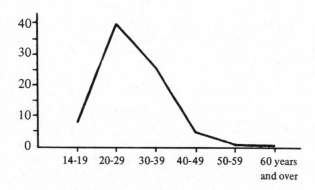

Figure 22

Average age indexes of the incidence of diseases of pregnancy, pathology of labor and the postnatal period in the population of five cities (number of admissions per year per 1,000 women of the corresponding age)

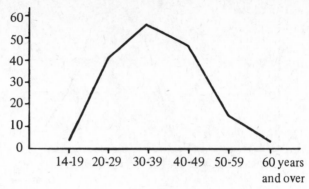

Figure 23

Incidence of inflammatory diseases of the uterus in women of different age groups (number of admissions per year per 1,000 women of the corresponding age)

Figure 23 shows the distribution of the group of inflammatory uterine diseases among women of the different age groups; they comprise over 30% of all gynecological diseases.

Benign neoplasms are most frequent at ages 40–50. At this age women most often come in for abnormalities in the position of the uterus and prolapse of the vaginal walls. Cervical erosions, which are regarded as a precancerous condition, are most often found from 20 to 49 years of age. This indicates the need to encourage women to undergo prophylactic gynecological examinations after the age of 18–20.

The age indexes for the sickness rate with regard to diseases of pregnancy, pathology of labor, and the postnatal period essentially parallel the features of the indexes for the class as a whole.

It should be stated that the indexes for the frequency of abortions given in Table 64 include all cases of induced and spontaneous interruptions of pregnancy recorded in the therapeutic-prophylactic institutions.

The greatest number of pregnancies (total of abortions and deliveries) occurs from 20 to 39 years of age. While at ages 20–29 the ratio of deliveries to abortions is 1:1, at 30–39 it is 1:2.5; at 40 to 49 there are many more abortions than deliveries and the ratio is now 1:6.

Participation in making the diagnosis does not define the amount of work by the obstetrician-gynecologist in the care of women. Nevertheless, the question of the amount of participation of physicians in the different specialties in making the diagnosis of diseases in the class of gynecological diseases, diseases of pregnancy, pathology of labor, and of the postnatal period is of indubitable interest (Table 65).

In 96.9% of the cases these diseases are diagnosed by the obstetrician-gynecologist, in only 3.1% by the other specialists (internists, surgeons, etc.).

Table 65

DISTRIBUTION OF DISEASES ACCORDING TO SPECIALTIES OF DIAGNOSING
PHYSICIANS (Stupino)

Disease	Proportion of diagnoses made by physicians in different specialties, in %					
	obstetrician-gynecologist	internist	surgeon	neuro-patho-logist	dermato-venereo-logist	pedia-trician
Diseases of the external genitals	100.0	—	—	—	—	—
Vaginitis (including trichonomal)	95.5	—	—	—	0.5	—
Diseases of the cervix	100.0	—	—	—	—	—
Uterine diseases	100.0	—	—	—	—	—
Oophoritis and salpingitis	94.1	2.2	1.5	—	1.5	0.7
Ovarian cysts	96.7	—	3.3	—	—	—
Parametritis	100.0	—	—	—	—	—
Menstrual disorders	95.7	2.6	—	—	—	1.7
Sterility	97.2	2.8	—	—	—	—
Other diseases of the female genitals	95.7	2.6	0.9	0.8	—	—
Toxemias of pregnancy	90.0	10.0	—	—	—	—
Mastitis	62.2	11.1	26.7	—	—	—

Incidence of Gynecological Diseases According to Data of Complete Medical Examinations

In making prophylactic checkups in Stupino, gynecologists detected 116.8 acute and chronic cases of gynecological diseases per 1,000 women examined.

Of all the diseases found during the prophylactic checkups only the chronic ones should be taken into account. The acute cases found by chance in small numbers should not be considered, because they do not represent the whole incidence of acute diseases, and give a picture of the day of the examination only. Adding them to the chronic diseases only distorts the picture of the incidence of the latter. Below, our analysis will be made from the calculation of only the newly detected chronic cases, which amounted to 86.6 per 1,000 persons examined (Table 66).

As is evident from Table 66, uterine diseases make up the principal group in disease incidence (35.8 per 1,000 women examined). In second place are diseases of the ovaries and tubes (19.5 per 1,000 examined); then come vaginal diseases, essentially vaginitis (14.2 per 1,000 persons examined). The group of neoplasms of the female genitals are in fourth place (11.1 per 1,000 women examined); abnormalities of position of the uterus and vagina are last (8.3 per thousand).

On more detailed acquaintance with diseases newly detected on complete medical examination it was possible to determine the following: the bulk (86.8%) of uterine

Table 66

INCIDENCE OF CHRONIC GYNECOLOGICAL DISEASES NEWLY DETECTED ON MEDICAL EXAMINATION (number of cases per 1,000 population—women, both sexes)

Disease	7–13 years		14–19 years		20–29 years		30–39 years		40–49 years		50–59 years		60 years and over		Total	
	women	both sexes	women	both sexes	women	both sexes	women	both sexes	women	both sexes	women	both sexes	women	both sexes	women	both sexes
1. Vaginitis	—	—	—	—	7.8	4.6	19.8	11.3	23.9	14.5	31.3	18.2	16.0	11.3	14.2	8.0
2. Uterine diseases	—	—	1.9	0.9	54.8	32.1	55.1	31.4	51.0	30.7	43.8	25.4	36.5	25.6	35.8	20.1
These include:																
cervicitis	—	—	1.9	0.9	2.6	1.5	11.2	6.4	5.0	3.0	1.6	0.9	—	—	3.9	2.2
erosions of the cervix	—	—	—	—	46.9	27.5	26.7	15.2	21.0	12.7	10.9	6.4	2.3	1.6	17.0	9.6
polyposis of the cervix	—	—	—	—	2.6	1.5	3.4	2.0	5.0	3.0	7.8	4.5	18.3	12.8	4.3	2.4
endometritis, metroendometritis and other inflammatory uterine processes	—	—	—	—	1.3	0.8	6.9	3.9	4.0	2.4	—	—	—	—	2.3	1.3
abnormalities of position of the genital organs	—	—	—	—	1.3	0.8	6.9	3.9	16.0	9.6	23.5	13.6	15.9	11.2	8.3	4.6
3. Diseases of the ovaries and tubes	1.6	0.8	—	—	22.2	13.0	48.3	27.5	26.9	16.3	10.9	6.4	4.6	3.2	19.5	10.8
These include: oophoritis and salpingitis	1.6	0.8	—	—	19.5	11.5	42.2	24.1	21.9	13.2	6.3	3.6	2.3	1.6	16.3	9.1
ovarian cysts	—	—	—	—	—	—	2.6	1.5	3.0	1.7	3.2	1.8	2.3	1.6	1.6	0.9
4. Other gynecological diseases	—	—	—	—	11.7	6.9	12.9	7.4	6.0	3.6	3.2	1.8	4.6	3.2	6.0	3.4
These include:																
parametritis	—	—	—	—	6.5	3.8	5.2	2.9	3.0	1.8	1.6	0.9	—	—	2.6	1.5
menstrual disorders	—	—	—	—	3.9	2.3	0.9	0.5	—	—	—	—	—	—	0.7	0.4
5. Malignant neoplasms of the female genitals	—	—	—	—	—	—	0.9	0.5	—	—	4.7	2.7	6.8	4.8	1.2	0.8
6. Benign neoplasms of the female genitals	—	—	—	—	5.2	3.1	11.2	6.4	28.9	17.5	12.5	7.3	4.6	3.2	9.9	5.6
Total for the group of female genital diseases	1.6	0.8	1.9	0.9	101.7	59.7	148.2	84.5	136.7	82.6	106.4	61.8	73.0	51.3	86.6	48.7

diseases is made up of diseases of the cervix (erosions, cervicitis, and polyposis).

Among the diseases of the ovaries and tubes the inflammatory conditions predominate (oophoritis and salpingitis), 16.3 per 1,000 women examined.

Among the other genital diseases the most common (43.3%) is parametritis, 2.6 per 1,000 women examined. At the same time, various menstrual disorders comprise only 11.7% (0.7 per 1,000 women examined).

The highest number of cases of gynecological diseases was detected in women from 30 to 39 years old (148.2 per thousand); at the ages of 40–49 they were found somewhat less often (136.7 per thousand). It should be noted that these diseases are quite numerous at the ages of 20–29 (101.7 per thousand). The lowest incidence of newly detected chronic cases is at the ages of 60 and over (73 per thousand).

The main group in all the chronic cases newly detected in the examination consisted of inflammatory processes of the female genitals.

In women from 20 to 29 years old the incidence of inflammatory processes detected on examination is 84.6 per thousand. In this group of cases there is a predominance of cervical erosions (46.9 per thousand).

In the next age group (30–39) the inflammatory diseases come to 112 per thousand, mainly due to salpingo-oophoritis, 42.2 per thousand.

At the ages of 40–49 the incidence of salpingo-oophoritis, cervical erosions, and vaginitis is about the same, with some predominance of vaginitis.

In the next age group the inflammatory diseases comprise 51.7 per thousand, over half of these cases being from vaginitis (60.5%).

Inflammatory gynecological disease comes to a total of 20.6 per thousand in women over 60. Among these diseases there is also a predominance of vaginitis (77.7 per thousand).

While inflammatory disease of female genital organs is essentially pathology of young women, and with increase in age its proportion gradually drops, such gynecological diseases as prolapse of the genitals, neoplasms as well as ovarian cysts, and polyps of the cervix progressively increase with age, both with regard to proportion and the frequency with which they are detected.

The data given above on the incidence of chronic diseases in the female genitals detected on medical examination are undoubtedly not representative of the entire amount of such pathology, since a considerable proportion of such cases is certainly found in women visiting the therapeutic-prophylactic institutions.

We established the fact that in 51% of the cases of chronic diseases of the female genitals the women had gone to gynecological consulting offices during the year in which the study of the population morbidity was made, and 49% of this pathology was detected on mass prophylactic examinations of the population.

This ratio undergoes considerable changes in accordance with the age of the women.

Most of the cases in young and middle-aged women (20–49) are determined by the sickness rate data. This is connected with the fact that disease associated with symptoms that cause the women to come to the physician (pain, disorders of secretory and menstrual function) is more characteristic of these ages. In addition, women of childbearing age come to the obstetrician-gynecologist for pregnancy more often, and thereby some gynecological pathology is detected. At the same time, in the older ages (50 and over) gynecological cases are detected more often on prophylactic gynecological examinations. This is explained by the fact that older women apply for gynecological care exceptionally rarely, even when they have a number of disease symptoms.

Therefore, it is perfectly obvious that, even with the maximum specialized gynecological care available to the population, the sickness rate data for women at the therapeutic-prophylactic institutions far from fully depict (particularly for the older age group) the prevalence of chronic gynecological diseases.

We attempted to remedy this underestimate of this pathology to a certain degree with data on the morbidity found from complete medical examination of the Stupino population.

Therefore, in calculations of the optimum level of the population requirement of obstetric-gynecologic care, it is essential to use data on the incidence of chronic gynecological cases detected as corrective factors for the morbidity data obtained from the admissions of women to the therapeutic-prophylactic institutions.

Attendance at Outpatient-Polyclinic Institutions by the Female Urban Population

There is an established relationship between the sickness rate of the population for gynecological disease and the amount of medical work by obstetrician-gynecologists in the outpatient-polyclinic institutions; this is characterized by the attendance rate of the women at the therapeutic institutions for these diseases.

Rendering therapeutic-prophylactic care to patients with female genital disease, however, does not cover the entire amount of work of the obstetrician-gynecologists in the care of the women. Consideration must also be given to medical consultations by obstetrician-gynecologists for other women's diseases treated chiefly by physicians of other specialties.

In addition, the participation of obstetrician-gynecologists in various types of prophylactic examinations of the female population should be taken into account. Naturally, the amount of this work is determined essentially by the official laws and directives of the Ministry of Health of the USSR.

In the present investigation we attempted to take into account all the essential components of the amount of therapeutic and prophylactic work by obstetrician-gynecologists working in the outpatient-polyclinic institutions (including house calls to women).

Table 67 shows the intensive indexes for attendance by the female urban population

Table 67

ATTENDANCE RATE AT OUTPATIENT-POLYCLINIC INSTITUTIONS FOR DISEASES AND PHYSIOLOGICAL STATES CHIEFLY UNDER THE CARE OF OBSTETRICIAN-GYNECOLOGISTS AS WELL AS MEDICAL CONSULTATION VISITS FOR OTHER DISEASES (number of visits per 1,000 women per 1,000 population of both sexes)

Disease and condition	Average number of visits (therapeutic, therapeutic-prophylactic, and medical consultation)											
	actually made				added by the experts				sum of those actually made and added by experts			
	physicians of all specialties		these include obstetrician-gynecologist		physicians of all specialties		these include obstetrician-gynecologist		physicians of all specialties		these include obstetrician-gynecologist	
	women	both sexes	women	both sexes	women	both sexes	women	both sexes	women	both sexes	women	both sexes
Vaginitis (including trichonomal)	41.6	23.2	40.4	22.6	12.3	6.8	10.5	5.8	53.9	30.0	50.9	28.4
Uterine diseases	67.2	37.5	66.7	37.2	14.0	7.7	12.5	6.9	81.2	45.2	79.2	44.1
These include: diseases of the cervix	50.9	28.3	50.7	28.2	10.8	6.0	9.7	5.4	61.7	34.3	60.4	33.6
Diseases of the ovaries and tubes	59.9	33.0	55.2	30.4	4.9	2.7	4.0	2.2	64.8	35.7	59.2	32.6
These include: oophoritis and salpingitis	37.5	20.9	33.9	18.9	2.7	1.5	2.2	1.2	40.2	22.4	36.0	20.0
Other diseases of the female genitals	25.8	15.0	23.6	13.7	6.6	3.6	5.3	2.9	32.4	18.6	28.9	16.6
Total for the class of gynecological diseases	194.5	108.7	185.9	103.9	37.8	20.8	32.3	17.8	232.3	129.5	218.2	121.7
Diseases of pregnancy	12.0	6.7	11.0	6.1	1.1	0.6	0.6	0.3	13.1	7.3	11.6	6.4
Pathology of labor	2.2	1.2	2.2	1.2	2.2	1.2	1.5	0.8	4.4	2.4	3.7	2.0
Diseases of the postnatal period	7.5	4.8	4.3	2.7	1.2	0.7	0.5	0.3	8.7	5.5	4.8	3.0
Total for the class of diseases of pregnancy, pathology of labor, and the postnatal period	21.7	12.7	17.5	10.0	4.5	2.5	2.6	1.4	26.2	15.2	20.1	11.4
Delivery	381.8	207.0	307.7	167.0	—	—	—	—	381.8	207.0	307.7	167.0
Abortions	112.1	61.0	110.2	59.9	14.8	8.2	13.4	7.6	126.9	69.2	123.6	67.5
Total for the group of diseases and conditions chiefly under the care of the obstetrician-gynecologist	710.1	389.4	621.3	340.8	57.1	31.5	48.3	26.8	767.2	420.9	669.6	367.6
Visits to the obstetrician-gynecologist for other diseases	—	—	64.0	30.8	—	—	43.5	22.9	—	—	107.5	53.7
Total of all visits to the obstetrician-gynecologist for therapeutic, therapeutic-prophylactic, and medical consultation purposes	—	—	685.3	371.6	—	—	91.8	49.7	—	—	777.1	421.3

at the outpatient-polyclinic institutions for therapeutic purposes for gynecological diseases, pathology of pregnancy, as well as for pathology of labor and the postnatal period.

The table has been made up with consideration of the data of the experts' estimate of outpatient attendance material.

This estimate permitted the determination of the number of additional therapeutic visits needed in the various diseases. Therefore, it became possible to determine the number of therapeutic visits that, in our opinion, provide the optimum amount of therapeutic care to be given by obstetrician-gynecologists to women with the most varied diseases, as well as the maximum amount of therapeutic care by physicians in other specialties for gynecological diseases.

The attendance rate for normal pregnancy ending in delivery was not subjected to statistical analysis. The average data on the actual attendance were used for the five cities.

Table 68

THE AVERAGE NUMBER OF VISITS FOR THERAPEUTIC AND THERAPEUTIC-PROPHYLACTIC PURPOSES FOR THE VARIOUS NOSOLOGIC ENTITIES IN THE GROUP OF DISEASES AND CONDITIONS TAKEN CARE OF CHIEFLY BY THE OBSTETRICIAN-GYNECOLOGIST

Disease and condition	Average number of therapeutic visits per case			
	actually made		including expert corrections	
	to all specialists	including obstetrician-gynecologists	to all specialists	including obstetrician-gynecologists
Vaginitis (including trichonomal)	2.8	2.7	3.6	3.4
Uterine diseases	2.3	2.3	2.8	2.7
These include: diseases of the cervix, endometritis, metroendometritis, and other inflammatory uterine diseases	3.1	3.1	3.7	3.6
	1.8	1.8	2.3	2.2
Abnormalities of position of the uterus and vagina	1.3	1.3	1.4	1.4
Diseases of the ovaries and tubes	2.5	2.3	2.7	2.4
These include: oophoritis and salpingitis	3.2	2.9	3.4	3.1
ovarian cysts	1.7	1.5	1.9	1.7
Other gynecological diseases	1.6	1.4	2.0	1.8
These include: parametritis	2.4	2.4	2.8	2.7
menstrual disorders	2.2	2.1	2.7	2.6
extrauterine pregnancy	1.4	1.3	2.0	1.7
Diseases of the postnatal period	2.8	1.6	3.2	1.8
These include: mastritis	2.5	1.3	3.0	1.5
Pregnancy ending in delivery	10.3	8.3	—	—
Pregnancy ending in abortion	1.8	1.8	2.1	2.0

The intensive indexes were calculated not only for women but also for the population of both sexes together, which was dictated, as has been mentioned above, by the need for determining the requirement of the entire urban population for various types of specialized medical care.

As is evident from Table 67, in the group of diseases and physiological conditions under study there are 767.2 visits during the year per 1,000 women; this includes 710.1 per 1,000 women actually made and 57.1 per 1,000 women added by experts. Of these the obstetrician-gynecologists must have taken care of 669.6 visits (including 621.3 according to the actual data and 48.3 added by the experts).

The total number of visits for medical consultations by obstetrician-gynecologists for the diseases whose observation and treatment were the responsibility mainly of physicians in other specialties was 64 per 1,000 women (including the data of the experts).

The material given permits us to conclude that for every 1,000 women there are 777.1 visits to obstetrician-gynecologists per year for therapeutic-prophylactic and medical consultation purposes, and for the entire population (both sexes together) 421.3 visits.

If we speak of the entire amount of visits for the group of diseases and physiological states cared for chiefly by the obstetrician-gynecologist, the therapeutic-prophylactic visits of healthy women in connection with normal pregnancies come to 66.3%.

The bulk of these visits (75.1%) are for pregnancies which end in deliveries. The number of visits connected with prophylactic gynecological examinations were not the subject for evaluation by the experts, because their number is determined chiefly by the official instructions and laws on prophylactic care of the urban population.

The average number of visits for therapeutic purposes per disease in the various nosologic entities as well as the number of therapeutic-prophylactic visits for normal pregnancies ending in term deliveries or abortions are shown in Table 68. It shows the data on the number of visits actually made as well as those determined with consideration of the corrections made by the experts.

Expert analysis of the attendance showed that the actual average number of therapeutic visits per disease for gynecological diseases is, by and large, close to the level necessary. The greatest corrections were made by the experts for the number of visits per case of vaginitis (the number of visits per case was increased by 25%), endometritis, metroendometritis, and other inflammatory processes of the uterus (the number of visits per case was increased by 21.7%), as well as for ovarian-menstrual disorders (increased by 21.3%).

As for diseases of pregnancy, the number of visits for extrauterine pregnancy was increased by one-third per case. For the entire group of diseases and conditions taken care of chiefly by the obstetrician-gynecologist, the actual number of therapeutic and therapeutic-prophylactic visits is 89.4% of the visits per case.

Table 69

AVERAGE AGE INDEXES OF ATTENDANCE BY WOMEN AT OUPATIENT-POLYCLINIC INSTITUTIONS FOR VARIOUS GYNECOLOGICAL DISEASES, DISEASES OF PREGNANCY, PATHOLOGY OF LABOR AND THE POSTNATAL PERIOD AS WELL AS FOR DELIVERY AND ABORTION (number of actual visits per 1,000 women and per 1,000 population of both sexes of the corresponding age)

Disease and condition	to 4 years		5-6 years		7-13 years		14-19 years		20-29 years		30-39 years		40-49 years		50-59 years		60 years and over	
	women	both sexes	women	both sexes	women	both sexes	women	both sexes	women	both sexes	women	both sexes	women	both sexes	women	both sexes	women	both sexes
1. Vaginitis (including trichonomal)	—	—	—	—	0.5	0.3	4.6	2.4	41.3	22.9	65.2	37.2	73.4	44.4	76.5	45.6	23.6	16.5
2. Uterine diseases	—	—	—	—	1.0	0.5	3.5	1.8	96.5	53.9	128.0	73.3	125.5	76.1	50.3	30.1	15.9	10.7
These include:																		
diseases of the cervix	—	—	—	—	1.0	0.5	3.5	1.8	80.3	44.7	93.4	53.2	92.8	56.2	39.4	23.6	12.5	8.3
endometritis, metroendo-metritis, and other inflammatory uterine diseases									11.5	6.5	29.1	17.0	22.1	13.4	7.3	4.3	—	—
abnormalities of position of the uterus and vagina							4.7	2.7	4.7	2.7	5.5	3.1	10.6	6.5	3.6	2.2	3.4	2.4
3. Diseases of the ovaries and tubes					0.2	0.1	4.6	2.3	93.4	53.4	137.1	80.6	90.1	54.9	16.4	9.7	3.8	2.4
Oophoritis and salpingitis							4.6	2.3	56.1	32.0	81.6	48.0	60.6	37.0	10.3	6.1	—	—
Ovarian cysts									9.5	5.5	15.8	9.4	6.0	3.7	—	—	—	—
4. Other diseases of the female genitals	5.1	2.4	2.4	1.1	1.8	0.9	7.9	3.9	29.8	16.7	46.4	26.8	40.4	24.4	29.3	17.5	5.4	3.6
Parametritis									2.5	1.5	6.4	3.7	7.6	4.6	4.5	2.6		
For the class of gynecological diseases (as a whole)	5.1	2.4	2.4	1.1	3.5	1.7	20.6	10.4	261.0	146.9	376.7	217.9	329.4	199.8	172.5	102.9	48.7	33.2
6. Diseases of pregnancy							2.2	1.1	33.5	19.0	25.3	14.7	4.6	2.8	0.3	0.2		
7. Pathology of delivery							0.5	0.3	6.6	3.6	3.3	1.8	0.9	0.5	3.2	1.9		
Diseases of the postnatal period							2.3	1.1	18.3	10.2	14.1	8.4	5.9	3.5	2.3	1.4		
For the class of diseases of pregnancy, pathology of delivery and the postnatal period (as a whole)							5.0	2.5	58.4	32.8	42.7	24.9	11.4	6.8	5.8	3.5		
8. Term deliveries							256.0	131.2	1,130.2	638.7	691.7	405.4	48.2	29.5	7.8	4.6	—	—
9. Abortions							27.1	13.9	228.2	129.0	308.2	180.6	53.2	32.5	3.4	2.0	1.3	0.9

The average age indexes for outpatient attendance by women for genital diseases, pathological pregnancy, delivery and the postnatal period are shown in Table 69.

In addition, Table 69 shows the intensive indexes of therapeutic-prophylactic visits of the group of healthy women for pregnancy. For convenience of presentation we are calling them "visits for term deliveries" and "visits for abortions."

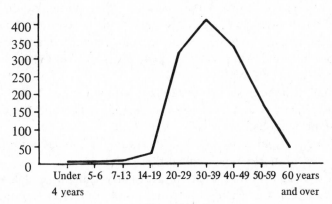

Figure 24

The average age indexes of outpatient attendance of the population for gynecological diseases, pregnancy, pathology of labor and the postnatal period (the number of visits for therapeutic purposes per 1,000 women of the corresponding age)

In Figure 24 the rate of visits by women of different ages for therapeutic purposes only is shown. The therapeutic-prophylactic visits for normal pregnancy (term delivery, abortions) are not depicted in the total number of visits, because the birthrate and particularly the number of abortions are less stable figures than the morbidity rate and its associated attendance.

The lowest attendance rate at the outpatient-polyclinic institutions for the treatment of gynecological diseases is noted in childhood.

At ages 14–19 the attendance rate rises sharply (by $5\frac{1}{2}$ times) and is equal to 25.6 visits for therapeutic purposes per 1,000 women of this age. At 20–29 years this figure reaches 319.4 per thousand.

The highest attendance rate by women at the outpatient-polyclinic institutions for the treatment of various gynecological diseases, as well as for pathological pregnancy and the postnatal period, is reached at ages 30–39 and 40–49 and comes to 419.4 and 340.8 per thousand, respectively.

At the subsequent ages there is a drop in the number of therapeutic visits, chiefly because of a reduction in the group of diseases of pregnancy, pathology of delivery and the postnatal period. At the age of 60 there are only 48.7 therapeutic visits per thousand women for the entire group of diseases under the care chiefly of obstetrician-gynecologists.

If we take into account also the number of therapeutic-prophylactic visits by healthy pregnant women to physicians, the attendance rate rises by more than 80 times at the age of 19 from the previous age group.

Among all the visits (both therapeutic for various gynecological conditions and therapeutic-prophylactic for normal pregnancies) the proportion of visits to gynecological consultation offices by pregnant women from 14 to 40 comprises 70–90%.

At 40–49 the number of visits associated with normal pregnancy is also quite high, 101.4 per thousand, which amounts to about 23% of all visits for the diseases and conditions which we studied.

In connection with the cessation of childbearing function, women over 50 scarcely ever apply to physicians in gynecological consulting offices for pregnancy, either physiological or pathological.

In the higher age groups women seek medical care for diseases or for prophylactic checkups by the obstetrician-gynecologist.

The attendance figures for diseases of pregnancy, pathology of labor, and the postnatal period undergo changes with age similar to those for the morbidity figures for this group of diseases.

The frequency of therapeutic-prophylactic visits by healthy pregnant women of different ages to obstetrician-gynecologists, as well as physicians in other specialties, is directly related to the number of normal deliveries and abortions.

The role of physicians in different specialties in the care of all types of visits by women in the outpatient-polyclinic institutions for diseases of the genital organs, pathological pregnancy, pathology of labor, and the postnatal period, as well as for pregnancy with a normal course, is shown in Figure 25.

As is seen in Figure 25, the bulk of all visits actually made (86.7%) is taken care of by the obstetrician-gynecologist. Participation in therapeutic and consultation work by physicians in other specialties is low (13.3%). Usually internists and dentists participate in the care of the women.

Table 70 shows the distribution of the outpatient visits among physicians of the various specialties for various diseases and pathological states that are the subject of our investigation.

Along with the visits made for therapeutic and therapeutic-prophylactic purposes, we took into consideration also the number of all prophylactic examinations of women by the obstetrician-gynecologist in Stupino during the year.

The following types of prophylactic examinations were defined: examinations of women working in industrial enterprises, public dining rooms and children's institutions; the issuance of various certificates; examinations at the time of being sent to the experts' commission for determining disability and for sanatorium-health resort

Table 70

DISTRIBUTION OF OUTPATIENT VISITS AMONG PHYSICIANS IN THE DIFFERENT
SPECIALTIES (including experts' corrections)

Disease	Proportion (in %) of visits to physicians in various specialties in % of total					
	obstetrician-gynecologist	internist	surgeon	neuro-patho-logist	dentist	other specialists
Vaginitis (including trichonomal)	94.4	2.1	0.7	1.1	—	1.7
Cervical erosions	98.6	—	—	—	—	1.0
Endometritis, metroendometritis, and other inflammatory uterine diseases	95.9	2.0	2.1	—	—	—
Abnormalities of position of the uterus and vagina	100.0	—	—	—	—	—
Oophoritis and salpingitis	89.8	6.7	2.2	0.8	—	0.5
Ovarian cysts	88.9	4.7	3.2	3.2	—	—
Parametritis	94.6	—	—	—	—	5.4
Menstrual disorders	95.6	2.2	0.7	—	—	1.5
Diseases of pregnancy	88.5	8.4	0.8	—	—	2.3
Diseases of the postnatal period These include:	55.2	4.6	40.2	—	—	—
mastitis	51.4	5.4	43.2	—	—	—
Pregnancy ending in delivery	80.6	9.7	—	—	9.7	—
Pregnancy ending in abortion	97.4	1.8	—	—	—	0.8
Total for the group of diseases and physiological conditions taken care of largely by obstetrician-gynecologists	87.3	6.2	0.8	0.2	4.8	0.7

Table 71

FREQUENCY OF PROPHYLACTIC VISITS BY THE OBSTETRICIAN-GYNECOLOGIST

Type of prophylactic visit	No. of visits per 1,000 population	
	women	both sexes
Examinations of workers of industrial enterprises	446.7	246.5
Examinations of public dining room workers and workers in children's institutions	12.8	7.1
Issuance of various certificates, examinations at the time of sending to the experts' commission for determining disability, and sanatorium-health resort treatment	1.3	0.7
Checkups while patients were under dispensary care	2.7	1.5
Other prophylactic visits	61.9	34.1
Total	525.4	289.9

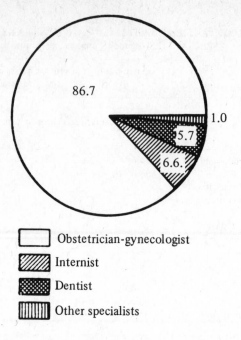

Obstetrician-gynecologist

Internist

Dentist

Other specialists

Figure 25

Participation of physicians in different specialties in the outpatient care of women for gynecological diseases, deliveries and abortions (in percentages of the total)

treatment, routine checks while the patients were under dispensary care, and other prophylactic visits.

Table 71 shows data on the number of prophylactic gynecological examinations of women actually made in Stupino during the year.

In our opinion, the frequency of the prophylactic gynecological examinations of workers in industrial enterprises, amounting to 446.7 per 1,000 women in Stupino, is somewhat high.

We believe that in determining the population requirement of prophylactic care by the obstetrician-gynecologist, it is most practical to use as a basis the calculations from the official instructions, laws, and directives of the Ministry of Health of the USSR concerning obligatory prophylactic care for certain groups of healthy and sick women.

We made a calculation of the frequency of prophylactic visits to obstetrician-gynecologists on the basis of official documents of public health agencies. It turned out that 486.9 prophylactic visits are needed per 1,000 women as against 266.9 per 1,000 population of both sexes.

Hospitalization of the Urban Population for Diseases of the Female Genital Organs, Term Deliveries, Abortions, as well as Pathological Pregnancies, Deliveries and Abortions

The average intensive indexes of hospitalization of the population of five cities for the group of diseases (physiological conditions) studied are shown in Table 72.

Calculation of the intensive indexes of hospitalization of the women was made (in a manner similar to the figures for morbidity and attendance) not only for the female population, but also for the population of both sexes.

The actual level of hospitalization of women for the group of diseases and physiological conditions cared for chiefly by obstetrician-gynecologists is quite high, 124.6 per thousand.

Most often women need hospital care for interruption of pregnancy (induced and spontaneous, 62.3 cases of hospitalization per 1,000 women per year) as well as in connection with delivery (36.9). In all, about 80% of all cases of hospital care in obstetrics and gynecology are for term deliveries and abortions.

Hospital care in almost 100% of the cases (99.8%) is rendered in the gynecology and obstetrics departments of the hospital for women hospitalized for induced interruption of pregnancy, term deliveries, various gynecological diseases (including tumors), as well as for pathological pregnancy, labor, and postnatal periods. Those hospitalized in the gynecological departments are mainly women who have been hospitalized for abortion (79.7%). Among the patients there is a predominance (26.1%) of women with pathological pregnancies. In second place (29.1%) are those with inflammatory diseases of the cervix, body of the uterus, parametritis, as well as oophoritis and salpingitis. In third place with regard to frequency of hospitalization in the gynecological department (10.3%) are women with various menstrual disorders. The proportion of patients with benign and malignant tumors of the female genitals is 8.9% of the total of all patients hospitalized in the gynecological department, i.e., with the exception of cases of abortion.

The average length of hospital treatment in the gynecological department (including cases hospitalized for induction of abortion) is 5.1 days. The highest proportion (87.2%) of those hospitalized in the obstetrics department is for deliveries. Of those hospitalized in the obstetrics department women with pathological pregnancy constitute 7.6%; those with pathological labor, 3.8%. The average length of stay in the obstetrics department (including hospitalization for delivery) is 10 days. The characteristics of hospitalization of women of different ages for gynecological diseases, pathology of pregnancy, labor, and the postnatal period are shown in Table 73 and Figures 26 and 27. The hospitalization rate of women for the diseases and physiological states which we studied ranges, at different ages, from 0.8 to 298 per 1,000 women of the corresponding age.

Most often, young women (20–29 and 30–39 years) are given hospital care.

Table 72

HOSPITALIZATION RATE OF THE URBAN POPULATION FOR PHYSIOLOGICAL PREGNANCIES, LABOR AND POSTNATAL PERIOD AND ABORTION AS WELL AS GYNECOLOGICAL DISEASES (No. of cases hospitalized per 1,000 population)

Disease and condition	No. of cases actually hospitalized						No. of cases hospitalized including additions by the experts						Average length of treatment in the hospital in days
	in all departments of the hospital		including the following departments				in all departments of the hospital		these include:				
			gynecological		obstetric				gynecological		obstetric		
	women	both sexes	women	both sexes	women	both sexes	women	both sexes	women	both sexes	women	both sexes	
I. Gynecological diseases	11.4	6.3	11.0	6.1	—	—	12.1	6.6	11.7	6.4	—	—	9.6
These include:													
1. Uterine diseases	3.1	1.7	3.1	1.7	—	—	3.1	1.7	3.1	1.7	—	—	9.3
These include:													
cervical erosions	0.4	0.2	0.4	0.2	—	—	0.4	0.2	0.4	0.2	—	—	9.9
abnormalities of the position of the uterus and vagina	0.02	0.02	0.02	0.02	—	—	0.02	0.02	0.02	0.02	—	—	20.0
2. Diseases of ovaries and tubes	4.6	2.5	4.4	2.4	—	—	4.9	2.6	4.7	2.5	—	—	10.7
These include:													
oophoritis and salpingitis	2.6	1.5	2.3	1.3	—	—	2.7	1.5	2.4	1.3	—	—	10.3
3. Other gynecological diseases	3.7	2.1	3.5	2.0	—	—	4.1	2.3	3.9	2.2	—	—	8.5
These include:													
parametritis	0.3	0.2	0.3	0.2	—	—	0.3	0.2	0.3	0.2	—	—	12.7
menstrual disorders	2.2	1.2	2.1	1.1	—	—	2.2	1.2	2.1	1.1	—	—	10.2
II. Diseases of pregnancy, pathology of labor and postnatal period	12.1	6.6	6.7	3.7	5.4	2.9	12.2	6.6	6.8	3.7	5.4	2.9	10.2
These include:													
toxemias of pregnancy	1.9	1.0	1.0	0.5	0.9	0.5	1.9	1.0	1.0	0.5	0.9	0.5	15.3
extrauterine pregnancy	0.9	0.5	0.9	0.5	—	—	0.9	0.5	0.9	0.5	—	—	12.6
mastitis	0.8	0.5	0.8	0.5	—	—	0.9	0.5	0.9	0.5	—	—	8.7
III. Neoplasms of the female genitals	1.9	1.1	1.8	1.1	—	—	1.9	1.1	1.8	1.1	—	—	16.7
These include:													
malignant	0.7	0.4	0.7	0.4	—	—	0.7	0.4	0.7	0.4	—	—	21.2
benign	1.2	0.7	1.1	0.7	—	—	1.2	0.7	1.1	0.7	—	—	14.7
IV. Deliveries	36.9	20.0	—	—	36.9	36.9	36.9	20.0	—	—	36.9	20.0	9.0
V. Abortions	62.3	33.8	61.6	33.4	0.7	0.4	62.7	34.0	62.0	33.6	0.7	0.4	3.4
Total for gynecological diseases, pathology of pregnancy, labor, postnatal period, deliveries and abortions	124.6	67.8	81.1	44.3	43.0	3.3	125.8	68.3	82.3	44.8	43.0	23.3	—

AVERAGE AGE INDEXES OF ACTUAL HOSPITALIZATION OF THE POPULATION OF FIVE CITIES FOR GYNECOLOGICAL DISEASES, DISEASES OF PREGNANCY, PATHOLOGY OF LABOR AND THE POSTNATAL PERIOD, ABORTIONS AND NORMAL DELIVERIES (No. of cases hospitalized per 1,000 women and 1,000 population of both sexes)

Disease and physiological condition	to 4 years		5–6 years		7–13 years		14–19 years		20–29 years		30–39 years		40–49 years		50–59 years		60 years and over	
Age groups	women	both sexes	women	both sexes	women	both sexes	women	both sexes	women	both sexes	women	both sexes	women	both sexes	women	both sexes	women	both sexes
I. Gynecological diseases	—	—	—	—	0.8	0.4	2.7	1.4	18.3	9.7	23.0	13.1	18.7	11.2	7.6	4.66	1.4	0.9
These include:																		
1. Vaginitis	—	—	—	—	—	—	0.7	4.6	2.4	7.5	4.1	5.1	0.1	0.1	0.2	0.1	0.4	0.3
2. Uterine diseases	—	—	—	—	—	—	0.2	0.1	2.3	1.2	3.2	1.7	3.0	1.6	0.96	0.4	—	—
These include:																		
diseases of the cervix	—	—	—	—	—	—	—	—	—	—	—	—	2.1	1.2	0.6	0.36	0.2	0.2
endometritis, metroendometritis, and other inflammatory uterine diseases	—	—	—	—	—	—	0.5	0.3	2.3	1.2	4.3	2.4	3.0	1.8	1.0	0.6	—	—
abnormalities of position of the uterus and vagina	—	—	—	—	—	—	—	—	—	—	—	—	—	—	—	—	0.2	0.1
3. Diseases of the ovaries and tubes	—	—	—	—	—	0.1	1.2	0.6	9.2	4.9	10.1	5.7	3.4	1.2	1.2	0.8	0.5	0.3
These include:																		
oophoritis and salpingitis	—	—	—	—	—	—	1.2	0.6	4.6	2.5	5.7	3.4	2.8	1.7	—	—	—	—
ovarian cysts	—	—	—	—	0.7	0.3	0.8	0.4	1.4	0.8	—	—	0.5	0.3	4.6	2.8	0.5	0.3
4. Other gynecological diseases	—	—	—	—	—	—	—	—	4.3	2.3	5.4	3.2	7.8	4.7	1.2	0.7	—	—
parametritis	—	—	—	—	—	—	—	—	0.6	0.3	0.9	0.5	0.4	0.3	0.2	0.2	—	—
menstrual disorders	—	—	—	—	—	—	—	—	2.2	1.6	4.1	2.4	6.8	4.0	0.1	0.1	—	—
II. Diseases of pregnancy, pathology of labor and the postnatal period	—	—	—	—	—	—	7.0	3.3	36.8	19.4	21.4	11.9	4.3	2.5	—	—	—	—
These include:																		
1. Diseases of pregnancy	—	—	—	—	—	—	4.0	1.9	25.5	13.4	17.1	9.6	3.3	1.9	—	—	—	—
These include:																		
toxemias of pregnancy	—	—	—	—	—	—	1.6	0.8	6.4	3.4	2.7	1.6	0.4	0.2	0.02	0.02	—	—
extrauterine pregnancy	—	—	—	—	—	—	0.06	0.02	1.7	0.8	2.7	1.5	0.2	0.1	0.08	0.04	—	—
2. Pathology of labor	—	—	—	—	—	—	1.9	0.9	8.6	4.6	3.3	1.8	0.7	0.4	0.1	0.1	—	—
3. Diseases of the postnatal period	—	—	—	—	—	—	1.1	0.5	2.7	1.4	1.0	0.5	0.3	0.2	—	—	—	—
These include:																		
mastitis	—	—	—	—	—	—	1.1	0.5	2.4	1.3	1.0	0.5	0.3	0.2	—	—	—	—
III. Neoplasms of the female genitals	—	—	—	—	—	—	—	—	0.7	0.4	2.1	1.1	6.6	3.9	4.3	2.7	1.24	0.92
These include:																		
malignant neoplasms	—	—	—	—	—	—	—	—	—	—	0.4	0.2	2.0	1.2	2.2	1.4	1.2	0.9
benign neoplasms	—	—	—	—	—	—	—	—	0.7	0.4	1.7	0.9	4.6	2.7	2.1	1.3	0.04	0.02
IV. Deliveries	—	—	—	—	—	—	31.8	15.5	109.0	55.9	70.7	39.7	5.8	3.5	0.8	0.5	—	—
V. Abortions	—	—	—	—	—	—	19.2	9.4	127.2	64.7	180.8	101.3	36.8	21.8	2.0	1.2	0.8	0.6
Total for the group of diseases and conditions chiefly under the care of the obstetrician-gynecologist	—	—	—	—	0.8	0.4	60.7	29.6	292.9	150.1	298.0	167.1	72.2	42.9	14.9	9.26	3.44	2.42

For every 1,000 women of these age groups there are, respectively, 292.9 and 298 cases hospitalized per year. (This is natural, because young women are often hospitalized for abortions and deliveries.)

If we speak of hospitalization solely for gynecological diseases (including benign and malignant neoplasms), the highest hospitalization rate (see Figure 26) is at 30–39 and 40– 49 years (25.1 and 25.3 per thousand, respectively). At 20–29 years it is also quite high and comes to 19.0 cases hospitalized per 1,000 women of this age.

From Figure 27 it is evident that the hospitalization rate for pathological pregnancy, labor and postnatal period is greatest at 20–29 years, 36.8 per thousand, and at 30–39 years, 21.4 per thousand (see Figure 27).

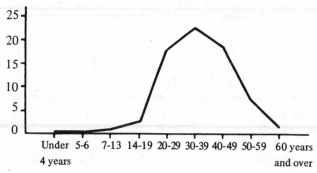

Figure 26

Average age indexes of hospitalization for gynecological diseases (No. of cases hospitalized per 1,000 women of the corresponding age)

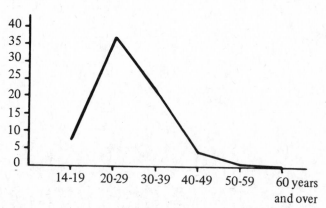

Figure 27

Average age indexes of hospitalization of women for diseases of pregnancy, pathology of labor and the postnatal period (No. of cases hospitalized per 1,000 women of the corresponding age)

Standards of Outpatient-Polyclinic Care in the Field of Obstetrics and Gynecology

In working out the standards of obstetric-gynecological care we proceeded on the basis that all women with various gynecological diseases who go to therapeutic-prophylactic institutions need to have therapeutic care to the degree determined by the actual data with consideration of the corrections of the experts.

The chronic cases of gynecological diseases newly detected on complete medical examinations in quite a large number for which the women did not seek gynecological care for various reasons during the year when the study of the morbidity (according to sickness rate) was made, even though they needed it, cannot be used fully in the calculation for determination of the standards of outpatient-polyclinic care for the next few years (1965–1970).

The amount of dispensary care of women with various chronic gynecological diseases is determined on the basis of data of the evaluation of morbidity data of the population by the experts with consideration of more complete coverage of these patients with dispensary observation than is actually the case at present in the majority of therapeutic-prophylactic institutions.

For calculations of dispensary care of women to be given by obstetrician-gynecologists, the number of cases according to sickness rate data and according to complete medical examinations were taken into account.

The volume of prophylactic examinations of women by gynecologists is determined in accordance with the existing directives and instructions on groups of the female population subject to regular prophylactic gynecological examinations.

Table 74 shows the standards of outpatient-polyclinic care in the field of obstetrics and gynecology with the existing morbidity rate (according to sickness rate) for gynecological diseases, pregnancy, pathology of labor, and the postnatal period with the existing birthrate and abortion rate, as well as for diseases chiefly under the care of physicians in other specialties.

In addition, this table shows data on the number of visits necessary for dispensary care of gynecological patients (specifically for the various nosologic entities). Finally, the number of regular prophylactic examinations by gynecologists is shown in the table with a breakdown according to types of examination.

The total number of therapeutic and therapeutic-prophylactic visits to obstetrician-gynecologists needed will come to 669.6 per 1,000 women (367.6 per thousand for the entire population as a whole).

Of these, 612.5 per thousand visits per 1,000 women were actually cared for by obstetrician-gynecologists (which amounted to 336.1 per thousand for the entire population as a whole) and 57.1 per 1,000 women (or 31.5 per thousand for the whole population) were added by the experts.

In addition, we are planning 107.5 visits to gynecologists per 1,000 women (or

53.7 per thousand for the entire population) for medical consultation work in caring for women with various extragenital diseases, which is usually accomplished by physicians in other specialties. Therefore, the total number of therapeutic, therapeutic-prophylactic and medical consultation visits to obstetrician-gynecologists will be 777.1 per 1,000 women, or 421.3 per thousand for the entire population.

Table 74

STANDARDS FOR OUTPATIENT-POLYCLINIC CARE OF THE

| Disease and condition | Average intensive indexes of morbidity (according to sickness rate) for five cities | | Average number of therapeutic and therapeutic-prophylactic visits to physicians in all specialties | | | | | | Average number of therapeutic and therapeutic-prophylactic visits to the obstetrician-gynecologist | |
| | | | actual | | added by the experts | | total of actual visits and those added by the experts | | | |
	women	both sexes	women	both sexes	women	both sexes	women	both sexes	women	both sexes
Vaginitis	15.1	8.4	41.6	23.2	12.3	6.8	53.9	30.0	50.9	28.4
Uterine diseases	28.9	15.9	67.2	37.5	14.0	7.7	81.2	45.2	79.2	44.1
These include: diseases of the cervix	19.1	10.5	50.9	28.3	10.8	6.0	61.7	34.3	60.4	33.6
Diseases of ovaries and tubes	24.4	13.3	59.9	33.0	4.9	2.7	64.8	35.7	59.2	32.6
These include: oophoritis and salpingitis	11.7	6.5	37.5	20.9	2.7	1.5	40.2	22.4	36.0	20.0
Other diseases of the female genitals	16.4	9.0	25.8	15.0	6.6	3.6	32.4	18.6	28.9	16.6
Total for the class of gynecological diseases	84.8	46.6	194.5	108.7	37.8	20.8	232.3	129.5	218.2	121.7
Diseases of pregnancy	9.6	5.3	12.0	6.7	1.1	0.6	13.1	7.3	11.6	6.4
Pathology of labor	2.6	1.4	2.2	1.2	2.2	1.2	4.4	2.4	3.7	2.0
Diseases of the postnatal period	2.7	1.5	7.5	4.8	1.2	0.7	8.7	5.5	4.8	3.0
Total for the class of diseases of pregnancy, pathology of labor, and the postnatal period	14.9	8.2	21.7	12.7	4.5	2.5	26.2	15.2	20.1	11.4
Deliveries	36.9	20.0	381.8	207.0	—	—	381.8	207.0	307.7	167.0
Abortions	61.2	33.2	112.1	61.0	14.8	8.2	126.9	69.2	123.6	67.5
Total for the group of diseases and conditions chiefly under the care of the obstetrician-gynecologist	—	—	710.1	389.4	57.1	31.5	767.2	420.9	669.6	367.6
Medical consultation visits to the obstetrician-gynecologist for other diseases (including neoplasms of the female genitals)	—	—	—	—	—	—	—	—	107.5	53.7
Total visits	—	—	—	—	—	—	—	—	777.1	421.3

We should dwell particularly on the subject of dispensary care of gynecological patients. Patients with precancerous conditions of the genitals (cervical erosions, polyposis, leukoplakia), inflammatory diseases of the female genital organs (in chronic and subacute stages as well as those with a tendency toward frequent exacerbations), benign tumors of the genitals, prolapse of the internal genital organs,

URBAN POPULATION FOR 1966–1970 (figures per 1,000 population)

| Average number of outpatient visit for dispensary care of patients with chronic diseases | | Total number of outpatient visits necessary for therapeutic purposes to the obstetrician-gynecologist | | Prophylactic checkups | | | | | | | | | | Total visits to the obstetrician-gynecologist (therapeutic and therapeutic-prophylactic institutions) | |
| | | | | of workers of industrial enterprises | | of workers in the public dining room system and children's institutions | | other | | total number of prophylactic visits | | | | | |
women	both sexes	women	both sexes	women	both sexes	women	both sexes	women	both sexes	women	both sexes	women	both sexes
—	—	50.9	28.4	—	—	—	—	—	—	—	—	—	—
111.4	61.6	109.6	105.7	—	—	—	—	—	—	—	—	—	—
101.0	55.6	161.4	89.2	—	—	—	—	—	—	—	—	—	—
39.8	22.2	99.0	54.8	—	—	—	—	—	—	—	—	—	—
30.8	17.2	66.8	37.2	—	—	—	—	—	—	—	—	—	—
10.4	6.0	39.3	22.6	—	—	—	—	—	—	—	—	—	—
161.6	89.8	379.8	211.5	—	—	—	—	—	—	—	—	—	—
—	—	11.6	6.4	—	—	—	—	—	—	—	—	—	—
—	—	3.7	2.0	—	—	—	—	—	—	—	—	—	—
—	—	4.8	3.0	—	—	—	—	—	—	—	—	—	—
—	—	20.1	11.4	—	—	—	—	—	—	—	—	—	—
—	—	307.7	167.0	—	—	—	—	—	—	—	—	—	—
—	—	123.6	67.5	—	—	—	—	—	—	—	—	—	—
161.6	89.8	831.2	457.4	—	—	—	—	—	—	—	—	—	—
47.6	26.2	155.1	79.9	—	—	—	—	—	—	—	—	—	—
209.2	116.0	986.2	537.3	408.2	223.6	12.8	7.0	65.9	36.3	486.9	266.9	1,473.2	804.2

and various menstrual disorders are subject to dispensary observation by obstetrician-gynecologists. ("Instructions on Organizational Methods for Obstetrician-Gynecologists in the Care of Female Workers at Industrial Enterprises", approved by the Ministry of Health of the USSR, January 10, 1959.)

In addition, in our opinion, it is necessary to determine the number of visits for dispensary care (not completely but in cooperation with oncologists) of patients with malignant tumors of the genitals after surgical or radiation treatment, as well as for symptomatic therapy (neglected forms, recurrences, metastases).

Naturally, if there is no oncological dispensary in the city, the dispensary observation of tumor patients is made entirely by gynecologists of the gynecological consultation offices in the district and city polyclinics.

Table 75 shows the calculations of the number of visits for dispensary observation of patients with various gynecological diseases by gynecologists.

The number of checkup visits by women to obstetrician-gynecologists was determined on the basis of morbidity data, as established according to sickness rate and complete medical examination data. The cases newly detected on medical examinations were considered only for the women who even now, in accordance with official

Table 75

CALCULATION OF OUTPATIENT VISITS FOR DISPENSARY OBSERVATION OF DISEASES BY GYNECOLOGISTS

Disease	Intensive morbidity indexes (according to sickness rate examinations) per 1,000 population		Average number of cases needing dispensary observation (per 1,000 population)		Proportion of patients with gynecological diseases needing dispensary observation in % of the number admitted	Frequency of checkups of patients under dispensary care per year	Average number of outpatient visits for dispensary care of patients with chronic diseases (per 1,000 population)	
	women	both sexes	women	both sexes	women	both sexes	women	both sexes
1. Cervical erosions	22.9	12.6	22.9	12.6	100.0	4	91.6	50.4
2. Polyposis of the cervix	4.7	2.6	4.7	2.6	100.0	2	9.4	5.2
3. Inflammatory gynecological diseases (of the uterus, ovaries, tubes and parametrium)	38.3	21.5	11.4	6.4	29.7	4	45.6	25.6
4. Ovarian cysts	4.5	2.5	4.5	2.5	100.0	2	9.0	5.0
5. Menstrual disorders	5.7	3.2	1.0	0.6	18.0	6	6.0	3.6
6. Malignant tumors of the genitals	1.4	0.7	1.4	0.7	100.0	2*	2.8	1.4
7. Benign tumors of the genitals	12.1	6.7	11.2	6.2	93.0	4	44.8	24.8
Total number of cases of gynecological diseases (including tumors)	155.0	85.8	57.1	31.6	36.8	3.7	209.2	116.0

*With simultaneous dispensary observation of the patient by the oncologist.

instructions, are subject to regular prophylactic checkups by obstetrician-gynecologists.

The total number of follow-up visits to gynecologists by this group of dispensary patients for 1966–1970 will come to 209.2 visits per 1,000 women.

As for the frequency of periodic visits by gynecological patients under dispensary observation of the gynecologist per year, the following figures are proposed by various authors (Table 76), not including outpatient visits for therapeutic purposes for exacerbations of chronic diseases.

The number of checkups of dispensary patients per year for the various diseases, which we adopted for determining the amount of dispensary care needed for gynecological patients (see Table 75), was the result of study of data in the literature on this

Table 76

AVERAGE NUMBER OF FOLLOW-UPS PER YEAR PER DISEASE FOR THE GROUP OF PATIENTS WITH GYNECOLOGICAL DISEASE NEEDING DISPENSARY OBSERVATION BY THE GYNECOLOGIST (according to data of various authors)

Disease	N.V.Kobozeva,* Leningrad, 1964	P.Ya.Lel'chuk, O.I.Barsukova,** Rostov-on-Don, 1964	Perm Medical Institute and City Health Department†	I.N. Zhelokhovtseva,†† Moscow, 1964
1. Cervical erosions (after removal by the conservative method, coagulation by diathermy, or surgical treatment)	No data	7–8	4	4
2. Polyposis of the cervix (after polypectomy)	1	2	4	1
3. Chronic inflammatory processes of the genitals (after treatment) which have frequent exacerbations	No data	2–4	2	2–4
4. Second- and third-degree prolapse of the uterus and vagina (operated and nonoperated)	No data	2	4	2–3
5. Ovarian cysts (after surgical treatment)	3–4	2	4	1
6. Menstrual disorders accompanied by hemorrhagic syndrome (after completion of combined drug-hormone treatment)	No data	4	No data	8–9
7. Malignant tumors of the female genitals (after completion of surgical or radiation therapy or with symptomatic treatment); with simultaneous dispensary observation by the oncologist	No data	No data	No data	1–2
8. Benign tumors of the female genitals (operated and nonoperated on)	3–4	4	4	4
9. After having had a hydatidiform mole	No data	12	No data	12

* In the book *Dispanserizatsiya gorodskogo naseleniya (Dispensary Care of the Urban Population)*, edited by Prof. S.Ya.Freidlin. Izdatel'stvo "Meditsina." Leningrad. 1964.

** *Zhenskaya konsul'tatsiya (osnovnye voprosy okhrany zdorov'ya zhenshchiny) (Gynecological Consultation (the Main Problems in Prophylaxis of Disease in Women))*, Rostovskoe knizhnoe izdatel'stvo. 1964.

† *Organization of Dispensary Care of the Population. Letter on Methods*. Perm. 1963.

Dlitel'nost' dispansernogo nablyudeniya ginekologicheskikh bol'nykh (skhema) (Duration of Dispensary Observation of Gynecological Patients (Outline)), Manuscript of the Institute of Obstetrics and Gynecology of the Ministry of Health of the USSR. Moscow. 1964.

subject, consultations with experienced gynecologists, and finally, study of the work experience of the leading therapeutic-prophylactic institutions. An average of 3.7 visits to the gynecologist per year was needed for gynecological diseases under dispensary care.

We deemed it more practical to consider the amount of outpatient-polyclinic care needed for healthy pregnant women as therapeutic-prophylactic visits for calculating the standards of the urban population requirement of therapeutic outpatient-polyclinic obstetric and gynecological care.

Therefore, in speaking of the dispensary care of the healthy female population, we shall mean only the amount of prophylactic gynecological examination necessary.

At the present time, the organized female population, mainly women working in industry, is subject to mass prophylactic gynecological examination, according to the official statutes ("Letter on Methods of Conducting Mass Prophylactic Gynecological Checkups of the Female Population," approved September 8, 1956, by the Ministry of Health of the USSR).

Prophylactically, examinations should be made of all married women beginning with the age of 18. Unmarried women are examined starting only at ages 30–35 or according to the indications. In the directive of the Minister of Health of the USSR dated September 7, 1957, No. 136, "Concerning Preliminary and Regular Medical Examinations of Workers," and in the "Instructions for Occupational Examinations of Workers Exposed to Loud Noises," approved by the Ministry of Health of the USSR, April 1, 1959, No. 287–59, mention is made of the need for prophylactic checkups by the gynecologist of women regularly working with pneumatic tools, exposed to loud noise in industry, working with radioactive agents and sources of ionizing radiation.

In addition, every year public dining room workers and workers in children's institutions should be checked by the gynecologist. Also all women should be examined when a card is made up for sanatorium-health resort treatment or for sending them to the Experts' Commission for Determining Disability.

Therefore, we determined the amount of prophylactic gynecological care separately for the group of women engaged in industry, for workers in the public dining rooms system and in children's institutions, and we also determined the number of "miscellaneous" prophylactic examinations (sending to the Experts' Commission for Determining Disability, for sanatorium treatment, etc.).

According to the data of the Central Statistical Administration of the Council of Ministers of the USSR (*SSSR v tsifrakh v 1963g. (The USSR in Figures for 1963)*, Izdatel'stvo "Statistika." Moscow, 1964), 46 % of the whole population engaged in industry are women. The number of women working in industry is 204.1 per 1,000 of the whole female population.

Therefore, with two examinations a year by the gynecologist of all women working in industry, the number of prophylactic examinations will come to 408.2 per 1,000 women, or 223.6 per 1,000 of the population as a whole.

The total number of women working at public dining room enterprises and in children's institutions is 12.8 per 1,000 of all women.

With one gynecological examination of these groups per year the number of prophylactic checkups will be 12.8 per 1,000 women, or 7 per 1,000 of the entire population.

For the group of "miscellaneous" prophylactic checkups we are planning 65.9 examinations per 1,000 women and 36.3 per 1,000 for the whole population for the next few years.

It should be mentioned that checkup clinics at the polyclinics have now become quite common in the cities; here prophylactic checkups of the women are made essentially by experienced midwives. Therefore, progressively broader coverage is being given to the "unorganized" female population by the examinations as well as to employees and those working in small businesses.

In a letter on methods of the Ministry of Health of the USSR (No. 06–14/16 dated October 2, 1964) concerning the organization of treatment of gynecological patients, there are recommendations on the need for expanding the prophylactic checkups of the "unorganized population" by physicians. Because of this the amount of prophylactic work done by obstetrician-gynecologists may be increased somewhat in the future.

In accordance with our calculations (see Table 74), with optimal outpatient-polyclinic care the total number of visits to obstetrician-gynecologists will amount to 1,473.2 per 1,000 female population and 804.2 per thousand for the entire population as a whole, including no fewer than 986.3 visits per 1,000 women (or 537.3 per thousand for the entire population as a whole) for therapeutic, therapeutic-prophylactic and medical consultation purposes, and 486.9 per thousand, respectively, for prophylactic purposes.

Standards of Hospital Care in the Field of Obstetrics and Gynecology

We calculated the standards of hospital care with consideration of the diseases of the female genital organs, for which the women came to gynecologists during the year in which the study of population morbidity according to sickness rate was made (Table 77) and using corrective factors determined on the basis of medical examination data.

Quite complete hospital care of the urban population can be provided if there are 82.3 cases hospitalized in the gynecological department and 43.0 cases in the obstetrics department per 1,000 women.

In the calculation for the entire population as a whole similar figures are equal, respectively, to 44.8 and 23.3 per thousand.

The average length of treatment in the gynecological departments of the hospitals of the cities we studied was 5.1 days. Pregnant women, parturients, and women in the

Table 77

STANDARDS OF HOSPITAL CARE OF THE URBAN POPULATION IN THE FIELD OF OBSTETRICS AND GYNECOLOGY FOR 1966–1970 (per 1,000 population)

Disease and condition	No. of cases of disease (sickness rate)		No. of cases of hospitalization						Average duration of hospitalization	No. of cases of hospitalization in different hospital departments					
			actual		added by the experts		total			gynecological		obstetric		other	
	women	both sexes	women	both sexes	women	both sexes	women	both sexes	women	women	both sexes	women	both sexes	women	both sexes
Gynecological diseases (for class as a whole)	84.8	46.6	11.4	6.3	0.7	0.3	12.1	6.6	9.6	11.7	6.4	—	—	0.4	0.2
These include uterine diseases	28.9	15.9	3.1	1.7	—	—	3.1	1.7	9.3	3.1	1.7	—	—	—	—
These include: cervical erosions	7.8	4.2	0.4	0.2	—	—	0.4	0.2	9.9	0.4	0.2	—	—	—	—
anomalies in position of uterus and vagina	3.3	1.7	0.02	0.02	0.3	0.1	0.02	0.02	0.02	0.02	0.02	—	—	—	—
Diseases of ovaries and tubes	24.4	13.3	4.6	2.5	0.3	0.1	4.9	2.6	10.7	4.7	2.5	—	—	0.2	0.1
These include: oophoritis and salpingitis	11.7	6.5	2.6	1.5	0.1	—	2.7	1.5	10.3	2.4	1.3	—	—	0.1	—
Other diseases of the female genitals	16.4	9.0	3.7	2.1	0.4	0.4	4.1	2.3	8.5	3.9	2.2	—	—	0.2	0.1
These include: parametritis	1.3	0.7	0.3	0.2	—	—	0.3	0.2	12.7	0.3	0.2	—	—	—	—
menstrual disorders	5.0	2.8	2.2	1.2	—	—	2.2	1.2	10.2	2.1	1.1	—	—	—	—
Disorders of pregnancy, pathology of labor and the postnatal period (for class as a whole)	14.9	8.0	12.1	6.6	0.1	—	12.2	6.6	10.2	6.8	3.7	5.4	2.9	—	—
Neoplasms of the femal genitals	5.9	3.1	3.1	1.1	—	—	1.9	1.1	16.7	1.8	1.1	—	—	—	—
These include: malignant	1.2	0.6	0.7	0.4	—	—	0.7	0.4	21.2	0.7	0.4	—	—	—	—
benign	4.7	2.5	1.2	0.7	—	—	1.2	0.7	14.7	1.1	0.7	—	—	—	—
Deliveries	36.9	20.0	36.9	20.0	—	—	36.9	20.0	9.0	—	—	36.9	20.0	—	—
Abortions	61.2	33.2	62.3	33.8	0.4	0.2	62.7	34.0	3.4	62.0	33.6	0.7	-0.4	—	—
Total for gynecological diseases, pathology of pregnancy, labor and the postnatal period, and for deliveries and abortions	—	—	124.6	67.8	1.2	0.5	125.8	68.3	—	82.3	44.8	43.0	23.3	—	—

puerpural period were in the obstetrics department an average of 10 days (the analogous figures for the RSFSR for 1963 are 4.3 and 9.4 days). With this hospitalization rate the number of obstetrics beds should be 0.8 per thousand of the whole population with an average duration of stay in the hospital of 10 days and of bed operation 300 days a year. The number of gynecological beds should be 0.7 per 1,000 of the whole population (with an average length of hospital treatment of 5.1 days and bed operation 330 days a year). Medical examinations have shown that for every 1,000 population an additional 2.8 cases of hospitalization are needed, and this leads to an increase in the number of gynecological beds by 0.1.

Standards of Therapeutic-Prophylactic Care of the Urban Population in the Field of Otorhinolaryngology

Incidence of Diseases of the Ear, Nose and Throat for the Urban Population (according to sickness rate data at the therapeutic-prophylactic institutions)

The average intensive indexes of the incidence (sickness rate) of ENT diseases are shown for the five cities in Table 78.

From Table 78 it is evident that for the group of ENT diseases under the care chiefly of otorhinolaryngologists there are 73 admissions per 1,000 urban population of both sexes (71.2 in men and 74.1 in women).

The population seeks treatment most often for diseases of the nasopharynx and pharynx (on the average 22.3 admissions per 1,000 population); this includes 11.9 for chronic tonsillitis. The proportion of nasopharyngeal and pharyngeal diseases among all cases included in the group of ENT diseases is 30.5%. Therefore, nasopharyngeal and pharyngeal diseases are the most common cause of visits to otorhinolaryngologists.

Diseases of the nose and sinuses are in second place (21.1%) in the group of ear, nose and throat diseases. The number of admissions per 1,000 population of both sexes amounts to 15.4. The number of admissions of the population for acute otitis is 12.6 per 1,000 inhabitants of both sexes.

The average age morbidity indexes of the population of both sexes are shown in Table 79.

The greatest prevalence of ENT diseases is noted in children under 13. In the other age groups this index is somewhat less; at the age of 60 and over ENT diseases are 50% as frequent as in children under 13.

Table 78
INTENSIVE AND STANDARDIZED INDEXES FOR THE INCIDENCE OF ENT DISEASES
(average data for the population of five cities)

Name of disease	No. of cases (admissions) per 1,000 population			Standardized indexes (per 1,000 population)		
	men	women	both sexes	men	women	both sexes
Acute otitis (media and without indications of location)	13.7	11.7	12.6	14.8	12.4	13.4
Chronic otitis	10.4	7.6	8.9	10.2	7.8	8.9
Other ear diseases	8.0	6.9	7.7	8.1	7.2	7.8
Laryngeal diseases	5.1	6.9	6.1	5.1	6.6	5.9
Diseases of the nasopharynx and pharynx	19.8	24.3	22.3	18.8	22.9	20.8
Chronic tonsillitis	11.6	12.3	11.9	10.7	10.8	10.8
Diseases of the nose and sinuses	14.2	16.3	15.4	14.1	15.9	15.0
Total for the group of ENT diseases	71.2	74.1	73.0	71.1	72.8	72.0
In addition:						
sore throats	59.6	55.7	57.4	58.7	51.4	54.5
common colds	198.4	146.7	169.4	204.5	146.3	171.2
influenza	94.5	75.3	84.0	94.4	75.1	83.8

Quite substantial differences are noted in the morbidity figures for the various nosologic entities in persons of different ages. These differences are particularly appreciable for acute otitis (Figure 28).

In the under-4 and 5–6-year-old age groups the incidence of acute otitis is the highest (51.9, or 34 per 1,000 of the child population of the corresponding age). Then

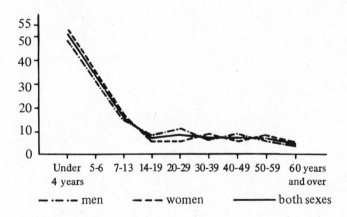

Figure 28

Average age indexes of the incidence (according to sickness rate) of acute otitis (number of admissions per 1,000 population of the corresponding age and sex) for five cities.

Table 79
AVERAGE AGE INDEXES OF THE INCIDENCE OF ENT DISEASES IN THE POPULATION OF FIVE CITIES (No. of admissions per 1,000 population of the corresponding age and sex)

Name of disease	men	women	both sexes	men	women	both sexes	men	women	both sexes
	under 4 years			5–6 years			7–13 years		
Acute otitis (media and without indications of location)	51.2	52.6	51.9	33.7	34.1	34.0	15.0	15.8	15.4
Chronic otitis	12.3	11.7	12.0	10.1	10.6	9.1	6.5	5.9	6.4
Other ear diseases	2.8	3.7	4.6	7.1	5.0	6.1	5.4	6.2	5.7
Laryngeal diseases	7.1	4.6	6.0	4.6	4.0	4.3	2.3	2.9	2.6
Diseases of the nasopharynx and pharynx	5.6	5.5	5.6	27.3	22.5	24.9	25.9	36.9	30.2
These include:									
chronic tonsillitis	4.0	1.7	2.8	16.3	16.3	16.3	18.5	27.1	23.6
diseases of the nose and sinuses	12.9	14.0	13.5	15.6	15.6	15.5	11.5	15.8	12.6
Total for the group of ENT diseases	91.9	92.1	93.6	98.4	91.8	93.9	66.6	83.5	73.9
In addition:									
sore throats	78.6	67.8	73.5	96.9	97.4	97.5	76.7	100.3	88.5
common colds	533.9	536.2	534.3	300.3	289.1	295.0	123.7	145.6	134.6
influenza	123.9	121.2	123.0	114.6	108.6	111.4	88.1	90.9	89.5
	14–19 years			20–29 years			30–39 years		
Acute otitis (media and without indications of location)	7.4	5.9	6.6	10.3	5.6	7.6	6.3	7.6	7.1
Chronic otitis	9.8	8.2	9.1	10.5	7.3	9.2	11.5	7.9	9.4
Other ear diseases	5.0	4.5	4.8	8.8	6.9	7.7	9.1	8.7	8.9
Laryngeal diseases	2.1	5.6	3.8	5.0	7.2	6.1	6.8	8.8	7.9
Diseases of the nasopharynx and pharynx	20.6	27.7	24.1	22.0	23.3	22.5	19.6	24.2	22.2
These include:									
chronic tonsillitis	16.5	20.1	18.2	14.8	14.2	14.1	9.1	10.2	9.8
diseases of the nose and sinuses	13.6	15.4	14.5	14.8	15.0	14.8	15.5	19.3	17.6
Total for the group of ENT diseases	58.3	67.3	62.9	71.4	65.3	67.9	68.8	75.5	73.1
In addition:									
sore throats	57.6	59.0	58.2	66.7	57.6	61.2	57.7	48.8	52.4
common colds	74.6	66.9	70.6	192.9	103.7	141.3	192.0	125.1	152.6
influenza	61.5	46.8	54.3	82.0	73.5	77.3	110.5	83.2	95.2
	40–49 years			50–59 years			60 years and over		
Acute otitis (media and without indications of location)	7.7	6.2	6.8	6.0	7.2	6.8	4.0	4.3	4.2
Chronic otitis	11.1	7.0	7.0	10.0	8.6	9.4	9.0	5.7	6.7
Other ear diseases	10.2	9.6	9.8	12.5	10.2	11.4	17.1	6.6	9.8
Laryngeal diseases	6.5	11.3	9.4	7.2	7.1	7.1	3.7	2.4	2.7
Diseases of the nasopharynx and pharynx	19.7	26.2	23.6	14.4	23.2	19.8	7.7	11.9	10.7
These include:									
chronic tonsillitis	5.7	5.3	5.6	2.6	2.4	2.7	0.8	1.8	1.4
diseases of the nose and sinuses	15.7	19.9	18.2	14.5	15.1	14.8	11.5	9.4	10.0
Total for the group of ENT diseases	71.9	80.2	77.5	65.4	71.4	69.3	53.0	40.3	44.1
In addition:									
sore throats	36.9	30.3	32.9	21.3	21.1	21.1	9.0	11.3	10.7
common colds	31.3	111.3	138.7	143.0	78.1	104.1	75.7	36.9	49.6
influenza	10.9	69.3	86.3	104.6	60.9	77.8	49.7	37.6	41.0

it drops, amounting to 15.4 at ages 7–13. In the remaining age groups the differences are no longer appreciable.

It should be noted that as a rule acute otitis causes the patient much suffering, depriving him of the ability to work, and for this reason induces every patient to come for medical help. We believe that sickness rate data for acute otitis most fully depict the actual morbidity of the population of different age groups.

The high incidence of acute otitis in children, as has already been noted, is explained not only by the structural characteristics of the anatomy of the ear in childhood but also by the fact that in early childhood frequent colds, influenza and other infectious diseases occur.

Different patterns of age indexes for morbidity may be noted in the group of other ear diseases. These figures are determined primarily by the sickness rate of the population for difficulty in hearing of different etiologies, chiefly caused by cochlear neuritis. We use this to explain the fact that the highest morbidity figure (11.4–9.8 per 1,000 population) for other ear diseases is revealed in persons in the older age groups (50–59, 60 and over); these persons suffer most often from difficulty in hearing, and in men an increase in the figures is noted beginning with the age range 20–29. Infants and children from 7 to 13 years old as well as persons in the 14–19-year age group come in for other ear diseases half as often (Figure 29). The incidence of nasopharyngeal and pharyngeal diseases in the population is determined chiefly by admissions for chronic tonsillitis, pharyngitis and adenoids.

The highest index for the sickness rate in these diseases is noted in children 7–13 years old (30.2 per 1,000 children of this age); girls become sick more often (36.9)

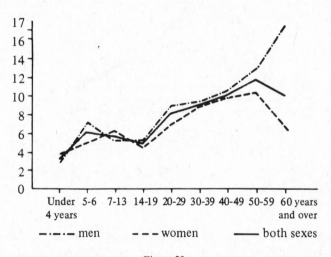

Figure 29

Average age indexes for the incidence (according to sickness rate) of other ear diseases in the population of five cities (No. of admissions per 1,000 population of the corresponding age and sex)

than boys (25.9). In children under seven years the highest proportion of chronic tonsillitis and adenoids is noted in the group of nasopharyngeal and pharyngeal diseases.

As is evident from Table 79, in children five to six years old and in the adult population the incidence of nasopharyngeal and pharyngeal diseases is also comparatively high (24.9–19.8), with the exception of the age group 60 and over, for which the indexes are considerably less than in the other groups.

It should also be noted that in the adult population, beginning with ages 40– 49, the proportion of admissions for chronic pharyngitis is predominant in the group of nasopharyngeal and pharyngeal diseases. The connection between age and the morbidity in chronic tonsillitis is particularly great (Figure 30).

The highest sickness rate for chronic tonsillitis is noted among children 5–6 years old, reaching a maximum at ages 7–13 (23.6 per 1,000 children), in adolescents and in young adults 20–29 years old. Beginning with the age of 30 the incidence of admissions for chronic tonsillitis falls off sharply, and beginning with the age group 50–59 these admissions are occasional (2.7 or 1.4 per 1,000 population). A very low incidence of chronic tonsillitis is noted also in children below the age of four (2.8 per 1,000 children). In some age groups of children and adults (7–13, 14–19, 30–39, 60 and over) the sickness rate for chronic tonsillitis is appreciably greater in women. In the other groups the morbidity figures are about the same for both sexes.

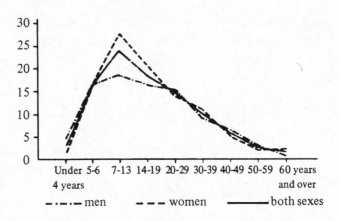

Figure 30

Average age indexes for the incidence (according to sickness rate) of chronic tonsillitis in the population of five cities (No. of admissions per 1,000 population of the corresponding age and sex)

Considering the tendency of some physicians toward making a diagnosis of sore throat when there is an exacerbation of chronic tonsillitis and a diagnosis of chronic tonsillitis when sore throat recurs frequently, we are presenting the sickness rate data for sore throat in the population (see Table 79).

The high incidence of sore throat in childhood is noteworthy, particularly at the ages of 5–6 and 7–13 (97.5–88.5 per 1,000 children of the corresponding age group). A high incidence of sore throat is also seen in adolescents and in middle-age groups (58.2–61.2 per 1,000). At 40–59 and 50–59 years a tendency is noted toward a reduction in the morbidity. At the age of 60 and over the incidence of sore throat decreases substantially.

The sickness rate for nasal and sinus conditions shows no essential variations in the various age groups.

Therefore, analysis of the age and sex characteristics of the incidence of ENT diseases in the population shows that the most prevalent diseases of this group (acute and chronic otitis, acute rhinitis, chronic tonsillitis as well as sore throat) are encountered chiefly in children, adolescents, and middle-aged persons. The persons in the older age groups most often seek treatment for other ear diseases (primarily cochlear neuritis), laryngeal diseases (chronic laryngitis), diseases of the pharynx (chronic pharyngitis) and nasal and sinus conditions (chronic rhinitis and sinusitis).

A direct relation is also seen between age and the incidence of common colds, influenza, and a number of diseases of the ear, larynx, pharynx, nose, and sinuses in the population.

In working up the standards for otorhinolaryngological care it is very important to take into account the distribution of all the patients with various diseases, according to the specialties of the physicians who must care for these patients in the polyclinic and the hospital. It is well known that some patients with diseases belonging to the ENT group are cared for not only by otorhinolaryngologists, but also by internists and pediatricians (for example, patients with chronic tonsillitis). At the same time, otorhinolaryngologists take care of a certain portion of the patients with diseases in other classes (for example, patients with sore throat, which belong to the "Infectious disease" class, patients with injuries to the ear, upper respiratory tract, esophagus, belonging to the class of "Injuries," etc.).

Using the data of Stupino, we calculated the indexes for admissions to otorhinolaryngologists by patients not only with ENT diseases but also other diseases belonging to various classes.

The proportion of visits to otorhinolaryngologists in all the visits for various nosologic entities is shown in Table 80.

The admissions to the otorhinolaryngologists in the group of ENT diseases are 84.8%; for all the other diseases, 15.2%.

Data on the seasonal variations in the sickness rate of the population with respect to different diseases (Table 81) are of definite interest.

The highest proportion of admissions for acute and some chronic diseases of the ear, nose and throat occurs in the cold season—the autumn, winter, and spring months. It should be noted that during the same periods of the year the population of Stupino most often sought treatment for influenza and common colds. As for

Table 80
PROPORTION OF ADMISSIONS FOR ENT DISEASES TO PHYSICIANS IN DIFFERENT
SPECIALTIES (in percent-age of the total number of admissions for these diseases)

Name of disease	% of admissions to physicians of different specialties			
	otorhino-laryngo-logists	internists	pediatricians	other specialists
Acute otitis media, and otitis without further description	78.4	2.2	19.1	0.3
Chronic catarrhal otitis media	94.3	1.1	4.6	—
Chronic purulent otitis media	90.1	0.8	7.6	1.5
Other ear diseases	94.5	2.7	2.8	—
Adenoids	86.8	2.6	10.6	—
Pharyngitis	98.0	9.3	1.3	0.3
Chronic tonsillitis	38.2	29.5	32.0	0.3
Laryngitis	58.7	28.1	13.2	—
Rhinitis (acute and chronic)	73.4	11.4	15.2	—
Sinusitis	61.1	29.6	5.6	3.7
Other diseases of the nose, pharynx, larynx and sinuses	75.6	12.2	12.2	—

chronic tonsillitis, the highest proportion of admissions occurs in January, February, and March, which most likely is connected with the hospitalization of students for this condition, chiefly during the winter and spring vacations.

Morbidity of the Urban Population (according to the data of complete medical examinations)

Medical examinations of the population are of great importance for the detection of chronic diseases and make it possible to work out correctly the therapeutic-prophy-lactic measures for controlling them.

For purposes of working out planning standards such examinations are particular-ly important, because by means of them data may be obtained that come close to the "exhaustive morbidity" of the population with respect to ENT diseases.

With complete and good-quality data collection available concerning the preva-lence of disease among the population, it is possible to determine the amount of the necessary therapeutic-health measures to be taken as well as to substantiate the optimum population requirement for therapeutic-prophylactic specialized care.

Study of the examination data shows that among the newly detected cases the comparatively mild cases that do not give rise to loss of the ability to work or serious disorders are of great importance. In this connection the question arises as to the

Table 81

SEASONAL VARIATIONS IN THE MORBIDITY OF THE POPULATION OF THE EXPERIMENTAL DISTRICTS OF STUPINO

(proportion of admissions in different months in the total number of admissions during the year)

Name of disease	Total number of admissions during the year	Jan.	Feb.	Mar.	Apr.	May	June	July	Aug.	Sept.	Oct.	Nov.	Dec.
Acute otitis media, and otitis with no further description	100.0	8.99	7.58	13.76	9.27	7.58	4.78	7.58	6.74	9.55	7.02	88.44	8.71
Chronic catarrhal otitis media	100.0	11.49	6.9	13.79	9.2	11.49	3.45	10.34	12.64	4.60	8.05	4.6	3.45
Chronic purulent otitis media	100.0	15.15	10.61	11.36	3.03	9.85	5.3	7.58	4.55	6.06	11.36	6.06	9.09
Other ear diseases	100.0	10.09	6.88	13.3	9.63	5.5	7.34	7.34		8.26	11.93	3.21	6.88
Adenoids	100.0	5.27	23.68	7.89	7.79	—	7.89	5.27	2.63	13.16	7.89	5.27	13.16
Pharyngitis	100.0	9.97	11.63	8.64	9.97	10.63	5.65	7.31	4.98	9.3	9.63	6.31	5.98
Chronic tonsillitis	100.0	13.73	12.79	9.2	—	7.8	5.93	7.8	5.3	7.34	8.27	8.11	5.93
Laryngitis	100.0	15.57	12.57	13.18	5.39	10.78	7.78	3.59	4.79	6.59	4.79	4.19	10.78
Rhinitis (acute and chronic)	100.0	10.11	8.57	10.11	10.77	7.03	4.62	6.37	5.28	10.11	11.87	7.47	7.69
Sinusitis	100.0	9.26	7.41	22.23	11.11	16.67	3.7	3.7	1.85	9.26	3.7	3.7	7.41
Other diseases of the nose, pharynx, larynx and sinuses	100.0	12.95	5.76	10.79	14.39	8.64	5.04	4.32	6.47	10.07	6.47	6.47	8.63
In addition:													
sore throat	100.0	8.76	8.47	8.83	7.89	7.31	6.44	7.67	6.51	10.2	9.98	8.90	9.04
common colds and influenza	100.0	9.7	9.4	10.6	8.7	15.8	5.0	4.6	4.8	8.3	7.0	8.3	7.8

methodically correct utilization of the medical examination data for working up the standards of therapeutic-prophylactic care.

First of all it is essential to determine the number of newly detected cases in which medical aid is actually required. Evaluation of the examination data by the experts, as well as the participation of physicians of different specialties in the examination, make it possible in a number of cases to evaluate the changes in the ENT organs as secondary, as the sequela of the main disease, and not requiring special treatment by the otorhinolaryngologist: for example, difficulty in hearing and dizziness in persons of advanced age or those who have had skull injury, subatrophic changes of the upper respiratory mucosa in chronic renal diseases, as well as, in elderly persons, changes in the pharynx (pharyngitis) in digestive diseases and otitis externa, of chronic type, in the exudative diathesis of children. In these cases we considered these local changes a disease, but in the calculations of standards we did not include them as additional work for the otorhinolaryngological service.

Table 82
INCIDENCE OF CHRONIC DISEASES NEWLY DETECTED ON EXAMINATIONS
(per 1,000 population of the corresponding age)

Name of disease	Age groups									Total
	under 2 years	3–6 years	7–13 years	14–19 years	20–29 years	30–39 years	40–49 years	50–59 years	60 years and over	
Chronic catarrhal otitis media	—	—	—	—	1.5	2.9	9.0	4.5	8.0	3.3
Chronic purulent otitis media	4.1	6.3	1.5	3.6	19.1	28.5	21.7	27.4	25.7	17.5
Other ear diseases	4.1	4.7	2.4	—	2.3	4.9	4.8	6.4	6.4	3.9
Adenoids	4.0	1.6	0.8	0.9	—	0.5	—	—	—	—
Pharyngitis	—	1.6	—	5.4	6.9	18.2	24.7	20.0	9.6	12.1
Chronic tonsillitis	4.0	32.8	47.4	33.5	42.1	32.0	22.3	13.6	6.4	29.4
Laryngeal diseases	—	—	—	0.9	1.5	5.9	4.2	3.6	—	2.6
Chronic rhinitis	—	7.8	2.4	3.6	6.5	8.8	7.8	5.5	3.2	6.4
Sinusitis	—	—	1.5	3.7	3.8	11.3	10.9	4.8	4.8	6.4
Other nasal and sinus conditions	—	—	—	1.8	2.3	7.9	11.5	20.9	27.3	7.9
Total for the group of diseases	16.2	54.8	56.0	53.4	85.6	120.9	116.9	110.1	91.4	89.5

Nor did we plan any therapeutic visits to otorhinolaryngologists for residuals of unilateral purulent otitis ending in cicatrization of the tympanic cavity. We adhered to the same principle for impacted wax, chronic catarrhal pharyngitis in smokers, conditions after operations on the middle ear or antrum with satisfactory results, adenoids, and first-degree hypertrophy of the tonsils (in which there were no obstructions to breathing through the nose or frequent sore throats in the history), and other pathological conditions requiring, as a rule, single visits to the otorhinolaryngologist usually for consultation rather than for therapeutic purposes.

All this made it possible to distinguish the group of conditions needing a certain amount of therapeutic care by otorhinolaryngologists from the group of all the chronic diseases and pathological conditions detected.

Data on the chronic diseases of ENT organs newly detected by medical examinations are shown in Table 82.

As is evident from the table, the total number of newly detected cases in which outpatient or hospital treatment or dispensary observation by the otorhinolaryngologist is required is 89.5 per 1,000 of the population of both sexes.

Among the diseases detected on examination needing various types of medical care, as might have been expected, there is a predominance of chronic tonsillitis and chronic otitis.

In all, for every 1,000 of the population, 29.4 cases of chronic tonsillitis were detected additionally through the medical examinations, whereas this figure is only 11.9 according to sickness rate data.

Approximately the same situation is noted for chronic otitis (catarrhal otitis media and chronic purulent otitis). The total sickness rate in chronic otitis is 8.9. In addition, 3.3 cases of chronic catarrhal otitis and 17.5 cases of purulent otitis media were detected by medical examinations. The considerable discrepancy between the sickness rate and medical examination data for the incidence of chronic tonsillitis and otitis speaks to some degree for the still unsatisfactory organization of dispensary care for those with these diseases.

The prevalence of the various diseases detected by medical examinations shows essential differences in the various age groups of the population. The majority of chronic cases is found in the adult population. Chronic tonsillitis is seen more often in 3–6-year-old children, younger schoolchildren, adolescents, and young adults, 20–29 years of age.

Therefore, the amount of otorhinolaryngological care for additionally detected cases is determined essentially by the considerable prevalence of chronic tonsillitis and chronic otitis.

Of definite interest are data of examinations on the prevalence of difficulty in hearing among the population. In all, per 1,000 population examined, 19.6 cases of hearing difficulty were detected (25.8 in men and 14.7 in women) (Table 83).

In the general distribution of the causes of hearing difficulty, cochlear neuritis constitutes 93.4%, chronic otitis, 3.6%, otosclerosis and adhesive otitis, 3%.

It should also be noted that the degenerative changes of the acoustic nerves with age, occupation, and cerebral contusion play an essential part among the factors causing cochlear neuritis.

In the various age and sex groups of the population there are essential differences in the prevalence of difficulty in hearing. Chiefly adults, beginning with age 20–29,

Table 83

PREVALENCE OF DIFFICULTY IN HEARING AMONG THE POPULATION
ACCORDING TO MEDICAL EXAMINATION FINDINGS (No. of cases per 1,000 population
of the corresponding age and sex)

Complaint	men	women	both sexes	men	women	both sexes	men	women	both sexes	men	women	both sexes
	under 14 years			15–19 years			20–29 years			30–39 years		
All types of hearing difficulty	1.4	—	0.7	—	4.3	2.1	7.4	11.7	9.9	25.2	9.5	16.2
	40–49 years			50–59 years			60 years and over			Total		
All types of hearing difficulty	36.5	13.0	23.4	87.0	17.2	46.4	107.5	86.8	92.9	25.8	14.7	19.6

suffer from hearing difficulty. The prevalence of difficulty in hearing reaches a maximum at age 50–59 (46.4 per 1,000 population, including 87 in men and 17.2 in women); at the age of 60 and over it is 92.9 (in men 107.5 and in women 86.8).

As has already been noted, the majority of persons suffer chiefly with mild difficulty in hearing, including the unilateral form, which does not cause any considerable difficulty in social communication and does not interfere with work. Of 19.6 persons detected per 1,000 population with difficulty in hearing, 3.2 needed a hearing aid, 0.2 needed a restorative operation for otosclerosis, 0.4 needed the same for adhesive otitis with a course similar to otosclerosis, and 0.3 needed outpatient treatment for the incipient forms of cochlear neuritis. Therefore, of the 19.6 cases of hearing difficulty only 4.1 per 1,000 population required various types of medical care.

Hospitalization of the Urban Population for ENT Diseases

The average hospitalization figures of the population of five cities are shown in Table 84. For every 1,000 inhabitants of cities in which the study was made, 5.3 cases of hospitalization were noted during the year, including 4.6 for ENT diseases and 0.7 for other diseases.

Among the patients hospitalized for ENT diseases those with diseases of the nasopharynx and pharynx were most common, 43.5%; this includes 37% with chronic tonsillitis. Second with regard to incidence of hospitalization are patients with diseases of the nose and sinuses (chronic sinusitis, deviations of the nasal septum, hypertrophic rhinitis and others) (23.9%). The hospitalization rate for acute and chronic otitis is about the same. The proportion of these patients is, respectively, 10.8 and 13%. The indexes of hospitalization of the population for laryngeal and miscellaneous ear diseases are equal, and the proportion of each group is 4.2%.

It should be noted that during the year there was 0.7 case in the ENT department

Table 84

HOSPITALIZATION RATE OF THE URBAN POPULATION FOR ENT DISEASES

(No. of cases hospitalized per 1,000 population)

Name of disease	No. of cases actually hospitalized			Added by the expert			No. of cases actually hospitalized plus those added by the expert			Average duration of treat- ment
	men	women	both sexes	men	women	both sexes	men	women	both sexes	
Acute otitis	0.8	0.4	0.5	0.1	—	0.1	0.9	0.4	0.6	9.6
Chronic otitis	0.6	0.4	0.6	—	—	—	0.7	0.4	0.6	14.8
Other ear diseases	0.2	0.2	0.2	—	—	—	0.2	0.2	0.2	14.5
Laryngeal diseases	0.4	0.2	0.2	—	—	—	0.4	0.2	0.2	8.4
Diseases of the nasopharynx and pharynx	2.1	1.9	2.0	0.9	1.5	1.3	3.0	3.4	3.3	8.3
These include: chronic tonsillitis	1.6	1.8	1.7	0.9	1.5	1.3	2.5	3.3	3.0	8.3
Diseases of the nose and sinuses	1.4	0.8	1.1	0.3	0.1	0.2	1.7	0.9	1.3	9.6
Total for the group of ENT diseases	5.6	3.9	4.6	1.3	1.6	1.6	6.9	5.4	6.2	9.5
For other diseases	0.8	0.6	0.7	0.4	0.3	0.3	1.1	0.9	0.1	9.5
Total	6.4	4.5	5.3	1.7	1.9	1.9	8.0	6.3	7.2	9.5

per 1,000 city dwellers hospitalized for various diseases, chiefly in the classes of "Injury," "Poisoning," and "Neoplasms."

In the group of ENT diseases men are hospitalized somewhat more often than women (5.6 and 3.9 per 1,000, respectively). No essential differences are seen in the hospitalization rate of the population of different sexes for other diseases.

The hospitalization rate for acute and chronic otitis, diseases of the larynx, nose, and sinuses in men is about twice as high as in women.

The actually obtained age indexes of hospitalization of the population of five cities are shown in Table 85 and Figure 31.

Most often children of all ages, adolescents, and young adults are hospitalized for ENT diseases. Among hospitalized infants and 5–6-year-old children, patients with acute otitis and chronic tonsillitis constitute the greatest number. In the subsequent age groups up to 40–49 the main causes of hospitalization are chronic tonsillitis and diseases of the nose and sinuses. From 40–49 and in elderly persons the most common cause of hospitalization is disease of the nose and sinuses.

The data of actual hospitalization rate, as pointed out above, were subjected to an evaluation by an expert. The total indexes of the actual hospitalization and indexes added by expert evaluation apparently are the optimal representation of the necessary hospitalization rate for the actual morbidity according to sickness rate data.

We added the largest number of cases needing hospitalization for chronic tonsillitis

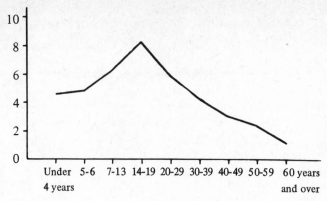

Figure 31

Average age indexes of hospitalization of the urban population for the group of ENT diseases
(No. of cases hospitalized per 1,000 population of the corresponding age)

Table 85

AVERAGE AGE INDEXES OF HOSPITALIZATION OF THE POPULATION OF FIVE
CITIES FOR ENT DISEASES (No. of cases hospitalized in the ENT department per 1,000 population)

Name of disease	Age groups									Total
	under 4 years	5–6 years	7–13 years	14–19 years	20–29 years	30–39 years	40–49 years	50–59 years	60 years and over	
Acute otitis	2.1	1.8	0.6	0.4	0.5	0.3	0.2	0.3	0.2	0.5
Chronic otitis	1.0	0.5	0.3	0.8	0.6	0.6	0.5	0.3	0.1	0.6
Other ear diseases	0.1	0.1	0.1	0.1	0.2	0.2	0.4	0.4	0.1	0.2
Laryngeal diseases	0.8	0.4	0.3	0.1	0.2	0.3	0.3	0.2	0.1	0.2
Diseases of the naso-pharynx and pharynx	0.2	1.5	4.1	5.1	2.5	1.5	0.5	0.5	0.2	2.0
These include: chronic tonsillitis	0.2	1.5	4.1	5.1	2.3	1.5	0.5	0.5	0.2	1.7
Diseases of the nose and sinuses	0.4	0.5	0.8	1.6	1.8	1.3	1.1	0.7	0.4	1.1
Diseases not included in the class of ENT diseases	4.1	0.7	1.1	—	1.6	0.4	0.3	1.0	—	0.7
Total for the group of diseases	8.7	5.5	7.3	8.1	7.4	4.6	3.3	3.4	1.0	5.3

(1.3 per 1,000 population). For acute otitis and sinusitis, respectively, 0.1 and 0.2 cases needing hospitalization per 1,000 inhabitants were added.

For diseases not included in the class of ENT diseases, according to the data of evaluation by the expert, additional hospitalization is also required, the level of which was, according to our data, 0.3 per 1,000 population.

The age indexes of additional cases of hospitalization of the population for ENT diseases are shown in Table 86.

Table 86
INCIDENCE OF ADDITIONAL CASES OF HOSPITALIZATION RECOMMENDED THROUGH EXPERT EVALUATION OF THE SICKNESS RATE DATA (No. of cases hospitalized per 1,000 population of the corresponding age)

Name of disease	Age groups									Total
	under 4 years	5–6 years	7–13 years	14–19 years	20–29 years	30–39 years	40–49 years	50–59 years	60 years and over	
Acute otitis	—	—	—	—	0.3	0.1	0.1	—	—	0.1
Diseases of the naso-pharynx and pharynx	—	1.3	2.2	1.6	1.0	1.8	1.0	0.5	—	1.3
These include: chronic tonsillitis	—	1.3	2.2	1.6	1.0	1.8	1.0	0.5	—	1.3
diseases of the naso-pharynx and sinuses	—	0.7	—	—	0.3	0.4	0.3	0.5	—	0.2
Diseases not included in the class of ENT diseases	—	—	—	0.3	0.3	0.9	—	—	—	0.3
Total for the group of diseases	—	2.0	2.2	1.9	1.9	3.2	1.4	1.0	—	1.9

The average duration of treatment (with consideration of corrections by the experts) in the otorhinolaryngological department was 9.5 days.

For a more complete characterization of the amount of work of otorhinolaryngologists in the outpatient care of patients it is necessary to consider the number of visits not only for the group of diseases suffered but also for a number of others, the so-called related diseases, in which there is a need for medical consultation with an otorhinolaryngologist (sore throat, injury to the upper respiratory tract, esophagus, etc.).

The sum of actual visits and those added by the expert, in our opinion, most fully represent the requisite volume of medical care for the actual morbidity rate according to sickness rate data for the population.

The average figures for attendance with the existing morbidity rate (sickness rate) of the population for ENT diseases are shown in Table 87.

As is evident from Table 87, there are 213 visits during the year per 1,000 population for the ENT disease group (this includes 132.8 actual visits and 80.2 added by the expert).

In addition, the total number of visits for medical consultations to the otorhinolaryngologist alone for diseases in various classes amounts to 61.7 per 1,000 population, 37.3 actual visits and 24.4 added by the expert.

The highest number of visits for treatment purposes is for pharyngeal and nasopharyngeal diseases—87 per 1,000 population, including 66.8 for chronic tonsillitis. About one-fifth of the total number of visits for the group of ENT diseases consists of visits for diseases of the nose and sinuses (44.1 per 1,000 population). There is also a considerable amount of therapeutic outpatient-polyclinic care for acute and chronic

Table 87

ATTENDANCE AT OUTPATIENT-POLYCLINIC INSTITUTIONS FOR THERAPY OF
VARIOUS ENT DISEASES (No. of visits per 1,000 population)

Name of disease	Average morbidity (according to sickness rate per 1,000 population)	No. of visits for treatment			Average No. of visits for treatment per case
		actual	added by the expert	sum	
Acute otitis	12.6	21.2	12.3	33.4	2.7
Chronic otitis	8.7	12.1	8.9	21.0	2.3
Other ear diseases	7.7	9.8	2.5	12.3	1.6
Laryngeal diseases	6.1	9.9	5.3	15.2	2.5
Diseases of the nasopharynx and pharynx	22.3	53.4	33.6	87.0	3.9
These include: chronic tonsillitis	11.9	40.5	22.3	66.8	5.6
Diseases of the nose	15.4	26.5	17.6	44.1	5.6
and sinuses	15.4	26.5	17.6	44.1	2.9
Total for the group of diseases	73.0	132.8	80.2	213.0	2.9
For other diseases		37.3	24.4	61.7	
Total		164.8	104.6	260.0	

Table 88

AVERAGE AGE INDEXES OF THE ACTUAL ATTENDANCE OF THE URBAN
POPULATION AT OUTPATIENT-POLYCLINIC INSTITUTIONS FOR ENT DISEASES
(No. of visits per 1,000 population of the corresponding age)

Name of disease	Age groups									Total
	under 4 years	5–6 years	7–13 years	14–19 years	20–29 years	30–39 years	40–49 years	50–59 years	60 years and over	
Acute otitis	96.7	65.8	27.9	9.9	13.4	12.6	10.3	16.0	5.93	21.1
Chronic otitis	26.9	20.1	5.9	9.2	7.6	13.8	16.7	11.2	10.0	12.1
Other ear diseases	4.1	9.4	9.2	3.7	9.0	11.2	13.9	13.2	12.0	9.8
Laryngeal diseases	8.8	7.2	4.3	6.5	8.1	12.1	17.4	15.4	4.2	9.9
Diseases of the naso-pharynx and pharynx	11.4	61.9	79.8	56.1	61.0	54.4	54.0	39.8	21.6	53.4
These include: chronic tonsillitis	8.6	50.3	73.4	53.5	53.5	39.5	21.5	10.1	4.4	40.5
Diseases of the nose and sinuses	25.4	30.1	24.1	22.2	22.7	30.0	34.4	30.4	14.9	26.7
Total for the group of ENT diseases	173.3	194.5	151.2	107.6	121.8	134.1	146.7	126.0	68.7	132.8

otitis (the number of visits is, respectively, 33.4 and 21 per 1,000 population). Some variations in the figures for the average number of visits per disease are explained by the frequency of exacerbations and the severity of the pathological process in various diseases.

In various age groups of the population there are essential differences in the attendance at outpatient-polyclinic institutions for treatment purposes. The average level of the age indexes of attendance of the urban population for the group of ENT diseases is shown in Figure 32 and Table 88.

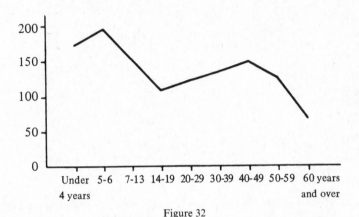

Figure 32

Average age indexes of attendance of the urban population for the ENT disease group (No. of outpatient-polyclinic visits for treatment purposes per 1,000 population of the corresponding age)

From Figure 32 and Table 88 it is evident that the highest number of visits for treatment purposes is noted in the youngest age groups of the population. Thus, in children under four and 5–6 years old the attendance figure is 173.3 and 194.5, respectively, per 1,000 children of the age indicated. In the next two age groups this figure is less: at the ages of 7–13 it is 151.2 visits per 1,000 inhabitants; in adolescents of 14–19 years, 107.6. Beginning with the 20–29-year-old age group the number of visits per 1,000 population increases somewhat in each successive age group to 50–59 inclusive. In these age groups the attendance figure ranges from 121.8 to 146.7 per 1,000 population. The lowest figure for attendance occurs in elderly persons (68.7 per 1,000 population).

For the purpose of determining the amount of outpatient care that is actually given by otorhinolaryngologists, it is very important to determine the proportion of treatment visits in the ENT disease group cared for by the otorhinolaryngologists alone and the proportion cared for by physicians in other specialties.

The distribution of the overall and age indexes of the actual outpatient attendance among physicians of different specialties is shown in Tables 89 and 90.

Table 89

DISTRIBUTION OF OUTPATIENT VISITS AMONG PHYSICIANS OF DIFFERENT
SPECIALTIES (including corrections by experts)

Name of disease	Proportion (in %) of visits to corresponding specialists				No. of visits per 1,000 population				
	otorhino-laryngo-logists	internists	pedia-tricians	other specialists	total visits	otorhino-laryngo-logists	internists	pedia-tricians	other specialists
Acute otitis media and otitis without further description	85.7	2.5	11.8	—	33.4	28.7	0.8	3.9	—
Chronic otitis	91.4	2.4	4.8	1.4	21.0	19.2	0.5	1.0	0.3
Other ear diseases	95.9	1.6	2.5	—	12.3	11.8	0.2	0.3	—
Laryngeal diseases	76.9	16.4	6.7	—	15.2	11.7	2.5	1.0	—
Pharyngeal and naso-pharyngeal diseases	55.7	18.4	25.7	0.2	87.0	48.4	16.0	22.3	0.2
These include: chronic tonsillitis	57.8	23.1	18.9	0.2	62.8	36.3	14.5	11.9	0.1
diseases of the nose and sinuses	83.4	8.4	6.8	1.2	44.1	36.8	3.8	3.0	0.5
Total for the disease group	73.6	11.1	14.8	0.5	213.0	156.7	23.8	31.5	1.0

From these tables it is seen that of the total number of all visits for the ENT disease group 73.6 % of the visits are covered by the otorhinolaryngologists alone; 26.4 % by physicians in other specialties, namely: internists, 11.1 %; pediatricians, 14.8 %; and other specialists, 0.5 %. In taking care of patients with chronic tonsillitis 57.8 % of visits are covered by otorhinolaryngologists.

It should also be noted that a considerable number of the visits were under the care of internists and pediatricians as district physicians for home coverage.

The age indexes of the additional visits of otorhinolaryngologists for purposes of medical consultations are shown in Table 91.

The total number of visits to otorhinolaryngologists for treatment (including corrections of the experts and with consideration of the visits to various specialists) amounts to 218.4 per 1,000 population at the existing morbidity rate (according to sickness rate); this includes 156.7 for the group of ENT diseases and 61.7 for other diseases.

Of all visits to otorhinolaryngologists for purposes of treatment the visits for the group of ENT diseases comprise 71.8; for the other diseases, 28.2.

As for the number of prophylactic visits to otorhinolaryngologists, these are determined by the existing laws and instructions for prophylactic care of the population. We took into account all cases of prophylactic visits, including regular house calls by physicians to children under the age of one, examinations of preschool children, dispensary care of 7-year-old children entering school, examinations of

Table 90

AVERAGE AGE INDEXES OF ATTENDANCE BY THE URBAN POPULATION AT OUTPATIENT-POLYCLINIC INSTITUTIONS FOR ENT DISEASES AND THEIR DISTRIBUTION AMONG PHYSICIANS OF DIFFERENT SPECIALTIES (No. of visits per 1,000 population of the corresponding age)

Name of disease	Visits for medical consultations	Age groups									Total
		under 4 years	5-6 years	7-13 years	14-19 years	20-29 years	30-39 years	40-49 years	50-59 years	60 years and over	
1. Acute otitis	*Total*	96.7	65.8	27.9	9.9	13.4	12.6	10.3	16.0	5.9	21.1
	This includes:										
	otorhinolaryngologist	43.4	52.6	24.8	9.5	12.6	12.1	10.0	14.3	4.2	16.4
	pediatrician	53.3	13.2	3.1	—	—	—	—	—	—	3.9
	internist	—	—	—	0.4	0.8	0.5	0.3	1.7	1.7	0.8
	other specialists	—	—	—	—	—	—	—	—	—	—
2. Chronic otitis	*Total*	26.0	20.1	5.9	9.2	7.6	13.8	16.7	11.2	10.0	12.1
	This includes:										
	otorhinolaryngologist	13.5	16.1	4.1	9.2	7.1	12.2	15.6	10.6	10.0	10.3
	pediatrician	13.4	4.0	1.8	—	—	—	—	—	—	1.0
	internist	—	—	—	—	0.4	1.6	1.1	—	—	0.5
	other specialists	—	—	—	—	0.1	—	—	0.6	—	0.3
3. Other diseases	*Total*	4.1	9.4	9.2	3.7	9.0	11.2	13.9	13.2	12.0	9.8
	This includes:										
	otorhinolaryngologist	2.1	4.0	7.3	3.7	8.7	10.4	12.7	13.2	11.0	9.3
	pediatrician	2.0	5.4	1.9	—	—	—	—	—	—	0.3
	internist	—	—	—	—	0.3	0.8	1.2	—	1.0	0.2
	other specialists	—	—	—	—	—	—	—	—	—	—
4. Laryngeal diseases	*Total*	8.8	7.2	4.3	6.5	8.1	12.1	17.4	15.4	4.2	9.9
	This includes:										
	otorhinolaryngologist	0.7	2.0	1.0	5.3	5.7	8.5	12.5	10.3	2.9	6.4
	pediatrician	8.1	5.2	3.3	0.4	—	—	—	—	—	1.0
	internist	—	—	—	0.8	2.4	3.6	4.9	5.1	1.3	2.5
	other specialists	—	—	—	—	—	—	—	—	—	—

Table 90 (continued)

Name of disease	Visits for medical consultations	under 4 years	5–6 years	7–13 years	14–19 years	20–29 years	30–39 years	40–49 years	50–59 years	60 years and over	Total
5. Nasopharyngeal and pharyngeal diseases	Total	16.4	61.9	79.8	56.1	61.0	54.4	54.0	39.8	21.6	53.4
	This includes:										
	otorhinolaryngologist	0.7	19.3	26.1	23.1	27.9	26.0	37.0	25.4	16.7	14.9
	pediatrician	10.7	42.6	54.3	21.1	—	—	—	—	—	22.3
	internist	—	—	—	11.9	32.5	28.2	15.9	13.1	4.9	16.0
	other specialists	—	—	0.3	—	0.6	0.2	1.1	1.3	—	0.2
These include: chronic tonsillitis	Total	8.6	50.3	73.4	53.5	53.5	39.5	21.5	10.1	4.4	40.5
	This includes:										
	otorhinolaryngologist	—	11.2	20.3	20.8	27.9	14.3	10.4	2.5	0.5	14.0
	pediatrician	8.6	39.1	52.8	20.9	—	—	—	—	—	11.9
	internist	—	—	—	11.8	25.0	25.1	11.0	7.6	3.9	14.5
	other specialists	—	—	0.3	—	0.6	0.1	—	—	—	0.1
6. Diseases of the nose and sinuses	Total	25.4	30.1	24.1	22.2	22.7	30.0	34.4	30.4	14.9	26.5
	This includes:										
	otorhinolaryngologist	2.4	15.0	19.3	17.6	15.3	22.9	26.5	24.3	14.9	19.2
	pediatrician	23.0	15.1	3.7	4.0	—	—	—	—	—	3.0
	internist	—	—	—	0.6	6.1	5.7	7.3	5.4	—	3.8
	other specialists	—	—	0.8	0.6	0.3	1.4	0.6	0.7	—	0.5
7. Total for the group of ear diseases	Total	173.3	194.5	151.5	107.6	121.8	134.1	146.7	126.0	68.6	132.8
	This includes:										
	otorhinolaryngologist	62.8	109.0	82.9	68.4	78.3	92.1	114.3	98.1	59.7	76.5
	pediatrician	110.5	85.8	67.2	25.5	—	—	—	—	—	31.5
	internist	—	—	1.1	13.7	42.5	40.4	30.7	25.3	8.9	23.8
	other specialists	—	—	—	—	1.0	1.6	1.7	2.6	—	1.0
8. Other diseases	To otorhinolaryngologists	33.1	52.7	97.5	21.0	55.2	57.4	52.6	38.0	22.8	37.3
Total	To otorhinolaryngologists	95.9	161.7	179.4	89.7	133.5	149.5	166.9	136.1	82.5	113.8

Table 91

AGE INDEXES OF THE VISITATION RATE TO OTORHINOLARYNGOLOGISTS FOR PURPOSES OF MEDICAL CONSULTATION (No. of visits per 1,000 population of the corresponding age)

Name of disease	Age groups									Total
	under 4 years	5–6 years	7–13 years	14–19 years	20–29 years	30–39 years	40–49 years	50–59 years	60 years and over	
Acute otitis	68.4	46.8	13.9	4.5	7.6	5.7	5.7	6.7	4.1	12.3
Chronic otitis	23.2	9.1	8.0	6.9	7.0	7.9	8.2	11.0	8.9	8.9
Other ear diseases	—	4.5	2.9	0.4	2.1	3.1	—	2.4	4.1	2.5
Laryngeal diseases	2.2	5.2	2.5	3.3	2.7	7.3	9.8	8.1	1.3	5.3
Pharyngeal and naso-pharyngeal diseases	5.5	35.1	59.2	38.3	31.8	33.2	32.9	23.1	15.2	33.6
These include:										
chronic tonsillitis	4.4	28.7	50.0	35.0	26.4	19.7	9.5	6.7	0.7	22.3
diseases of nose and sinuses	16.6	20.8	18.8	23.4	9.8	18.1	18.1	21.1	8.9	17.6
Total for the group of ENT diseases	115.9	121.5	105.3	76.8	61.0	75.3	75.2	72.4	42.5	80.2
Other diseases	33.1	8.5	21.7	17.3	19.3	20.9	16.5	21.7	53.9	24.4
Total	149.0	130.0	127.0	94.1	80.3	96.2	91.7	94.1	96.4	104.6

Table 92

FREQUENCY OF PROPHYLACTIC VISITS TO OTORHINOLARYNGOLOGISTS

Prophylactic visits	No. of visits to oto-rhinolaryngologists per 1,000 population
House calls by otorhinolaryngologists to children aged up to 1 year	0.2
Examinations of preschool children	0.3
Dispensary care of children entering school (7-year-old children)	1.5
Examinations of schoolchildren	18.8
Prophylactic checkups of workers	10.4
Examinations of adolescent workers	3.0
Examinations of workers in the public dining room system and children's institutions	0.4
Issuance of various examination certificates at the time of sending to the Experts' Commission Determining Disability and sanatorium-health resort treatment	0.5
Periodic checks during the dispensary care of patients	0.2
Other prophylactic visits	27.2
Total	62.5

schoolchildren, examinations of workers including adolescent workers and public dining room workers, visits for the purpose of receiving various kinds of certificates, examinations of the patient for sending to the Experts' Commission for Determining Disability and for sanatorium-health resort treatment, as well as patients' appointments during dispensary care and other visits. The data of actual prophylactic visits to the otorhinolaryngologist are shown in Table 92.

Therefore, the total number of prophylactic visits to and by otorhinolaryngologists amounts to 62.5 per 1,000 population. The amount of prophylactic work of the otorhinolaryngologists in Stupino cannot be considered satisfactory, and therefore in determining the population requirement of prophylactic care for the next few years a calculation is needed of the requisite level of prophylactic visits, based on existing instructions, laws, and directives of the Ministry of Health of the USSR concerning compulsory prophylactic care of certain population groups.

Standards for the Urban Population's Requirement of Therapeutic-Prophylactic ENT Care

On the basis of the sickness rate data it is possible to gain a sufficiently complete concept of only the acute and a certain portion of the chronic cases of ENT diseases that have a definitely expressed clinical picture and produce frequent exacerbations.

For a certain number of chronic cases, as has already been noted above, the population does not actually apply to the otorhinolaryngologist, though some patients must have been to the ENT clinic by way of dispensary care. Therefore, in working out the standards of therapeutic-prophylactic care for the next few years, consideration should be given to a certain portion of the chronic cases detected on medical examinations and subject to dispensary care at present. An additional amount of therapeutic-prophylactic care should be calculated for this group of diseases.

Standards of Outpatient-Polyclinic Care for the Urban Population (1966–1970)

In calculations of the need for ENT care for the next few years we used as a basis the average figures for the morbidity rate and the related hospitalization and attendance at outpatient-polyclinic institutions, including corrections by the experts and with consideration of the distribution of the visits for treatment purposes among physicians of different specialties. In determining the amount of dispensary care of patients during the same periods with the sickness rate data, certain corrections were introduced with consideration of the data of complete medical examinations. In connection with the fact that otorhinolaryngologists must, according to existing directives and instructions, conduct a dispensary observation of all patients with chronic tonsillitis and chronic purulent otitis, the need for dispensary care of this category of patients was planned on the basis of morbidity rates taken from medical examination data. It was taken into consideration that optimal medical care (including corrections by the experts) had been rendered to patients for chronic tonsillitis and chronic purulent otitis during the year of the investigation, and we considered it practical to plan an additional amount of care for them, particularly periodic checks of patients by way of dispensary service. At the same time it was assumed that all persons with chronic tonsillitis and chronic purulent otitis detected on examination had been registered at different times when they visited therapeutic institutions or at the time of prophylactic checkups, but they had not been put on the dispensary records; therefore, we planned for an additional amount of medical care (dispensary care and hospitalization) for these persons.

In calculating the need for medical care by the population for acute otitis, it was taken into consideration that all those with acute otitis need therapeutic care to the degree shown by the sickness rate (taking account of corrections by the experts). The number of cases of acute otitis per 1,000 population is 12.6. The number of visits, according to sickness rate data for acute otitis, is 33.4 per 1,000 population per year (visits to and by otorhinolaryngologists 28.7).

The number of cases of chronic otitis is 8.9 per 1,000 inhabitants according to sickness rate, while the number of visits, according to sickness rate data for chronic otitis, is 21 per 1,000 population (taking account of corrections by the experts), including 19.2 to otorhinolaryngologists. Aside from treatment during a period of exacerbation, patients with chronic purulent otitis media, as is well known, need dispensary observation. Data on the amount of dispensary care of this group of patients will be given below.

The following were included in the group of miscellaneous ear diseases, for which we are calculating the amount of therapeutic care needed: otosclerosis, adhesive otitis, the incipient forms of cochlear neuritis (presbyacusis), as well as all cases of hearing difficulty in which there is a need for a hearing aid, and external otitis. The total number of treatment visits, according to sickness rate data, will be 12.3 per 1,000 population for this group of diseases, including 11.8 visits to otorhinolaryngologists.

In this group of patients we distinguish those who need a hearing aid. Their number is 3.2 per 1,000 population. The number of visits connected with selection of hearing aids for this category of patients was included in the total number of visits for treatment.

The number of treatment visits for laryngeal diseases is determined essentially by the visits for acute laryngitis. The total number of visits for treatment for laryngeal diseases will come to 15.2, including 11.7 visits per 1,000 inhabitants to otorhinolaryngologists. In nasopharyngeal and pharyngeal diseases the number of cases of disease is 48.5 per 1,000 population, including 38.1 cases for chronic tonsillitis.

The total number of visits for treatment in the group of pharyngeal and nasopharyngeal diseases is 87 per 1,000 population, including 66.8 for chronic tonsillitis.

Table 93

NUMBER OF VISITS FOR MEDICAL CONSULTATIONS TO PHYSICIANS OF DIFFERENT SPECIALTIES WITH CONSIDERATION OF THE CORRECTIONS BY THE EXPERTS PER 1,000 POPULATION OF THE CORRESPONDING AGE

Name of disease	Visits for medical consultations	Age groups									Total
		under 4 years	5–6 years	7–13 years	14–19 years	20–29 years	30–39 years	40–49 years	50–59 years	60 years and over	
Acute otitis	*Total*	164.1	112.6	41.8	14.4	21.0	18.3	16.0	22.7	10.0	33.4
	This includes:										
	otorhinolaryngologist	111.8	99.4	38.7	14.0	20.2	17(8	15.7	21.0	8.3	28.7
	pediatrician	53.3	13.2	3.1	—	—	—	—	—	—	3.9
	internist	—	—	—	0.4	0.8	0.5	0.3	1.7	1.7	0.8
	other specialists	—	—	—	—	—	—	—	—	—	—
Chronic otitis	*Total*	50.1	29.1	13.9	16.1	14.6	21.7	24.9	22.2	18.9	21.0
	This includes:										
	otorhinolaryngologist	36.7	25.2	12.1	16.1	14.1	20.1	13.8	21.6	18.9	19.2
	pediatrician	13.4	4.0	1.8	—	—	—	—	—	—	1.0
	internist	—	—	—	—	0.4	1.6	1.1	—	—	0.5
	other specialists	—	—	—	—	0.1	—	—	0.6	—	0.3
Other ear diseases	*Total*	4.1	13.9	12.1	4.1	11.1	14.3	13.9	15.6	16.1	12.3
	This includes:										
	otorhinolaryngologist	2.1	8.5	10.2	4.1	10.8	13.5	12.7	15.6	15.1	11.8
	pediatrician	2.0	5.4	1.9	—	—	—	—	—	—	0.3
	internist	—	—	—	—	0.3	0.8	1.2	—	1.0	0.2
	other specialists	—	—	—	—	—	—	—	—	—	—
Laryngeal diseases	*Total*	11.0	12.4	6.8	9.8	10.8	19.4	27.2	23.5	5.5	14.2
	This includes:										
	otorhinolaryngologist	2.9	7.2	3.5	8.6	8.4	15.8	22.3	18.4	4.2	11.7
	pediatrician	8.1	5.2	3.3	0.4	—	—	—	—	—	1.0
	internist	—	—	—	0.8	2.4	3.6	4.9	5.1	1.3	2.5
	other specialists	—	—	—	—	—	—	—	—	—	—

Nasopharyngeal and pharyngeal diseases										
Total	16.9	97.0	138.0	94.4	92.8	87.6	86.9	62.9	36.8	87.0
This includes:										
otorhinolaryngologist	6.2	54.4	85.3	61.4	59.7	59.2	69.9	48.5	31.9	48.5
pediatrician	10.7	42.6	53.4	21.1	32.5	28.2	15.9	13.1	—	22.3
internist	—	—	—	11.9	0.6	0.2	1.1	1.3	4.9	16.0
other specialists	—	—	0.3	—	—	—	—	—	—	0.2
These include: chronic tonsillitis										
Total	13.0	79.0	123.4	88.5	79.9	59.2	31.0	16.8	5.1	66.8
This includes:										
otorhinolaryngologist	4.4	39.9	70.3	55.8	54.3	34.0	20.0	9.2	1.2	36.3
pediatrician	8.6	39.1	52.8	20.9	—	—	—	—	—	11.9
internist	—	—	—	11.8	25.0	25.1	11.0	7.6	3.9	14.5
other specialists	—	—	0.3	—	0.6	0.1	—	—	—	0.1
Diseases of the nose and sinuses										
Total	42.0	50.9	42.9	45.6	32.5	48.1	52.5	51.5	23.8	44.1
This includes:										
otorhinolaryngologist	19.0	35.8	38.1	41.0	26.1	41.0	44.6	45.4	23.8	36.8
pediatrician	23.0	15.1	3.7	4.0	—	—	7.3	5.4	—	3.0
internist	—	—	—	0.6	6.1	5.7	0.6	0.7	—	3.8
other specialists	—	—	0.8	—	0.3	1.4	—	—	—	0.5
Total for the group of ENT diseases										
Total	289.2	316.0	256.5	184.4	182.8	209.4	221.9	198.4	111.1	213.0
This includes:										
otorhinolaryngologist	178.7	230.5	188.2	145.2	139.3	167.4	189.5	170.5	102.2	156.7
pediatrician	110.5	85.5	67.2	25.5	—	40.4	30.7	25.3	—	31.5
internist	—	—	—	13.7	42.5	1.6	1.7	2.6	8.9	23.8
other specialists	—	—	1.1	—	1.0	—	—	—	—	1.0
Other diseases										
To otorhinolaryngologists alone	66.2	61.2	119.2	38.3	74.5	78.3	69.1	59.7	86.7	61.7

The visits to otorhinolaryngologists alone in these diseases come to 48.5 per 1,000 population; for chronic tonsillitis, 36.3.

In addition, for the care of patients with chronic tonsillitis we provided the requisite number of visits by way of dispensary observation (Table 93).

For diseases of the nose and sinuses the number of visits for medical consultations is 44.1 per 1,000 population, including 36.8 to otorhinolaryngologists.

From what has been stated, it is evident that the number of visits to various specialists for therapeutic and consultation purposes in the group of ENT diseases comes to 213 per 1,000 population.

The greatest amount of outpatient-polyclinic care is for the care of patients with nasopharyngeal and pharyngeal diseases. The proportion of visits by these patients in the total number of visits for the ENT disease group is 40.8%.

As has been pointed out above, the visits for treatment in the ENT disease group are distributed essentially among the physicians of three specialties: otorhinolaryngologists, internists, and pediatricians. This applies particularly to visits for chronic tonsillitis, in which internists and pediatricians take care of a little less than half of the visits.

The total number of visits to otorhinolaryngologists in the group of ENT diseases is 156.7 per 1,000 population.

In addition, otorhinolaryngologists take care of a number of cases including those in different classes of disease: injuries to the ear, upper respiratory tract and esophagus and neoplasms in the same location, as well as those of some patients with sore throat, influenza, and other diseases.

The number of visits (taking account of corrections by the experts) to otorhinolaryngologists for these diseases is 61.7 per 1,000 population, as the calculations indicated.

Therefore, the total number of visits for medical consultation purposes to otorhinolaryngologists for all diseases will come to 218.4 per 1,000 population (Table 94). The number of visits to various specialists for medical consultations on account of ENT diseases is shown in Table 93.

At the Fifth All-Union Congress of Otorhinolaryngologists in 1958 it was recognized that dispensary care of those with chronic tonsillitis is one of the most important measures in the prophylaxis of sore throat. The work experience of Leningrad otorhinolaryngologists (S. Ya. Freidlin: *Dispanserizatsiya gorodskogo naseleniya (Dispensary Care of the Urban Population)*, Leningrad, 1964) shows that systematically formulated and planned general hygienic and therapeutic measures lead to a reduction in the incidence of sore throats, chiefly among the groups under dispensary care.

At the same congress the need was emphasized for the most active participation by physicians of various specialties in the control of chronic tonsillitis, chiefly internists, pediatricians and otorhinolaryngologists. All this indicates that the work in the

Table 94

STANDARDS OF OUTPATIENT-POLYCLINIC CARE OF THE URBAN POPULATION IN THE FIELD OF OTORHINOLARYNGOLOGY FOR 1966–1970 (per 1,000 population)

Name of disease	Average intensive morbidity figures for five cities	Average number of visits for treatment per 1,000 population			Average number of visits for treatment per case	Incidence of cases needing dispensary observation by the oto-rhinolaryngologist detected by medical examinations	Total number of outpatient visits to the otorhinolaryngologist needed for treatment purposes	Dispensary care of patients with ear and pharyngeal diseases	Prophylactic checkups				Total number of prophylactic visits	Total visits (therapeutic and prophylactic)
		actual	added by the experts	sum					of workers in industrial enterprises	of adolescents (15–18 years old)	of preschool children	of others		
Acute otitis	12.6	21.1	12.3	33.4	2.7	—	28.7	—	—	—	—	—	—	—
Chronic otitis	8.9	12.1	8.9	21.0	2.3	17.3	19.2	34.6	—	—	—	—	—	—
Other ear diseases	7.7	9.8	2.5	12.3	1.6	—	11.8	—	—	—	—	—	—	—
Laryngeal diseases	6.1	9.9	5.3	15.2	2.5	—	11.7	—	—	—	—	—	—	—
Nasopharyngeal and pharyngeal diseases	22.3	53.4	33.6	87.0	3.9	26.3	48.5	52.4	—	—	—	—	—	—
These include:														
chronic tonsillitis	11.9	37.3	22.3	62.8	5.0	26.2	36.3	52.4	—	—	—	—	—	—
Diseases of the nose and sinuses	15.4	26.5	17.6	44.1	2.9	—	36.8	—	—	—	—	—	—	—
Total for the group of ENT diseases	73.0	132.8	80.2	213.0	2.9	43.5	156.7	—	—	—	—	—	—	—
Diseases not included in the ENT disease group	—	37.3	24.4	61.7	—	—	61.7	—	—	—	—	—	—	—
Total							218.4	87.0	32.0	69.0	19.7	38.6	159.3	464.7

dispensary care of patients with chronic tonsillitis should be done by the otorhino-laryngologists in contact with the district and shop physicians (internists) and pediatricians (school physicians or physicians covering nurseries and kindergartens).

As for the number of periodic checks, we use as a basis the experience of dispensary care of patients in Leningrad.

An analysis of the work volume in the dispensary care of patients in some districts of Leningrad shows that in chronic tonsillitis (as well as in chronic purulent otitis media) the number of follow-ups during the year ranges from two to four. We are calculating the requisite work volume in dispensary care on the basis of two obligatory checkups per year.

In determining the requirement of dispensary care for chronic tonsillitis by the population we did not plan any visits for cases known from sickness rate data, because we believed that five visits (including the experts' corrections) for every case admitted for chronic tonsillitis fully provide for the outpatient care of this group of patients. The dispensary visits were planned for cases of chronic tonsillitis detected on examinations, with the exception of those for which hospitalization had been provided during the year. Of the group of cases detected, the annual hospitalization rate per 1,000 population for chronic tonsillitis is 3.3. Therefore, of the total number of cases detected, 26.2 cases of chronic tonsillitis need dispensary observation. The total number of visits per year by way of dispensary observation of the patients with chronic tonsillitis will come to 52.4 per 1,000 population.

The total number of cases of chronic purulent otitis for which we are planning dispensary care comes to 17.3 per 1,000 population. For the rest of the cases detected on examinations (0.2 per thousand) hospital care has been planned.

With two follow-ups a year the number of visits for the dispensary care of the patients with chronic purulent otitis will come to 34.6 per 1,000 population.

Therefore, the work volume in the dispensary care of patients with chronic tonsillitis and chronic purulent otitis by the otorhinolaryngologists has been found to be 87 visits per year per 1,000 population.

Provision has also been made for the regular observation of a certain group of the healthy population with the aim of timely detection of the initial stages of the diseases. In determining the work volume for care of prophylactic visits we considered the existing directives of the Ministry of Health of the USSR as well as instructions on methods and instructions on annual prophylactic checkups by physicians of different specialties (with participation of otorhinolaryngologists) among the various groups of the healthy population constituted according to type of work or age.

In accordance with directive No. 321 of the Ministry of Health of the USSR dated July 20, 1960, "Concerning the Status and Measures for the Further Improvement of Outpatient-Polyclinic Care of the Urban Population," seven-year-old children should have dispensary examinations by physicians of the various specialties. This is the first mass examination of children by otorhinolaryngologists before entering school. The number starting school every year is 19.6 per 1,000 urban population. Therefore, the number of prophylactic visits for preschool children should be 19.7 per 1,000 population.

According to a directive of the Ministry of Health of the USSR (No. 354 dated July 30, 1963), "Concerning Measures for the Further Improvement of Medical-Health Care of Adolescents," adolescent clinics should make regular medical examinations of adolescents once a year, using physicians of the limited specialties, including otorhinolaryngologists. It is mentioned in this directive that specialists of polyclinics and hospital should also be used for medical and health care of 15–18-year-old adolescents working at occupational training, students of technical education or occupational training, students of technical schools, and students in the 9th to 11th grades of secondary schools. Therefore otorhinolaryngologists must yearly examine all adolescents from 15 to 18 years of age. For every 1,000 urban population, according to the data of the 1959 census, the group of students and adolescents 15–18 years old numbers 69. Therefore the number of visits to otorhinolaryngologists for dispensary care of this population group should also number 69 per 1,000 population. In the Soviet Union special attention is given to the medical care of workers in various branches of industry. Participation of the otorhinolaryngologist in the regular medical checkups of workers engaged in enterprises in which there is intense noise, in "hot" shops, as well as at work whose conditions require constant stability of the vestibular apparatus and normal hearing, has been provided by Directive No. 136 of the Ministry of Health of the USSR dated September 7, 1957, concerning prophylactic checkups by physicians of workers engaged in various branches of industry. The number of workers subject to annual prophylactic checkups by otorhinolaryngologists, according to the 1959 census, is 32 per 1,000 city population. Therefore, the total number of prophylactic visits to the otorhinolaryngologist by way of dispensary care of industrial workers should be 32 per 1,000 population.

We also took into account the amount of prophylactic care derived from regular examinations by otorhinolaryngologists of those receiving licenses to drive cars, motorcycles, buses, streetcars, as well as those engaged in servicing railroad and water transportation, in construction and assembly work at heights, and others.

For convenience in calculations we combined this category of persons into the general group of "miscellaneous," which comes to 38.6 per 1,000 urban population. With a single annual examination of the "miscellaneous" group, the number of prophylactic visits to the otorhinolaryngologist should be 38.6 per 1,000 population.

Therefore with optimal outpatient-polyclinic care, the total number of visits by the urban population to otorhinolaryngologists should come to no fewer than 464.7 per 1,000 inhabitants during the year (including 218.4 visits for treatment and 246.3 for prophylactic purposes).

The numerical data given above are presented in the summarizing tables 94 and 95.

Table 95

AGE INDEXES OF THE NEED FOR OUTPATIENT-POLYCLINIC CARE OF THE POPULATION BY OTORHINOLARYNGOLOGISTS (No. of visits per 1,000 population of the corresponding age)

Type of outpatient-polyclinic care	Age groups									Total
	under 4 years	5–6 years	7–13 years	14–19 years	20–29 years	30–39 years	40–49 years	50–59 years	60 years and over	
Visits for therapeutic purposes	224.9	291.7	307.4	183.5	213.8	258.6	230.2	230.2	188.9	218.4
Dispensary care of the patients	8.2	72.0	82.2	61.6	111.8	115.2	86.8	82.0	64.2	87.0
Prophylactic checkups	—	126.6	126.0	1,031.9	84.6	88.2	82.6	51.0	5.2	159.3
Total	257.5	490.3	515.6	1,277.0	410.2	449.1	428.0	363.2	258.3	464.7

Standards of Hospital Care in the Field of Otorhinolaryngology

In determining the population need for hospital care for the next few years, we used the actual hospitalization rate in the ENT departments according to sickness rate data (taking account of the corrections made by the experts).

Included in the hospitalization figures for sickness rate are corrections made to account for selection of persons for hospital treatment from the group of those with chronic purulent otitis and chronic tonsillitis kept on dispensary records. The additional amount of hospital treatment for this group of patients has been established on the basis of data of the complete medical examinations of the Stupino population.

The number of cases hospitalized according to sickness rate data (taking account of corrections by the experts) in the ENT department, on the average for five cities, was 7.2 per 1,000 population. Of these 0.6 was for acute otitis, 0.6 for chronic otitis, 0.2 for other ear diseases, 0.2 for laryngeal diseases, 3.3 for nasopharyngeal and pharyngeal diseases, 1.3 for diseases of the nose and sinuses, and 1 for diseases included in different classes (injuries, foreign bodies in the upper respiratory tracts and esophagus, benign tumors, etc.). Through medical examinations it was additionally demonstrated, that of the group of those with chronic tonsillitis and chronic purulent otitis, 16.4 need hospital treatment for chronic tonsillitis and 1.1 per 1,000 population for chronic purulent otitis complicated by cholesteatoma, polyps and osteomyelitis.

Therefore, for all the newly detected chronic cases of ENT disease the amount of hospital care should be doubled by comparison with that existing now.

It would be an error, however, to provide an additional amount of hospitalization every year with reference to the morbidity established from a single examination of the population. Patients with chronic diseases of the ear, nose and throat, needing hospital therapy have accumulated in the population for years, and not just because of an inadequacy of beds but also on account of the small amount of current dispensary care of the healthy population, which makes it possible to detect chronic diseases only in that part of the population given annual prophylactic examinations.

Table 96
AGE INDEXES OF THE POPULATION REQUIREMENT OF HOSPITAL TREATMENT
(No. of cases hospitalized per 1,000 inhabitants of the corresponding age group)

Name of disease	Age groups									Total
	under 4 years	5–6 years	7–13 years	14–19 years	20–29 years	30–39 years	40–49 years	50–59 years	60 years and over	
Acute otitis	2.1	1.8	0.6	0.4	0.8	0.4	0.3	0.3	0.2	0.6
Chronic otitis	1.0	0.5	0.3	0.8	1.4	1.1	0.5	0.3	0.1	0.8
Other ear diseases	0.1	0.1	0.1	0.1	0.2	0.2	0.4	0.4	0.1	0.2
Laryngeal diseases	0.8	0.4	0.3	0.1	0.2	0.3	0.3	0.2	0.1	0.2
Nasopharyngeal and pharyngeal diseases	4.2	5.9	14.1	13.0	8.0	5.9	2.1	1.0	0.2	6.5
These include: chronic tonsillitis	4.2	5.9	14.1	13.0	7.8	5.9	2.1	1.0	0.2	6.2
Diseases of the nose and sinuses	0.4	1.2	0.8	1.6	2.1	1.7	1.4	1.2	0.4×	1.3
Other diseases	4.1	0.7	1.1	0.3	1.9	1.3	0.3	1.0	—	1.0
Total	12.7	10.6	17.3	16.3	14.6	10.9	5.3	4.4	1.1	10.6

Table 97
STANDARDS OF HOSPITALIZATION OF THE URBAN POPULATION IN THE FIELD OTORHINOLARYNGOLOGY (1966–1970)

Name of disease	Per 1,000 population					
	No. of cases of disease (according to sickness rate data and data of medical examinations)	actually hospitalized	added by the expert	No. of cases of annual hospitalization out of No. of those attending for examination	total hospitalization requirement	average duration of treatment
Acute otitis	12.6	0.5	0.1	—	0.6	9.6
Chronic otitis	29.7	0.6	—	0.2	0.8	14.8
Other ear diseases	11.6	0.2	—	—	0.2	14.5
Laryngeal diseases	8.7	0.2	—	—	0.2	8.4
Nasopharyngeal and pharyngeal diseases	64.3	2.0	1.3	3.2	6.5	8.3
These include: chronic tonsillitis	41.3	1.7	1.3	3.2	6.2	8.3
Diseases of the nose and sinuses	35.6	1.1	0.2	—	1.3	9.6
Total for group of diseases	162.6	4.6	1.6	3.4	9.6	9.2
For other diseases	—	0.7	2.3	—	1.0	9.2
Total		5.3	1.9	3.4	10.6	9.2

It is also important to note that the chronic cases subject to hospital treatment require surgery, after which recovery usually occurs. Therefore, in the planning of ENT beds the current hospitalization rate should be used as a basis, with consideration of the corrections made by the experts (7.2 per 1,000 population), and an additional number of beds should be provided annually for five years, amounting to one-fifth of the total number of patients with chronic tonsillitis and chronic purulent otitis detected on the examinations who need hospitalization, i.e., 3.4 beds per 1,000 population. With this selection indicated of patients for hospital treatment from the group detected on examinations, there is a change in the composition of the group of patients hospitalized, in connection with which the average length of treatment in the ENT department will drop from 9.5 (with actual hospitalization) to 9.2 days.

Therefore the urban population requirement of hospital treatment may be optimally satisfied with an annual hospitalization rate of 10.6 per 1,000 population, when the average length of the patient's stay in bed is 9.2 days and the beds are in operation 340 days a year. The age and overall indexes for the population requirement of hospital treatment are shown in Tables 96 and 97, respectively.

Standards of Therapeutic-Prophylactic Care of the Urban Population in the Field of Ophthalmology

Total Morbidity of the Urban Population (according to sickness rate at therapeutic-prophylactic institutions)

The average intensive indexes of the incidence of eye diseases for five cities are shown in Table 98.

From Table 98 it is evident that per 1,000 urban population of both sexes there are 39 admissions (40.3 for men and 37.9 for women) for the diseases in the "Eye disease" class. Eye injuries, including foreign bodies, are in the class of "Injuries," but are dealt with, as a rule, by ophthalmologists alone. Therefore, the column "Total" of Table 98 includes eye injuries. The sickness rate for eye diseases thereby rises substantially and reaches 47.4 in the population for both sexes. For a more detailed study of some of the nosologic entities in the "Eye disease" class we distinguished the following: conjunctivitis, glaucoma, cataract, malignant progressive myopia, as well as refractive errors. Moreover, we kept in mind the fact that some of the patients with these diseases should be treated on an outpatient basis, and some in the hospital. As is evident from Table 98, the population of the cities studied seeks treatment most often for conjunctivitis (on the average 19.8 admissions per 1,000 population for both sexes).

The incidence of glaucoma (according to sickness rate) is 0.5 per 1,000 population; it is higher in women.

The number of cases of injury with a foreign body in the eye is over three times higher in men than in women (13.9 cases per 1,000 men and 4.1 per 1,000 women). This may be explained by the fact that men most often work in the most hazardous occupations. Superficial eye injuries (contusions of the lids, wounds of the lids and

213

Table 98
AVERAGE INTENSIVE INDEXES OF THE TOTAL INCIDENCE OF EYE DISEASES IN
THE POPULATION OF FIVE CITIES

Disease	Number of admissions (per 1,000 population)			Standardized indexes		
	men	women	both sexes	men	women	both sexes
Glaucoma	0.5	0.6	0.5	0.6	0.7	0.6
Foreign bodies	13.9	4.1	8.4	13.7	3.5	7.8
Conjunctivitis	20.7	19.1	19.8	21.6	19.5	20.3
Other eye diseases	19.2	18.2	18.7	19.4	18.1	18.7
According to class of eye disease	40.3	37.9	39.0	41.6	38.3	39.6
Total (including injury)	54.2	42.0	47.4	55.3	41.8	47.4
In addition: Refractive and accommodation errors	6.5	7.6	7.1	6.4	7.1	6.6

conjunctivitis, burns, etc.) are of great importance, together with foreign body cases. They come to 2.1 % of the total number of eye injuries.

Refractory and accommodation errors, which, strictly speaking, should not be classed among the diseases, are most often seen in women. According to sickness rate data, refractive and accommodation errors come to 7.1 per 1,000 population (6.5 for men and 7.6 per 1,000 population for women).

The age indexes of the population morbidity are shown in Table 99 on the average for five cities.

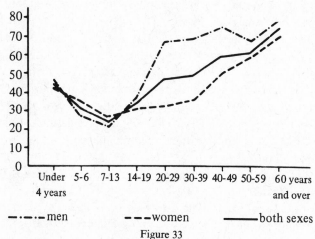

Figure 33
Average age indexes of incidence of eye diseases in the population of five cities (No. of admissions per 1,000 population of the corresponding age and sex)

Table 99

AVERAGE AND AGE INDEXES FOR THE INCIDENCE OF EYE DISEASES IN THE POPULATION OF FIVE CITIES

(No. of cases per 1,000 population of the corresponding age and sex)

Disease	Age groups								
	men	women	both sexes	men	women	both sexes	men	women	both sexes
	under 4 years			5–6 years			7–13 years		
Foreign bodies	0.3	0.5	0.4	1.2	0.3	0.8	2.3	1.5	1.9
Conjunctivitis	37.5	36.8	31.1	20.3	24.8	22.4	13.5	15.1	14.3
Glaucoma	—	—	—	—	—	—	—	—	—
Other eye diseases	7.3	6.3	6.9	7.4	10.1	8.6	8.9	9.9	9.4
Class of eye diseases	44.8	43.1	44.0	34.9	30.9	22.4	25.0	25.0	23.7
Total	45.1	43.6	44.4	28.9	35.2	31.7	24.7	26.5	25.6
Refractive and accommodation errors	—	—	—	—	1.3	0.6	7.8	3.8	5.9
	14–19 years			20–29 years			30–39 years		
Foreign bodies	7.7	3.9	6.7	26.2	6.0	14.3	23.5	4.5	12.5
Conjunctivitis	11.6	10.7	11.1	19.1	10.2	15.9	26.4	16.4	18.1
Glaucoma	—	—	—	0.3	0.1	0.2	0.3	0.2	0.2
Other eye diseases	16.0	16.7	16.4	20.0	13.2	16.2	22.7	14.1	17.9
Class of eye diseases	27.6	27.4	27.5	39.4	27.1	32.3	43.6	30.6	36.1
Total	35.3	31.3	34.2	65.6	33.1	64.6	67.1	35.1	48.6
Refractive and accommodation errors	10.4	7.6	9.1	1.8	3.9	3.0	3.4	6.1	4.9
	40–49 years			50–59 years			60 years and over		
Foreign bodies	18.0	4.8	10.0	19.4	3.4	6.2	4.2	2.3	2.9
Conjunctivitis	26.6	19.1	22.1	25.3	24.2	24.7	25.3	25.7	25.5
Glaucoma	0.8	0.5	0.6	1.0	1.6	1.4	5.5	4.1	4.5
Other eye diseases	28.3	24.2	25.9	34.0	28.9	29.3	42.7	39.9	40.8
Class of eye diseases	55.7	43.8	48.6	56.3	54.7	55.4	73.4	68.7	71.0
Total	73.7	48.6	58.6	66.7	58.1	61.6	77.6	72.0	73.9
Refractive and accommodation errors	14.1	15.4	14.9	14.5	16.0	15.4	5.1	6.6	6.2

The prevalence of eye diseases is relatively high among children under 4 (Figure 33). Then the incidence gradually drops, reaching a minimum at 7–13 years of age. Beginning with the 14–19-year-old group, the indexes gradually rise. The highest incidence is noted in the group of 60 years and over. In various age groups there are substantial variations in the figures for men and women.

Considerable variations in the intensive morbidity indexes were noted for persons of different age according to the various nosologic entities also. The differences in

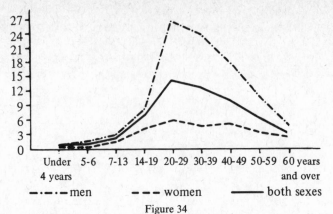

Figure 34

Prevalence of eye injuries with foreign bodies (No. of injuries per 1,000 population of the corresponding age and sex)

the incidence of injury to the eye by a foreign body were particularly great among persons of different age and sex (Figure 34).

Many cases of eye injury occur during the period of most active work. In all age groups, with the exception of the under-4 age group, the rate of injury is higher in men than in women.

Essential differences in the morbidity figures of the population of different age groups were also shown for conjunctivitis. The highest incidence is noted under the age of 4, (37.1 per 1,000 children) (Figure 35).

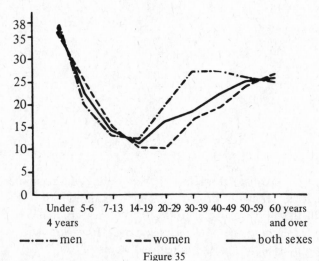

Figure 35

Age indexes for the incidence of conjunctivitis in the urban population (number of cases per 1,000 population of the corresponding age and sex)

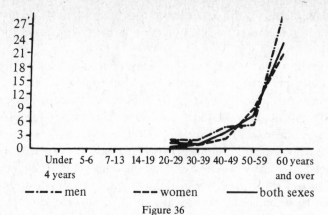

Figure 36

Age indexes for the incidence of glaucoma in the urban population (No. of admissions per 1,000 population of the corresponding age and sex)

The prevalence of glaucoma depends to a high degree on the age (Figure 36). The highest incidence of glaucoma in the population is seen at the age of 60 and over. Cases of senile cataract are encountered beginning with ages 50–59. In the younger age groups cataracts are most often of traumatic origin and are found only in men.

Aside from eye diseases, workup of the data on refractive errors, which we did not include in the eye disease group, is of great importance for determining the outpatient work volume of ophthalmologists. Refractive and accommodation errors are found relatively rarely in younger children (Figure 37). However, beginning

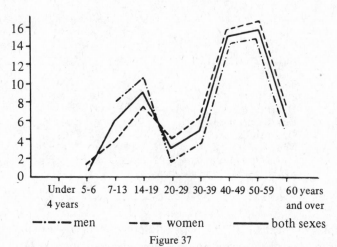

Figure 37

Age indexes for the incidence of refractive and accommodation errors in the urban population (average age and sex)

with school age, the figures for refractive errors in children rise. This is evidently associated with the fact that medical attention is better organized for school-age children.

In the age group from 20 to 29 the incidence of refractive errors drops to one-third of that in the previous group. At 30–39 it rises somewhat, and beginning with age 40 the number of admissions for refractive errors again increases because of incipient presbyopia in many. At the ages of 50 to 59 the figure for refractive errors remains at almost the same level as at 40 to 49. However, in the oldest age group it again drops sharply. Apparently this is connected with the fact that most of those needing glasses had already acquired them in previous years. Therefore we see two rises in the figures for the incidence of sickness rate for refractive errors: the first at school age, the second with the appearance of presbyopia in older persons and the associated need for glasses.

In the work of determining the standards of ophthalmological care, the distribution of all patients with various diseases according to specialties of the physicians who are to take care of them in the polyclinic and hospital is very important. Thus, some patients with eye diseases are treated not only by ophthalmologists but also by surgeons (for example, some types of injuries) and pediatricians (for example, conjunctivitis), etc.

The proportion of diagnoses made by ophthalmologists is shown in Table 100.

Table 100
PROPORTION OF ADMISSIONS FOR EYE
DISEASES TO OPHTHALMOLOGISTS
(in % of the total number of admissions for these
diseases)

Disease	% of admissions to ophthalmologists
Conjunctivitis	96.2
Cataract	100
Glaucoma	100
Malignant progressive myopia	100
Retinal detachment	100
Other eye diseases	92.76
In addition:	
Foreign bodies in the eye	94.66
Refractive and accommodation errors	98.13

Ophthalmologists deal with 2.96% of all admissions for disease, including 2.74% for the group of eye diseases and injuries, and the remaining 0.22% for diseases treated by physicians in other specialties.

Incidence of Eye Diseases among the Urban Population According to the Data of Complete Medical Examinations

Data on the incidence of chronic cases newly detected on medical examination are shown in Table 101.

As is evident from Table 101, the number of cases of eye diseases newly detected on medical examinations is 41.5 per 1,000 population (34.3 among men and 47.2 among women). However, the composition of the diseases newly found during medical examinations is substantially different from the morbidity distribution obtained from analyzing the sickness rate data. During medical examinations mainly chronic cases in the early stages were found, while the prevalence of the various diseases determined on examination was sometimes higher than from the sickness rate.

The incidence of cataracts, according to the examination data, is 10 per 1,000 population, whereas from the sickness rate it is 1.3; the incidence of glaucoma is 5.3 and 0.5, respectively.

Through the examinations quite a considerable number of persons (5.7 per 1,000 population) were found to have concomitant strabismus.

The figures for the prevalence of malignant progressive myopia are comparatively high (3.6 per 1,000 population). We included in this group patients with a high degree of myopia of a progressive nature and associated with changes in the fundus (myopic chorioretinitis, retinal detachment, etc.).

We put those with a high degree of myopia with no tendency toward progression and unaccompanied by changes in the fundus in the group with refractive errors, and they were not included among the patients with eye diseases.

The data on the prevalence of refractive errors among the population are of great interest, because fitting glasses for refractive errors considerably increases the amount of outpatient work by ophthalmologists. According to the examination data, the figure for the prevalence of refractive errors is 246.4 per 1,000 population.

The figures for the prevalence of various eye diseases shown on medical examinations are essentially different in the various age and sex groups of the population; however, their main patterns are essentially the same as those determined from the sickness rate data, and for this reason we are not dwelling on them in detail here. However, we should analyze the age and sex characteristics of the prevalence of concomitant strabismus, malignant progressive myopia, and refractive errors.

It should be noted that in the children's groups concomitant strabismus and a high degree of progressive myopia are the basic forms of pathology found on examination; these account for from 50 to 90% of the cases in children of different ages. Thus, the number of cases of concomitant strabismus per 1,000 children of the 7–12 age group is 8.6; in the 3–6-year-old group, 9.4; and at 1–2 years, 8.1.

Of considerable interest are the data on the prevalence of progressive malignant

Table 101

CHRONIC EYE DISEASE CASES NEWLY DETECTED BY COMPLETE MEDICAL EXAMINATIONS (No. of cases per 1,000 population)

Name of disease	both sexes	men	women	both sexes	men	women	both sexes	men	women
	under 1 year			1–2 years			3–6 years		
Class of eye diseases (total)	—	—	—	16.2	23.1	8.6	12.5	13.4	11.9
This includes:									
cataracts	—	—	—	—	—	—	1.6	3.3	—
glaucoma	—	—	—	—	—	—	—	—	—
malignant progressive myopia	—	—	—	—	—	—	—	—	—
concomitant strabismus	—	—	—	8.1	15.4	—	9.4	6.7	11.9
Other eye diseases	—	—	—	8.1	7.7	8.6	1.5	3.4	—
	7–12 years			13–15 years			14–19 years		
Class of eye diseases (total)	9.4	13.8	4.7	19.2	14.7	24.8	10.4	12.2	8.5
This includes:									
cataracts	0.8	1.5	—	—	—	—	—	—	—
glaucoma	—	—	—	—	—	—	—	—	—
malignant progressive myopia	—	—	—	9.2	8.8	10.6	2.1	—	4.3
concomitant strabismus	8.6	12.3	4.7	8.0	3.4	14.2	—	—	—
Other eye diseases	—	—	—	1.6	2.9	—	8.3	12.2	4.2
	20–29 years			30–39 years			40–49 years		
Class of eye diseases (total)	19.8	20.4	19.6	31.9	38.9	26.6	48.8	42.6	52.9
This includes:									
cataracts	0.7	1.9	—	2.0	2.3	1.7	2.4	1.5	3.0
glaucoma	—	—	—	2.0	4.6	—	5.4	9.1	3.0
malignant progressive myopia	2.3	1.8	2.6	1.0	1.1	0.9	10.9	9.1	11.2
concomitant strabismus	6.1	7.4	5.2	2.9	1.1	4.3	3.6	—	6.0
Other eye diseases	10.7	9.3	11.8	4.9	4.6	5.1	3.6	3.1	4.0
	50–59 years			60 years and over			total		
Class of eye diseases (total)	63.7	54.4	70.4	214.7	155.9	239.7	41.5	34.3	47.2
This includes:	0.9	—	1.5	1.6	5.4	—	1.1	1.1	1.1
glaucoma	12.7	6.5	17.2	115.4	69.9	134.7	10.0	6.4	12.9
malignant progressive myopia	12.8	13.0	12.5	30.4	48.4	22.8	5.3	5.0	5.5
concomitant strabismus	5.5	4.4	6.3	12.8	5.3	16.0	3.6	1.8	5.0
Other eye diseases	3.6	2.2	4.7	8.0	5.4	9.1	5.7	5.7	5.7

myopia among the population. Those persons in whom there were various eye complications of progressive myopia were put into this group on examination. There were 3.6 per 1,000 population examined in this group. In the various age groups the figures for the prevalence of this type of pathology vary. The highest figures for the incidence of progressive malignant myopia are noted in the age groups of 13–15 years (9.6 per 1,000 population of this age), and 60 years and over (12.8). In all the age groups the figure for the prevalence of progressive malignant myopia is higher in women than in men.

For the purpose of determining the additional amount of outpatient work by ophthalmologists the age and sex indexes for the prevalence of the various types of refractive errors among the population are significant; these are presented in Table 102.

About half of all cases of refractive errors are from hypermetropia, the prevalence of which is 132.6 per 1,000 population. Among women the number with hypermetropia is 147.1 per 1,000; among men it is 114. The number of persons with myopia is 79.1. For completeness of characterization of the prevalence of refractive errors, the number of patients with malignant progressive myopia, categorized among the eye diseases, was put in this group. The number of persons with astigmatism is 34.7 per 1,000 population, while about one-fourth of the cases are from myopic astigmatism, and three-fourths from hypermetropic astigmatism.

The figures for the various types of refractive errors, according to the medical examination data for the population, are different in the various age groups. For example, the number of cases of myopia per 1,000 children aged 3–6 is 9.4. In the 7–12 age group the number with myopia rises by more than four times from the previous age group and is 39.7 per 1,000 population. In the age group from 13 to 15 the number with myopea reaches 110.6 per thousand, which is 12 times higher than the similar figures for 3–6-year-old children.

The highest figure for the prevalence of mypoia is noted in the age group from 16 to 19 (147.6 per 1,000 population, in young men 117.8, in young women 178.8).

Beginning with the age group 20–29 these figures gradually drop in each successive age group.

Let us look at the prevalence of the various degrees of myopia among the population (Table 103). According to the classification adopted in the USSR, we divided all cases of myopia found on examination into three degrees: mild, up to 3.0 diopters; medium, from 3.0 to 6.0 diopters; severe, 6.0 diopters or more. In Table 103 we have the age and sex figures for the prevalence of the different degrees of myopia among the population (number of cases per 1,000 population of the corresponding age and sex).

From Table 103 it is evident that the mild form of myopia is found most often among the population (58.9 cases per 1,000 population). This form of myopia is seen more often among women than among men (66.1 and 49.6, respectively).

The number of cases of moderate myopia per 1,000 population is 10.5; it is almost

Table 102

AGE AND SEX INDEXES FOR PREVALENCE OF VARIOUS TYPES OF REFRACTIVE ERRORS AMONG THE POPULATION

(No. of cases detected on medical examinations per 1,000 population of the corresponding age and sex)

Age group	Myopia of all degrees			Hypermetropia of all degrees			Astigmatism					
							myopic			hypermetropic		
	men	women	both sexes	men	women	both sexes	men	women	both sexes	men	women	both sexes
Under 1 year	—	—	—	74.1	178.6	127.3	—	—	—	—	—	—
1–2 years	—	—	—	184.5	162.4	174.1	—	2.9	1.5	10.0	3.0	6.3
3–6 years	10.0	8.8	9.4	237.5	264.7	251.9	3.1	6.3	4.7	23.0	30.1	26.5
7–12 years	39.8	39.6	39.7	125.7	128.2	126.9	11.7	3.5	8.1	17.6	14.1	16.0
13–15 years	105.6	116.6	110.6	41.1	60.0	49.7	8.1	12.8	10.4	12.2	42.5	27.0
16–19 years	117.8	178.8	147.6	20.4	29.8	25.0	18.5	9.1	13.0	5.6	23.5	16.0
20–29 years	87.0	152.1	119.4	9.2	24.8	18.3	9.1	10.3	9.8	33.2	28.4	20.5
30–39 years	60.5	108.5	88.5	12.6	20.7	17.2	4.6	20.0	13.9	35.0	40.9	38.6
40–49 years	59.3	103.8	86.1	94.2	125.2	113.2	6.5	4.7	5.5	23.9	42.2	34.5
50–59 years	43.5	75.2	62.0	315.2	441.3	388.5	10.8	4.5	6.4	32.3	25.1	27.3
60 years and over	75.3	84.6	81.7	440.8	365.3	387.8	—	—	—	—	—	—
Total	60.4	93.5	79.1	114.0	147.1	132.6	7.7	9.4	8.6	22.4	29.0	26.1

Table 103

AGE AND SEX INDEXES OF THE PREVALENCE OF DIFFERENT DEGREES OF MYOPIA IN THE POPULATION (No. of cases per 1,000 population of the corresponding age and sex)

Age groups	Mild myopia (under 3.0 diopters)			Moderate myopia (from 3.0 to 6.0 diopters)			Severe myopia (over 6.0 diopters)		
	men	women	both sexes	men	women	both sexes	men	women	both sexes
Under 1 year	—	—	—	—	—	—	—	—	—
3–6 years	10.0	5.9	7.8	—	—	—	—	2.9	1.6
7–12 years	38.3	34.8	36.6	1.5	3.2	2.3	—	1.6	0.8
13–15 years	79.2	91.9	84.9	11.7	14.1	12.8	14.7	10.6	12.9
16–19 years	77.2	114.9	95.6	32.5	46.8	39.5	9.1	17.1	12.5
20–29 years	70.4	96.5	85.7	9.2	28.7	20.7	7.4	16.9	13.0
30–39 years	52.6	75.9	65.9	5.7	15.5	11.4	2.2	18.1	11.2
40–49 years	51.7	75.8	66.3	6.1	12.0	9.6	1.5	16.0	10.2
50–59 years	39.1	51.7	46.4	—	9.4	5.5	4.4	14.1	10.1
60 years and over	48.4	57.1	54.5	16.1	2.3	6.4	10.8	25.2	20.8
Total	49.6	66.1	58.9	6.8	13.4	10.5	4.1	14.0	9.7

twice as high in women (13.4) as in men (6.8). The number with severe myopia is 9.7 per 1,000 population, while the figure for women (14) is almost $3\frac{1}{2}$ times higher than for men (4.1). This pattern is noted in all age groups. Although myopia is not classed as a disease, in a number of cases it contributes to severe functional disorders of the eye that are of a progresssive nature. Therefore, a comparison of the prevalence of severe myopia and its malignant forms is interesting.

From Table 104 it is seen that the number of cases of malignant progressive myopia is 3.6 per 1,000 population, of severe myopia, 9.7 cases. The figure for incidence of malignant progressive myopia is 2.7 times greater in women (5) than in men (1.8). Therefore, in 1.8 cases out of 4.1 in men and 5 out of 14 in women, severe myopia is associated with severe changes in the eye or has a steadily progressive nature. Patients with malignant progressive myopia are encountered even in the 13–15-year age group. In this group the number of patients with malignant progressive myopia is 9.6 per 1,000 persons of this age; of all those with severe myopia, 12.9. This confirms the opinion of a number of workers who point out that progression of myopia occurs during the school years.

Malignant progressive myopia is found most often among women. From the data given it is evident that the figures for the prevalence of myopia in all age groups are quite high, but particularly high among schoolchildren. So far medical science has not conclusively elucidated the reasons for the occurrence and development of myopia. To date, it is also difficult to explain the difference in the prevalence of severe myopia between men and women.

Table 104

PREVALENCE OF SEVERE MYOPIA AND MALIGNANT
PROGRESSIVE MYOPIA AMONG THE POPULATION OF
DIFFERENT AGES AND SEXES

(No. of cases per 1,000 population of the corresponding age and sex)

Age groups	No. of cases of severe myopia			No. of cases of malignat progressive myopia		
	men	women	both sexes	men	women	both sexes
Under 1 year	—	—	—	—	—	—
1–2 years	—	—	—	—	—	—
3–6 years	—	2.9	1.6	—	—	—
7–12 years	—	1.6	0.8	—	—	—
13–15 years	14.7	10.6	12.9	8.8	10.6	9.6
16–19 years	8.1	17.1	12.5	—	4.3	2.1
20–29 years	7.4	16.9	13.0	1.9	2.6	2.3
30–39 years	2.2	18.1	11.2	1.1	4.3	2.9
40–49 years	1.5	16.0	10.2	—	6.0	3.6
50–59 years	4.4	14.1	10.1	4.4	6.3	5.5
60 years and over	10.8	25.2	20.8	5.4	16.0	12.8
Total	4.1	14.0	9.7	1.8	5.0	3.6

Important for determining the standards are the data on the prevalence of hypermetropia among the population obtained on the basis of data of complete medical checkups.

The medical examinations showed that in the children's groups the prevalence of hypermetropia is relatively high. Thus, in the 3–6 age group 251.9 cases of hypermetropia per 1,000 persons examined were detected. In the age group from 7 to 12 the number with hypermetropia drops to 126.9; at 13–15, to 49.7. At 16–19, 20–29, and 30–39 years a further reduction in the incidence of hypermetropia is noted. This is explained by the fact that in these age groups refraction was determined without the instillation of cycloplegics. Because of this no cases of latent hypermetropia could be found, but only those with overt hypermetropia were detected whose disease could not be covered up by straining the accommodation. Latent hypermetropia was therefore not completely determined.

The prevalence of hypermetropia rises again sharply in the 40–49 age group (113.2 per 1,000 population of this age). At 50–59 all the hypermetropia is completely detected and the figures rise to 388.5 per 1,000 population. For purposes of planning standards a certain degree of incompleteness of data on hypermetropia in younger persons (due to facultative hypermetropia) is not of essential importance, because for practical purposes those with hypermetropia in these age groups do not go to the physician to obtain glasses. It is also important to take into consideration the amount of outpatient work required for care of those with refractive errors. With this aim in view, all cases of hypermetropia were divided into two groups, under 3.0 diopters and over 3.0 diopters. From data in the literature and observations of practicing physicians and investigators (A. V. Khvatova, E. M. Belostotskii and others) it is well known that children with hypermetropia under 3.0 diopters do not need to wear glasses when there is no concomitant strabismus, vision is good, and there are no signs of asthenopia. Therefore they do not need to visit the oculist for glasses.

The prevalence of hypermetropia of different degrees among the population is shown in Table 105.

Table 105
PREVALENCE OF DIFFERENT DEGREES OF HYPERMETROPIA
(No. of cases per 1,000 population of the corresponding age and sex)

Age groups	Hypermetropia under 3.0 diopters			Hypermetropia over 3.0 diopters		
	men	women	both sexes	men	women	both sexes
Under 1 year	74.1	178.6	127.3	—	—	—
1–2 years	179.6	162.4	179.0	7.6	—	4.1
3–6 years	217.4	252.9	236.3	20.1	11.8	15.6
7–12 years	115.0	117.1	116.0	10.7	11.1	10.9
13–15 years	35.2	45.9	40.1	5.9	14.1	9.6
16–19 years	16.3	29.8	22.9	4.1	—	2.1
20–29 years	9.2	24.8	18.3	—	—	—
30–39 years	91.9	124.7	111.4	3.0	1.0	1.8
40–49 years	12.6	20.7	17.2	—	—	—
50–59 years	310.9	427.2	378.5	4.3	14.1	10.0
60 years and over	440.8	353.9	379.8	—	11.4	8.0
Total	109.2	141.8	127.5	4.8	5.3	5.1

As is evident from the table, the figures for the prevalence of hypermetropia are 132.6 per 1,000 population (114 for men and 147.1 for women). A mild hypermetropia (less than 3.0 diopters) is most common; it comes to 127.5 per 1,000 population. The prevalence of higher degrees of hypermetropia is only 5.1 cases per 1,000 population. It should be noted that the study of refraction by instillation of cycloplegics in the age group under one year was not accomplished in all children because of the toxicity of homatropine for infants; instillation was accomplished only in children over six months of age.

Hospitalization of the Urban Population for Eye Diseases

The average figures for the hospitalization rate of the urban population for eye diseases are given in Table 106.

Table 106

HOSPITALIZATION RATE OF THE URBAN POPULATION FOR EYE DISEASES

(No. of cases hospitalized per 1,000 population of each sex)

Name of disease	No. of cases actually hospitalized			No. of cases added by experts			No. of cases actually hospitalized plus those added by experts		
	men	women	both sexes	men	women	both sexes	men	women	both sexes
Conjunctivitis	0.2	0.1	0.2	0.2	—	0.1	0.4	0.1	0.3
Glaucoma	0.1	0.1	0.1	—	0.1	0.04	0.1	0.2	0.14
Other eye diseases	1.0	0.8	0.9	0.2	0.1	0.2	1.2	0.9	1.1
These include:									
cataract	0.3	0.1	0.2	—	—	—	0.3	0.1	0.3
Class of eye diseases	1.3	1.0	1.2	0.4	0.2	0.3	1.7	1.2	1.5
In addition:									
Foreign bodies in the eye	0.2	—	0.1	—	—	—	0.2	—	0.1
Refractive and accommodation errors	0.2	0.1	0.1	—	—	—	0.2	0.08	0.1
Total	1.7	1.1	1.4	0.4	0.2	0.34	2.1	1.38	1.74

For every 1,000 inhabitants there are 1.4 cases hospitalized (in men, 1.7; in women, 1.1); this includes, for the other eye diseases, 0.9; for conjunctivitis 0.2 (for men 0.2, for women 0.1), glaucoma, 0.1; injury with foreign body in the eye, 0.1; refractive and accommodation errors, 0.1.

Only men were hospitalized for injury to the eye involving foreign body.

In the various age groups the hospitalization rates are different. The average age indexes for hospitalization of the population of five cities are shown in Table 107 and in Figure 38.

The hospitalization rate of the population for eye diseases varies in the different age groups from 0.2 to 5.7 per 1,000 population of each age group.

The lowest hospitalization rate on the average for five cities is noted in the age group 5–6 (0.2), the highest at 60 and over (5.7 per 1,000 population).

To the actual hospitalization rate (1.4 cases per 1,000 population) we have added another 0.34 cases per 1,000 population, including 0.1 for conjunctivitis, 0.04 for glaucoma, and 0.2 for the other eye diseases. The actual hospitalization rate data and material of the expertise (number of additional cases of hospitalization recommended) are, in our opinion, a quite complete representation of the population requirement of hospital care for this sickness rate.

The average figures for the visitation rate to ophthalmological institutions of various cities with the existing incidence (sickness rate) of eye diseases in the population is shown in Table 108.

Table 107

AGE INDEXES OF HOSPITALIZATION RATE OF THE POPULATION OF FIVE CITIES

(No. of cases hospitalized per 1,000 population of the corresponding age and sex)

Name of disease	Age groups								
	men	women	both sexes	men	women	both sexes	men	women	both sexes
	under 4 years			5–6 years			7–13 years		
Foreign bodies	—	—	—	0.1	—	0.1	0.2	—	0.1
Conjunctivitis	1.2	0.7	1.0	0.1	0.1	0.1	0.1	0.04	0.1
Glaucoma									
Other eye diseases	—	0.6	0.3	0.1	0.08	0.1	0.1	0.5	0.3
Total	1.2	1.3	1.3	0.3	0.18	0.3	0.4	0.54	0.5
	14–19 years			20–29 years			30–39 years		
Foreign bodies	—	—	—	0.2	—	0.1	0.4	0.1	0.2
Conjunctivitis	0.04	0.04	0.04	0.4	0.05	0.2	0.1	0.2	0.1
Glaucoma									
Other eye diseases	1.1	0.5	0.8	1.0	0.6	0.8	0.7	0.4	0.6
Total	1.14	0.54	0.84	1.6	0.65	1.1	1.2	0.5	0.9
	40–49 years			50–59 years			60 years and over		
Foreign bodies	0.2	—	0.1	0.1	—	0.1	—	—	—
Conjunctivitis	0.1	—	0.1	0.1	0.05	0.08	0.5	—	0.2
Glaucoma	0.4	0.1	0.2	0.1	0.6	0.4	1.5	1.9	1.7
Other eye diseases	1.9	0.5	1.0	1.9	1.6	1.7	3.8	3.8	3.8
Total	2.6	0.6	1.4	2.2	2.2	2.2	5.8	5.7	5.7

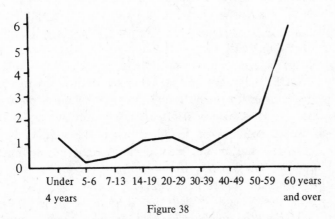

Figure 38

Age indexes of hospitalization rate of the urban population for eye diseases and injuries (No. of cases hospitalized per 1,000 population of the corresponding age)

Table 108
VISITATION RATE TO OUTPATIENT-POLYCLINIC INSTITUTIONS FOR THERAPEUTIC
PURPOSES FOR VARIOUS EYE DISEASES
(No. of visits for therapeutic purposes per 1,000 population)

Name of disease	Women			Men			Both sexes		
	actually made	added by experts*	total	actually made	added by experts*	total	actually made	added by experts*	total
Foreign bodies in the eye	3.2	0.4	3.6	21.5	2.6	24.1	11.9	1.4	13.3
Class of eye diseases	53.7	20.3	74.0	69.3	32.1	92.4	60.4	21.4	81.8
These include:									
conjunctivitis	32.1	11.9	35.0	30.9	12.3	43.2	26.5	12.1	38.6
glaucoma	1.2	0.6	1.8	1.3	0.4	1.7	1.2	0.5	1.7
other eye diseases	29.4	7.8	37.2	37.1	10.4	47.5	32.7	8.5	41.2
Refractive and accommodation errors	8.8	3.0	11.8	8.2	4.2	12.4	8.6	3.5	12.1
Total	65.7	23.7	89.4	99.0	29.9	128.8	80.9	26.3	107.2

* Corrections by the experts were introduced only for the nosologic entities mentioned in the table. For all other diseases the number of visits added by the experts rises to 47.5 per 1,000 population.

As is evident from the table, the average number of visits for eye diseases, injuries with the incorporation of foreign bodies, and refractive and accommodation errors is 80.9 per 1,000 population with the incorporation of foreign bodies, and refractive and accommodation errors (99 in men and 65.7 in women). However, it should be noted that with evaluation by the experts in various cases a definitely inadequate number of visits for a number of diseases, as well as refractive and accommodation errors, was found. Cases existed in which glasses were fitted on children without preliminary atropinization in the presence of eye injuries in which there were foreign bodies and acute conjunctivitis. Not uncommonly the patients came in only once.

In the different age and sex groups of the population there are essential differences in the visitation rate to the outpatient-polyclinic institutions for treatment.

The average age indexes for the visitation rate of the population to ophthalmologists for eye diseases are shown in Table 109 and Figure 39.

From Table 109 and Figure 39 it is evident that in the younger age groups the figures for the visitation rate for treatment purposes are relatively high. However, the highest figures for visitation rate are noted in the age groups 50–59 (118.7 per 1,000 population of this age) and 60 and over (117).

In the majority of the age groups (with the exception of the groups under 4 and 5–6 years old) men visited the ophthalmologist more often than women.

Most often the population comes to ophthalmological institutions for conjuncti-

Table 109
AVERAGE AGE INDEXES OF VISITATION RATE OF THE POPULATION TO OPHTHALMOLOGISTS FOR EYE DISEASES (No. of visits per 1,000 population)

Name of disease	men	women	both sexes	men	women	both sexes	men	women	both sexes
	___								
	under 4 years			5–6 years			7–13 years		
Foreign bodies	0.3	—	0.2	1.2	—	0.7	3.0	1.7	2.3
Class of eye diseases	66.6	74.9	70.5	40.8	63.1	50.8	43.3	38.5	40.8
Conjunctivitis	51.6	63.8	57.4	30.4	47.2	38.0	30.0	26.9	28.4
Glaucoma									
Other eye diseases	15.0	11.2	13.1	10.4	15.9	12.8	13.3	11.6	12.4
Refractive and accommodation errors	—	—	—	—	2.7	1.3	11.3	3.8	7.7
All visits including class of eye diseases, injuries and refractive and accommodation errors	66.9	74.9	70.7	42.0	65.8	52.8	57.6	44.0	50.8
	14–19 years			20–29 years			30–39 years		
Foreign bodies	8.9	2.0	5.3	46.3	3.4	20.8	36.7	4.2	17.4
Class of eye diseases	32.2	32.3	32.6	73.0	29.4	47.6	76.4	46.2	58.7
Conjunctivitis	11.3	8.7	10.0	29.7	13.1	20.0	28.1	16.2	21.1
Glaucoma				1.1	0.2	0.6	1.2	0.6	0.8
Other eye diseases	21.0	23.6	22.6	42.2	16.1	27.0	47.1	29.5	36.8
Refractive and accommodation errors	12.9	9.3	11.1	3.1	4.6	3.8	4.9	8.1	6.7
All visits including class of eye diseases, injuries and refractive and accommodation errors	54.0	43.6	49.0	122.4	37.4	72.2	118.0	58.0	82.8
	40–49 years			50–59 years			60 years and over		
Foreign bodies	28.9	5.2	14.6	15.5	4.2	8.9	4.7	2.0	2.9
Class of eye diseases	91.4	64.0	74.4	109.0	80.4	92.5	109.4	105.0	106.5
Conjunctivitis	36.2	22.9	28.0	42.7	29.5	34.8	37.0	33.0	34.5
Glaucoma	1.5	0.3	0.8	2.0	4.7	3.6	11.2	6.4	7.8
Other eye diseases	53.7	40.8	45.6	65.0	46.2	54.0	61.2	65.6	64.2
Refractive and accommodation errors	16.5	16.0	16.2	15.7	18.4	17.3	5.1	8.5	7.6
All visits including class of eye diseases, injuries and refractive and accommodation errors	120.8	85.2	105.2	140.9	103.0	118.7	119.2	115.5	117.0

Age groups

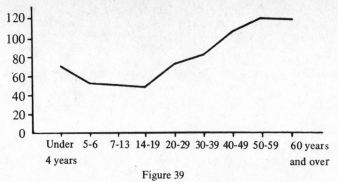

Figure 39

Age indexes for visitation rate of the urban population for eye disease and injury, refractive and accommodation errors (No. of visits per 1,000 population of the corresponding age)

vitis, which accounts for 33.1% of the visits. Patients with conjunctivitis, foreign bodies in the eye, and refractive errors are responsible for 57.6% of the visits.

In order to determine the population requirement of ophthalmological care, a record of all visits to ophthalmologists, made not only for eye diseases but also for other diseases largely treated by physicians in other specialties by way of medical consultation care, is of great importance. It is also necessary to determine the fraction of visits made for eye diseases to the physicians of other specialties. The proportion of visits to ophthalmologists for eye diseases is shown in Table 110.

The number of visits for medical consultation to ophthalmologists for other diseases is 11.8 per 1,000 population. It should be stated that this number of visits is definitely inadequate for complete care of patients with the various eye diseases. The number of visits recommended by the experts for the other diseases was 16.4 per

Table 110
PROPORTION OF VISITS TO OPHTHAL-
MOLOGISTS FOR EYE DISEASES (in percentages
of the total number of visits for these diseases)

Name of disease	% of visits to ophthalmologists
Foreign bodies	92.8
Conjunctivitis	93.5
Cataract	100.0
Glaucoma	100.0
Malignant progressive myopia	100.0
Retinal detachment	100.0
Other eye diseases	94.21
Refractive and accommodation errors	98.1
Total	94.1

1,000 population. Therefore, the total number of visits needed should be 28.2 per 1,000 population.

Ophthalmologists are responsible for 94.1% of the visits made for eye diseases.

Some of the patients visited physicians in other specialties for eye diseases. The fraction of visits to pediatricians noted was 4.2%; to internists, 0.8%; to surgeons, 0.2%; to neuropathologists, 0.2%; to phthisiologists, 0.1%; to other specialists, 0.4%. Therefore, the number of visits to ophthalmologists for eye diseases is 100.2 per 1,000 population.

Table 111
FREQUENCY OF PROPHYLACTIC VISITS TO THE
OPHTHALMOLOGIST (No. of visits per 1,000 population)

Type of prophylactic visit	Including visit to the ophthalmologist
Regular home visits by physicians to children under 1 year of age	0.2
Examinations of schoolchildren	0.5
Dispensary care of children entering school (7-year-old children)	3.2
Examinations of schoolchildren	37.1
Prophylactic checkups of workers	5.8
Examinations of adolescent workers	3.21
Examinations of pregnant women	0.2
Examinations of workers in the public dining room system, in children's institutions, municipal enterprises	0.1
Issuance of various certificates	1.0
Periodic checkups during dispensary care	1.0
Other prophylactic visits	27.8
Total	62.5

Along with the visits for treatment it is exceedingly important to take into account also the visits for prophylactic purposes. Among the prophylactic visits we included regular house calls to children under the age of one year, examinations of preschool children, dispensary care of children entering school (7-year-old children), prophylactic checkups of schoolchildren, adolescent workers, examinations of pregnant women, of public dining room system workers, workers in children's institutions, municipal enterprises, visits for the purpose of obtaining various kinds of certificates, checkups made during dispensary care of patients, and other prophylactic visits. The data of the prophylactic visits actually made are shown in Table 111.

The number of prophylactic visits to ophthalmologists is 62.5 per 1,000 population. The amount of prophylactic work in Stupino is small in the field of ophthalmology.

Therefore, in determining the requirement of ophthalmological care these data should be varied in accordance with the existing instructions, laws and directives of the Ministry of Health of the USSR.

Standards of Therapeutic-Prophylactic Care of the Urban Population in the Field of Ophthalmology

A comparison of the figures for the sickness rate and the frequency of detection of chronic cases in complete medical examinations is shown in Table 112.

From the table it is evident that during the course of medical examinations a considerable number of chronic cases were detected for which in the previous year the population had not sought medical care.

It should be pointed out, however, that not all the newly detected cases need the amount of hospital and outpatient care given for the same conditions as judged by sickness rate. For example, elderly persons with concomitant strabismus do not need repeated visits for treatment. They require only advice during the prophylactic visits, the frequency of which increases from year to year. The same may be said about various types of refractive and accommodation errors in different age groups of the population.

In calculations of the amount of therapeutic-prophylactic care for the next few years we did not take into consideration all the cases found by examinations. In the next few years the annual prophylactic examinations will not cover the whole population of the country, but only certain groups of it. Therefore, not all chronic cases of eye disease which are not clinically manifest, can be detected at present.

Table 112
PREVALENCE OF EYE DISEASES AND REFRACTIVE AND ACCOM-
MODATION ERRORS AMONG THE URBAN POPULATION ACCORDING
TO SICKNESS RATE DATA AND DATA OF COMPLETE MEDICAL
EXAMINATIONS

Name of disease	Per 1,000 population	
	average intensive indexes of population sickness rate in 5 cities	number of chronic cases detected on medical examinations for which no admissions had been recorded in the previous year
Conjunctivitis	19.8	1.1
Glaucoma	0.5	5.3
Other eye diseases	18.7	18.2
Total for the class of eye diseases	39.0	24.6
Foreign bodies	8.4	—
Refractive and accommodation errors	7.1	246.4

According to the existing directives and instructions, ophthalmologists should participate in the annual prophylactic examinations of preschool children, schoolchildren from 7–14 years, adolescents 15–18 years old, and workers in some branches of industry.

According to our data, in the age groups under 19 the number of newly detected chronic cases is 4.8 per 1,000 population, including chronic conjunctivitis 0.1, glaucoma 0.6, cataract 0.1, malignant progressive myopia 0.8, concomitant strabismus 2.4, and other eye diseases 0.8.

In calculating the population requirement of outpatient-polyclinic visits, we used as a basis the fact that all patients with conjunctivitis need therapeutic care to the same degree as applied to the sickness rate (with consideration of corrections made by the experts). The number of cases of conjunctivitis is 19.9 per 1,000 population (of these 19.8 were previously known from admissions to the institutions and 0.1 per 1,000 population were newly detected in the age groups under 19). The number of visits, according to data of admissions for conjunctivitis, is 38.6 per 1,000 population. The number of additional treatment visits for the newly detected cases is 0.2 per 1,000 population. Therefore the total number of necessary visits for conjunctivitis will be 38.8 per 1,000 population per year.

By a similar method the number of additional visits was determined for taking care of the population, both in the other age groups and for other diseases detected through examinations.

The number of persons under 19 needing annual visits for refractive and accommodation errors, of the group of all the newly detected cases, is 43.6 per 1,000 population, including mild myopia 15.1, medium degree of myopia 3.0, and severe myopia 0.9; with myopic astigmatism 1.7; with hypermetropia over 3.0 diopters, 3.2; with hypermetropic astigmatism, 6.1; with hypermetropia under 3.0 diopters, 14.6.

Therefore, the number of persons needing annual visits for refractive and accommodation errors is 50.7 per 1,000 population, and the number of visits should be 3.2 for each case admitted.

According to the sickness rate data, there are 12.1 visits per 1,000 population. Therefore the total number of visits needed for refractive and accommodation errors should amount to 136.77 per 1,000 population.

In determining the amount of work in dispensary care of patients and in the prophylactic checkups of the population performed by ophthalmologists the following considerations were used as a basis. At present, patients with glaucoma, tuberculosis of the eye, children with malignant progressive myopia, severe myopia and concomitant strabismus, and patients with eye tumors need dispensary care by ophthalmologists.

In calculations of the need for visits by patients with concomitant strabismus, we used as a basis data in the literature and material that the Department of Children's

Eye Safety of the Helmholtz State Scientific Research Institute of Eye Diseases has at its disposal.

Many authors distinguish between accommodative and nonaccommodative strabismus. In the opinion of the majority of them (I. L. Smol'yaninova, A. V. Khvatova, E. M. Belostotskii, E. S. Avetisov and others), accommodative strabismus is corrective through permanent wearing of glasses, not only cosmetically but also functionally (that is, the visual acuity is increased, the deviation decreases or disappears, and binocular vision is restored). According to their data, approximately one-fourth of the patients in this group who do not need special types of treatment fall into this category. Functional treatment is needed for the majority of the patients. In the calculations it should be taken into consideration that in children with concomitant strabismus under the age of 6, usually no functional treatment is given because of the considerable difficulties associated with the children's forgetting the tasks assigned during the functional treatment. In early childhood the basic treatment method is the constant wearing of glasses (E. M. Belostotskii, 1960).

The number of children with concomitant strabismus under 6 years of age, according to our data, is 0.8 per 1,000 population. At this age, as has already been pointed out, functional treatment is not given, but children with this defect need frequent visits because of amblyopia, which is found in 70% of them. These children should visit the therapeutic-prophylactic institutions every 10 days, on the average.

The number of children with concomitant strabismus and reduced vision, according to our data, is 0.56 per 1,000 of the whole population. Recovery of vision through functional treatment at this age (mainly through occlusion) occurs after long treatment. The minimum treatment period for children with amblyopia under 6 years of age with the use of occlusions is four months. Recently, in the Department for Children's Eye Safety of the Helmholtz State Scientific-Research Institute of Eye Diseases, treatment was given to 51 children under the age of 6 with concomitant strabismus associated with reduction in vision: for 23 patients, 22 weeks were needed for recovery of vision; for seven patients, 28 weeks; for four patients, 30 weeks; for 17 patients, 26 weeks. Therefore, on the average, the duration of treatment was about 20 weeks (19.8 weeks), i. e., about 140 days.

During the period in which the occlusion is accomplished the patients should visit the ophthalmologist, on the average, once every 10–14 days to check on the state of vision. Therefore, with an average duration of therapy equal to 140 days and the number of visits equal to 14 (they are provided every 10 days), the number of visits needed is 7.84.

For children with concomitant strabismus not associated with reduction of vision (without amblyopia), for which the main type of treatment is the constant wearing of glasses, seven visits are provided for each child. We used as a basis the fact that they need glasses fitted after 10 days of atropinization, for which four visits are needed. Repeated visits, for the purpose of checking on the state of vision and the degree to which the glasses prescribed correct the existing ametropia, are provided once every four months (that is, three subsequent visits per year).

Therefore, for each 1,000 of the whole population there is 0.24 person with concomitant strabismus needing 1.68 visits to the ophthalmologist. The total number of visits by children under 6 for concomitant strabismus is 9.52 per 1,000 population. In the 7–15 age group the prevalence of concomitant strabismus is 1.4 per 1,000 of the whole population. At this age the orthoptic exercises are possible. According to the data of a number of authors, over two-thirds of the children with concomitant strabismus need functional treatment, primarily for the existing amblyopia, which is found in 70% of them. The course of treatment of amblyopia consists of 20 exercises. The number needing functional treatment at this age is 0.98 per 1,000 of the whole population.

The orthoptic exercises should be supervised by specially trained nurses. During this period the children with concomitant strabismus should visit the physician after 10 exercises have been done. Therefore, each child visits the physician three times a year (the first visit, before the exercises are started; the second, after the first 10 exercises; and the third, after the completion of the exercises).

In 25% of the children with concomitant strabismus unstable fixation is found. According to our data, these patients amount to 0.24 per 1,000 population. Therefore, the number of additional visits is 0.96 per 1,000 population (0.24 × 4).

The course of treatment of amblyopia conducted once, however, does not give a satisfactory result in 50% of the patients. This group of patients needs repeated courses every three to four months (20 exercises in each). Therefore, the total number of additional visits for treatment for this group is 4.32 (0.48 × 9).

Patients with concomitant strabismus unassociated with amblyopia constitute 30% of the total. It has already been mentioned that children from 7 to 15 years old with concomitant strabismus constitute 1.4 per 1,000 population. Therefore, the number of children with concomitant strabismus without reduction of vision is 0.42 per 1,000 population. This group of patients needs preoperative and postoperative orthoptic treatment (30 exercises before operation and 30 after it). The total number of visits needed for children with concomitant strabismus without reduction of visual acuity is 3.36 per 1,000 population (0.42 × 8).

Therefore the total number of visits by physicians to children under 15 with concomitant strabismus for purposes of ophthalmological treatment is 21.1 per 1,000 population.

In the older age groups the basic type of treatment of these patients is operation, in which a cosmetic effect is achieved. Only in childhood is it possible to attain the principal goal, the restoration of binocular vision, in correcting concomitant strabismus. In the older age groups it is no longer possible to restore the visual functions in this category of patients.

In determining the number of dispensary visits for glaucoma, the instructions and

Directive No. 753 of the Ministry of Health of the USSR dated August 27, 1952, as well as data in the literature, were made the basis of the determination.

According to the data of the majority of investigators, each person given dispensary care for glaucoma should visit the eye clinic once a month on the average.

Therefore, we determined the fact that the number of visits for dispensary care of patients with glaucoma should be 4.3 per 1,000 population.

At present children under 14 years of age, young persons 15–19 years old, and patients with malignant progressive myopia should be covered by dispensary care. The number of these patients is 0.7 per 1,000 population. According to the clinical experience gained at the present time, such patients require two to three courses of treatment of a general tonic nature. Before beginning these courses and after conducting them, outpatient visits are required (about six to eight per patient). With the average number of visits which we adopted for the calculations equal to 7, the number of visits needed is 4.9 per 1,000 population. The same principle is used for determining the number of dispensary visits for severe myopia unassociated with changes in the optic fundus and with no tendency toward rapid and steady progression. The number of cases of severe myopia among persons under 19 is 0.9 per 1,000 population. With a number of visits equal to 7, the number of visits needed is 6.3 per 1,000 population. The number of visits needed for the dispensary care of patients for tuberculosis of the eye (0.3 case per 1,000 population) will be 2.1 per 1,000 population when the number of visits is 7. In these calculations we are using as a basis the need to give two courses of specific antituberculosis treatment during the year; visits are needed before they are begun and after they are finished. The number of dispensary visits for tumors is 1.2.

In the opinion of ophthalmologists of the Ukraine, at present all students with moderate degrees of myopia, that is with myopia which, in the opinion of a number of ophthalmologists, A. I. Dashevskii and others, belongs to the progressive group, should be given dispensary care. The number of persons with moderate degrees of myopia under the age of 19 is 3 per 1,000 of the whole population.

The fact should also be taken into account that, in schoolchildren with an increased strain on the eyes, mild degrees of myopia can also progress. According to the data of the majority of investigators, the progression of myopia occurs until the fourth to sixth grade (that is, until the age of 13 to 15). The number of persons with mild degrees of myopia under the age of 15, according to our data, is 10.5 per 1,000 population. In addition to the visits connected with the fitting of glasses these children need dispensary visits twice to three times a year. The total number of visits of this group of children will be 31.5 per 1,000 population.

Therefore in our calculations of the amount of outpatient ophthalmological care required by the urban population for 1965–1970, main attention is paid to the care of children and young people with various eye diseases, as well as adults with severe eye diseases leading to loss of the visual functions.

From all the considerations we have given, it follows that the total number of visits in the dispensary care of patients is 71.4 per 1,000 population. Dispensary care, as has already been pointed out, implies, along with care of the patients, regular observation of certain categories of healthy persons for the purpose of detecting the initial forms of disease and preventing them. In determining the population requirement of prophylactic visits we used the existing directives of the Ministry of Health of the USSR and the instruction on methods of taking care of the various groups of the healthy population, combined according to the work they do.

In the calculations of the need for prophylactic care of the population, the age and sex and social composition of the population of the USSR according to the All-Union Census of 1959 were used as a basis.

On February 16, 1957 (No. 236/57) the Ministry of Health of the USSR published instructions on methods, "Concerning Measures for Prevention of Visual Disorders in Preschool Children and Schoolchildren." It was pointed out in them that prophylaxis of visual disorders may be effective only when hygienic and ophthalmologic measures are taken at the same time. The number of children 4–5 years old is 19.2 per 1,000 population, while the number of those of 6–7 years entering school every year is 19.7 per 1,000 population. Therefore the total number of prophylactic visits for preschool children should be 38.9 per 1,000 population. Studies of vision in school-age children should be conducted yearly by oculists or school physicians. The latter should check only visual acuity, and if visual acuity less than 20/20 is found the children should be sent to the ophthalmologist. It is recommended that refraction be accomplished with particular care and refractive errors be corrected (after 10 days of atropinization) in schoolchildren in the fourth to sixth grades, because myopia appears and develops usually at this age. The number of children from 8 to 15 is 134.1 per 1,000 population. Investigation of schoolchildren permits timely detection of children with refractive errors, which constitutes the basic measure for the prevention of progression of the myopia. Therefore the number of prophylactic visits by school ophthalmologists is 134.1 per 1,000 population.

Along with dispensary care of schoolchildren in the Soviet Union great attention is being given to dispensary care of adolescent workers.

In connection with the existing serious defects in the dispensary care of adolescents working in industrial enterprises, engaged in agriculture, studying in occupational and technical schools, as well as other 15–18-year-olds the Minister of Health of the USSR issued Directive No. 354 dated 30 July 1963, "Concerning Measures for the Further Improvement of Medical Care of Adolescents." According to this directive, beginning with 1963, adolescents' clinics should make regular medical examinations of the adolescents once a year, using specialists in the more limited specialties. For medical care of adolescents 15–18 years old working in industry, students in the occupational and technical schools, technical schools, schoolchildren in the 9th to 11th grades, and three-year secondary schools, the polyclinic and hospital specialists should be used. The number of persons in the 15–18-year-old group, according to

Table 113

STANDARDS OF OUTPATIENT-POLYCLINIC CARE OF THE URBAN POPULATION IN THE FIELD OF OPHTHALMOLOGY FOR 1965–1970 (per 1,000 population)

| Name of disease | Average intensive morbidity indexes for 5 cities | Average number of treatment visits per 1,000 population | | | Average number of treatment visits per disease | Frequency of chronic cases needing treatment in children and adolescents newly detected by medical examinations | Number of additional treatment visits for newly detected cases | Total morbidity figures (according to sickness rate and according to medical examination data) | Total number of outpatient visits for treatment | Dispensary care of patients | Prophylactic care | | | | | Total visits (therapeutic and prophylactic) |
		actual	added by the experts	total							of industrial workers	of adolescents (15–18 years old)	of preschool children	of school-children	of workers in the public dining room system	total number of prophylactic visits	
Conjunctivitis	19.8	26.5	12.1	38.6	1.8	0.1	0.2	19.9	38.8								
Glaucoma	0.5	1.2	0.5	1.7	3.4	0.6	2.0	1.1	3.7								
Other eye diseases	18.7	32.7	8.5	41.2	2.1	4.1	8.61	22.8	49.8								
Class of eye diseases	39.0	60.4	21.1	81.5	—	4.8	10.80	43.8	92.3								
In addition:																	
Foreign bodies in the eye	8.4	11.9	1.4	13.3	1.4	—		8.4	13.3								
Refractive and accommodation errors	7.1	8.6	3.5	12.1	1.7	43.6	124.7	50.7	136.8								
Medical consultative visits to ophthalmologists in connection with other diseases									26.6								
Total									269.0	71.4	12.2	69.0	38.9	134.1	38.6	292.8	633.22

the 1959 census, is 69 per 1,000 population. The number of visits of the ophthalmologists, connected with the dispensary care of this population group, is 69 per 1,000 population.

In accordance with Directive No. 136 of the Minister of Health of the USSR dated September 7, 1957, concerning obligatory preliminary examinations at the time of beginning work and regular medical checkups of workers in the various branches of industry, ophthalmologists should participate in prophylactic checkups of the workers in industries producing arsenic and its compounds, fluorine and its derivatives, methyl alcohol, and antibiotics, as well as of those engaged in work with considerable visual strain, work in servicing and operating electrical engineering plants, work with radioactive agents and sources of ionizing radiation. The number of workers subject to annual prophylactic examination by the ophthalmologist, according to the 1959 census, is 12.2 per 1,000 population. The need for prophylactic examinations by ophthalmologists for industrial workers should be 12.2 visits per 1,000 population.

Consideration was also given to the additional need for prophylactic care of transport workers.

Therefore complete outpatient-polyclinic care of the urban population in the field of ophthalmology can be assured with 633.22 visits per year per 1,000 population, including 269.02 treatment visits and 364.2 visits for prophylactic and dispensary purposes combined.

In composite form all the numerical data are given in Table 113.

Standards of Hospital Care in the Field of Ophthalmology

The data of the total morbidity according to the population sickness rate is the basic form for determining the standards of the need for hospital care by the population. Making complete medical examinations made it possible to demonstrate the additional number of persons needing hospital care in the group of those with previously unknown chronic illnesses. The number of cases hospitalized in the ophthalmological department in these cities was 1.2 per 1,000 population (including 0.2 for conjunctivitis, 0.1 for glaucoma, 0.9 for other eye diseases). In addition, patients are hospitalized in the ophthalmological department for eye injuries. The number of cases hospitalized for injuries amounted to 0.1 per 1,000 population. The hospitalization rate for refractive errors was 0.1 per 1,000 population.

Through a carefully made experts' examination an additional 0.3 cases of hospitalization per 1,000 population was determined (including 0.1 for conjunctivitis and 0.2 for other eye diseases).

Therefore, the number of cases hospitalized in the eye departments (with consideration of corrections made by expert analysis) is 1.7 per 1,000 population.

Carrying out complete medical examinations of the population made it possible to

Table 114

STANDARDS OF HOSPITAL CARE FOR THE URBAN POPULATION IN THE FIELD OF OPHTHALMOLOGY

Disease	No. of cases of disease (according to sickness rate data and data of medical examinations)	Per 1,000 population				
		No. of cases hospitalized		No. of cases hospitalized among the newly detected cases	total	average length of treatment (in days)
		actual	added by the experts			
Conjunctivitis	20.9	0.2	0.1	—	0.3	3.9
Glaucoma	5.8	0.2	—	0.6	0.8	20.4
Other eye diseases	36.9	0.8	0.2	3.8	4.8	14.3
Total eye disease	63.6	1.2	0.3	4.4	5.9	13.2
Foreign bodies	8.4	0.1	—	—	0.1	38.0
Refractive and accommodation errors	105.5	0.1	—	—	0.1	2.0
Malignant tumors of the eye (skin cancer)	0.1			0.1	0.1	24.6
Total					6.2	14.5

demonstrate that of the group of patients with previously unknown chronic eye diseases 4.5 per 1,000 population need ophthalmological hospital treatment; this includes 0.6 for glaucoma, 3.8 for other eye diseases, and 0.1 for eye tumors. The total number of cases in which hospital care is required is 6.2 per 1,000 population.

All the data given above are presented in Table 114.

The average length of treatment in the ophthalmological department was the following: 17.4 days in Stupino, 13.8 in Dneprodzerzhinsk, 12.3 in Rubezhnoe, and 14.5 days, on the average, for these cities. We consider that these figures can be adopted for calculations for the next few years (1965–1970).

Standards of Therapeutic-Prophylactic Care of the Urban Population in the Field of Neurology

The average intensive total morbidity, hospitalization rate, and outpatient visitation rate of the population, calculated from the data of five cities with populations of less than 1,500,000 persons and with consideration of the corrections made on the basis of data from complete medical examinations in Stupino, have been made the basis of calculations for the determination of standards of therapeutic-prophylactic care of the urban population in the field of neurology.

The use of data from statistical research conducted in the field of neurology in previous years by a number of authors (A. Ya. Dorsht, M. I. Lyapides, S. A. Safonov, E. A. Osipov, T. I. Gol'dovskaya and others) is complicated by the fact that the figures for the population morbidity that they established are, as a rule, presented in their extensive distribution and do not cover the entire list of nervous diseases.

Total Morbidity of the Urban Population at Therapeutic-Prophylactic Institutions (according to sickness rate)

The figures for the population morbidity of five cities according to sickness rate data at the therapeutic-prophylactic institutions are shown in Table 115.

As seen from the average indexes, 56.8 per 1,000 urban population suffer from diseases of the nervous system (53.8 men and 59.4 women).

Most often the population of the cities studied seeks treatment for lumbosacral radiculitis, neuritis, and sciatica, on the average of 21.9 admissions per 1,000 population of both sexes. The proportion of these diseases among all the nervous system diseases is a little less than half. Men come to the physician for lumbosacral radiculitis (26 admissions per 1,000 men) more often than women (18.5).

241

Table 115
INTENSIVE INDEXES OF THE INCIDENCE OF NERVOUS DISEASES IN THE URBAN
POPULATION (according to sickness rate data)

Name of disease	No. of cases per 1,000 population					
	actual figures			standardized indexes		
	both sexes	men	women	both sexes	men	women
Cerebral arteriosclerosis and other vascular lesions of the brain, with the exception of hypertension with cerebral hemorrhage	5.2	4.0	6.2	5.8	4.4	6.9
Epilepsy	0.9	1.0	0.8	0.9	1.0	0.8
Hereditary, familial and other CNS diseases	2.6	2.8	2.4	2.4	2.6	2.2
Lumbosacral radiculitis, neuritis and sciatica	21.9	26.0	18.5	20.4	25.1	16.6
Other nerve diseases	9.1	8.6	9.6	8.9	8.6	9.4
Neuroses and psychoneuroses	17.2	11.4	21.9	16.0	11.0	20.3
Total	56.8	53.8	59.4	54.4	52.7	56.2

Another common group of diseases are the neuroses, 17.2 per 1,000 population. In this group of diseases the figures for women (21.9 per 1,000 persons) are almost twice as high as for men (11.4).

The figures for morbidity in the various cities are at about the same level. Of considerable interest are the age indexes of morbidity shown in Table 116.

Differences in the age indexes of morbidity are noted in all disease groups. The incidence of lumbosacral radiculitis, neuritis, and sciatica is low in children under 14 (from 0.1 to 0.5 case per 1,000 children). The highest rise in morbidity is seen from 40 to 59 years of age (from 49.4 to 52.6 cases per 1,000 population of this age). In

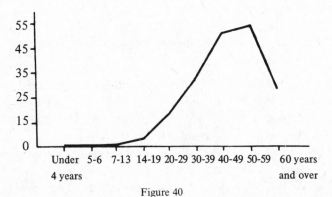

Figure 40
Age indexes of the incidence of lumbosacral radiculitis, neuritis and sciatica (No. of cases per 1,000 population of the corresponding age)

Table 116

AVERAGE AGE INDEXES OF INCIDENCE OF CNS DISEASES IN THE POPULATION OF FIVE CITIES (No. of cases of disease per 1,000 population of different age and sex groups)

Name of disease	under 4 years			5–6 years			7–13 years			14–19 years			20–29 years		
	both sexes	men	women	both sexes	men	women	both sexes	men	women	both sexes	men	women	both sexes	men	women
Cerebral arteriosclerosis and other vascular lesions of the brain, with the exception of hypertension with cerebral hemorrhage	0.1	—	0.1	—	—	—	0.1	—	0.3	0.5	0.5	0.4	0.8	0.4	1.1
Epilepsy	0.2	0.3	0.1	0.8	1.1	0.6	0.6	0.8	0.4	0.8	0.5	1.1	1.0	0.8	1.2
Hereditary, familial and other CNS diseases	0.4	0.8	0.2	1.5	1.8	1.1	1.4	1.6	1.4	1.4	1.5	1.3	2.0	2.9	1.3
Lumbosacral radiculitis, neuritis and sciatica	0.1	0.2	—	0.1	—	0.3	0.5	0.7	0.4	2.7	3.5	1.9	13.8	20.4	8.2
Other nerve diseases	1.0	0.9	1.2	0.9	0.8	1.2	1.1	1.4	0.9	2.9	2.6	3.3	7.5	8.8	6.5
Neuroses	1.5	1.2	1.7	2.2	2.7	1.6	3.2	2.6	3.8	4.4	3.5	5.4	15.0	12.4	17.8

Name of disease	30–39 years			40–49 years			50–59 years			60 years and over			total		
	both sexes	men	women	both sexes	men	women	both sexes	men	women	both sexes	men	women	both sexes	men	women
Cerebral arteriosclerosis and other vascular lesions of the brain, with the exception of hypertension with cerebral hemorrhage	1.2	1.0	1.4	5.1	4.0	6.0	21.6	21.9	21.4	36.6	37.5	36.0	5.2	4.0	6.2
Epilepsy	1.3	1.8	1.0	1.5	1.8	1.8	0.4	0.5	0.3	0.4	1.1	0.2	0.9	1.0	0.8
Hereditary, familial and other CNS diseases	3.5	3.0	3.9	4.1	4.7	3.7	2.9	4.0	2.2	3.3	3.7	3.3	2.6	2.7	2.4
Lumbosacral radiculitis, neuritis and sciatica	29.0	40.1	21.0	49.4	64.2	39.5	52.6	69.5	41.4	25.7	35.6	20.9	21.9	26.0	18.5
Other nerve diseases	12.6	13.2	12.3	18.0	18.1	18.0	18.5	15.2	20.9	12.8	17.6	11.2	9.1	8.6	9.6
Neuroses	31.5	23.0	38.3	36.3	44.4	23.5	13.0	30.3	5.7	4.9	6.0	17.2	11.4	11.4	21.9
Total	79.3	81.9	77.9	114.5	117.1	112.9	119.6	124.1	116.7	84.6	100.2	77.6	56.8	53.8	59.4

those aged 60 and over this figure begins to fall again (Figure 40). Similar patterns, particularly of the age distribution of morbidity rates, are also noted for other nervous system diseases.

An important factor in the work of determining the standards for neurological care is the distribution of all the patients with various diseases according to the specialties of the physicians who must take care of these patients in the polyclinic and in the hospital.

Thus, some patients with diseases of the nervous system are treated not only by the neuropathologists but also by surgeons (for example, injuries to the brain, spinal cord and peripheral nerves) or by internists (for example, nervous system lesions in essential hypertension, rheumatic lesions of the nervous system), etc.

According to the data from Stupino, figures for the admission rate of the population taken care of by neuropathologists for certain diseases were worked out.

The proportion of diagnoses made by the neuropathologists (in % of the number of all admissions for the given nosologic entity) is shown in Table 117.

Table 117
PROPORTION OF ADMISSIONS TO
NEUROPATHOLOGISTS FOR DISEASES OF THE
NERVOUS SYSTEM (in % of total No. of admissions for
these diseases)

Name of disease	% of admissions to neuro- pathologists
Cerebral arteriosclerosis and other vascular lesions of the brain, with the exception of hypertension with cerebral hemorrhage	23.6
Epilepsy	59.1
Hereditary, familial and other CNS diseases	65.1
Lumbosacral radiculitis, neuritis and sciatica	36.3
Other nerve diseases	37.3
In addition: logoneuroses	61.5

Morbidity of the Urban Population According to Data of Complete Medical Examinations

The morbidity data of the population as judged by sickness rate figures, obtained even with neurological care completely available, cannot give an exhaustive idea of the prevalence of the various diseases of the CNS in the population. The morbidity figures as judged by sickness rate approach the "exhaustive morbidity" only in cases of acute diseases and injuries. In the chronic diseases the admissions to neuropathologists are only for cases which are manifested quite well clinically, with appreciable functional disorders of the nervous system. A number of nervous diseases (cerebral arteriosclerosis, neuroses) in the initial stages of the disease do not give manifest subjective sensations, and the patients come to the physician often in the late stages of the disease, when a considerable functional derangement of the nervous system has taken place. One of the principal measures for controlling and preventing these diseases is the early detection of patients, at a time when the pathological process has not yet led to marked disorders and loss of work fitness and when timely treatment permits the prevention of serious sequelae in the majority of cases.

All these data attest to the fact that complete medical examinations are an exceptionally valuable method for detection of patients with many latent nervous diseases in the initial stages. For purposes of planning standards such examinations are particularly important, because they make it possible to obtain material about the "exhaustive morbidity" of the population.

Complete medical checkups of the population permit supplementing the total morbidity data (as judged by sickness rate) with data on the prevalence of chronic diseases for which the population has not sought medical assistance, although it was needed.

Data on the prevalence of chronic cases newly detected in medical examinations are shown in Table 118.

As is evident from Table 118, the number of cases of nervous diseases newly detected during the medical examinations is 90.9 per 1,000 population (90.1 for men and 90.8 for women). The nature of the cases newly detected during the examinations is different from the nature of the morbidity according to sickness rate data. In the medical examinations chiefly chronic cases were detected in the early stages, while the prevalence of the various diseases demonstrated during examinations proves to be higher than is shown by the sickness rate data. The incidence of cerebral arteriosclerosis and other vascular lesions of the brain, according to the examination data, is 9.3 per 1,000 population, whereas it is 5.8 from the sickness rate; 2.6 and 0.9, respectively, for epilepsy; and 8.2 and 8.4 for hereditary, familial, and other CNS diseases, etc.

The prevalence of neuroses is particularly high according to the examination data: 32.9 per 1,000 population as against 16 for the sickness rate. However, it should be pointed out that not all the chronic nervous disease cases demonstrated at examinations require medical care to the same extent.

Hospitalization of the Urban Population for Nervous Diseases

Data of hospitalization of the population in the various cities for nervous diseases are shown in Table 119.

As is evident from Table 119, the number of cases hospitalized for nervous diseases per 1,000 population is 5.8 for persons of both sexes, 7.6 for men and 4.5 for women.

Table 118

CHRONIC CASES NEWLY DETECTED IN MEDICAL EXAMINATIONS IN STUPINO
(per 1,000 population)

Age groups

Name of disease	under 1 year			1–2 years			3–6 years			7–12 years			13–15 years			16–19 years		
	both sexes	men	women	both sexes	men	women	both sexes	men	women	both sexes	men	women	both sexes	men	women	both sexes	men	women
Cerebral arteriosclerosis and other vascular lesions of the brain, with the exception of hypertension with cerebral hemorrhage	—	—	—	—	—	—	—	—	—	—	—	—	—	—	—	—	—	—
Epilepsy	—	—	—	—	—	—	6.3	10.0	2.9	5.4	4.6	6.3	1.6	—	3.5	—	—	—
Hereditary, familial and other CNS diseases	—	—	—	12.2	15.4	8.5	—	—	—	—	—	—	3.2	5.9	—	—	—	—
Lumbosacral radiculitis, neuritis and sciatica	—	—	—	—	—	—	7.8	6.7	8.8	16.4	23.0	9.5	16.0	11.7	21.3	6.2	8.1	4.3
Other nerve diseases	—	—	—	—	—	—	—	—	—	—	—	—	—	—	—	—	—	—
Neuroses	—	—	—	—	—	—	6.1	3.3	3.0	6.2	6.1	6.3	8.0	8.8	7.0	14.6	4.1	25.5
Stammering	—	—	—	—	—	—	9.4	13.4	5.9	28.9	42.9	14.3	19.3	26.4	10.6	24.9	28.5	21.3
Total	—	—	—	12.2	15.4	8.5	29.6	33.4	20.6	56.9	76.6	36.4	48.1	52.8	42.4	45.7	40.7	51.1

Name of disease	20–29 years			30–39 years			40–49 years			50–59 years			60 years and over			total		
	both sexes	men	women	both sexes	men	women	both sexes	men	women	both sexes	men	women	both sexes	men	women	both sexes	men	women
Cerebral arteriosclerosis and other vascular lesions of the brain, with the exception of hypertension with cerebral hemorrhage	2.3	3.7	—	0.5	—	0.8	7.2	7.6	7.0	36.4	47.8	28.2	62.5	80.7	54.8	9.3	9.5	9.0
Epilepsy	—	—	1.3	2.0	4.6	—	1.2	3.0	—	1.8	—	3.1	3.2	—	4.6	2.6	3.6	1.8
Hereditary, familial and other CNS diseases	4.6	7.4	2.6	6.9	10.3	4.3	6.0	3.0	8.0	3.6	6.5	1.6	8.6	26.9	2.3	8.2	10.9	6.0
Lumbosacral radiculitis, neuritis and sciatica	3.8	3.7	3.9	15.7	20.6	12.1	39.2	51.7	30.9	35.6	43.5	29.7	17.7	10.7	20.5	15.1	17.2	13.5
Other nerve diseases	3.1	1.8	3.9	8.4	8.6	8.0	19.9	28.9	14.0	16.4	17.4	15.7	11.2	10.7	11.4	7.8	8.4	7.4
Neuroses	19.9	13.0	24.8	57.7	34.3	75.0	61.5	25.8	84.8	52.8	23.9	73.5	9.6	5.4	11.4	32.9	17.0	45.5
Stammering	19.9	37.0	7.8	15.7	24.0	9.5	8.4	13.7	5.0	8.2	15.2	3.1	4.8	16.1	—	15.0	24.5	7.6
Total	53.6	66.6	44.3	106.7	101.8	110.3	143.4	133.7	149.7	154.8	154.3	154.9	118.6	150.5	105.0	90.9	91.1	90.8

Table 119

AVERAGE INTENSIVE INDEXES OF HOSPITALIZATION OF THE POPULATION OF FIVE CITIES FOR NERVOUS DISEASES (No. of cases hospitalized per 1,000 population)

Name of disease	No. of cases actually hospitalized			Added by the experts			No. of cases actually hospitalized plus those added by experts		
	men	women	both sexes	men	women	both sexes	men	women	both sexes
Cerebral arteriosclerosis and other vascular lesions of the brain with the exception of hypertension with cerebral hemorrhage	0.5	0.36	0.4	0.2	0.1	0.1	0.7	0.42	0.5
Epilepsy	0.3	0.4	0.3	0.1	0.3	0.2	0.4	0.7	0.5
Hereditary, familial and other CNS diseases	1.0	0.6	0.7	—	—	—	1.0	0.6	0.7
Lumbosacral radiculitis, neuritis and sciatica	4.1	1.5	2.7	0.2	—	0.1	4.3	1.5	2.8
Other nerve diseases	0.6	0.6	0.6	—	—	—	0.6	0.6	0.6
Neuroses and psychoneuroses	1.1	1.1	1.1	—	0.4	0.2	1.1	1.5	1.3
Nervous diseases	7.6	4.5	5.8	0.5	0.8	0.6	8.1	5.36	6.4

The most common causes of hospitalization were lumbosacral radiculitis, neuritis, and sciatica (2.6 per 1,000 population). In second place with regard to hospitalization rate were neuroses and psychoneuroses (1.1 per thousand).

For hereditary, congenital, and other CNS diseases 0.7 person per 1,000 population was hospitalized.

Table 120

AVERAGE HOSPITALIZATION RATES OF THE POPULATION OF FIVE CITIES (No. of hospitalized cases per 1,000 population)

Name of disease	Actual average figures		
	men	women	both sexes
Cerebral arteriosclerosis and other vascular lesions of the brain, with the exception of hypertension with cerebral hemorrhage	0.5	0.36	0.4
Epilepsy	0.3	0.4	0.3
Hereditary, familial and other CNS diseases	1.0	0.6	0.7
Lumbosacral radiculitis, neuritis and sciatica	4.1	1.5	2.7
Other nerve diseases	0.6	0.6	0.6
Neuroses and psychoneuroses	1.1	1.1	1.1
Nervous diseases	7.6	4.5	5.8

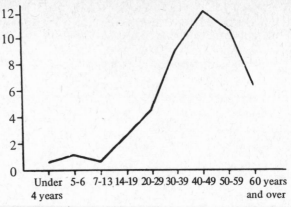

Figure 41

Average age indexes of hospitalization of the population for nervous diseases (No. of cases hospitalized per 1,000 population of the corresponding age)

The hospitalization rate for men (7.6) is higher than for women (4.5). This difference is particularly pronounced for cases of lumbosacral radiculitis, in which the hospitalization rate for men is 4.1 per thousand, for women 1.5.

The average age indexes for hospitalization rate of the population of five cities are shown in Tables 120 and 121, and in Figure 41.

The hospitalization rate of the population of the different age groups shows major variations. The lowest hospitalization rate is seen under the age of 4 and at 7-13 years (0.7 cases per thousand), while comparatively high figures are seen at 40-49 (12.3) and 50-59 years (10.6 cases).

The hospitalization rate for the various age groups varies in accordance with the group of nervous disease. Thus, the highest rate for lumbosacral radiculitis is noted at 40–49 years (6.4 cases per thousand) and at 50–59 years (5.5 cases), i.e., over twice as much as the average for all ages (2.7).

Persons 50-59 years old (1.8) and 60 and over (2.2) are most often hospitalized for arteriosclerosis, i. e., 4-5 times as often as the average for all ages (0.4).

The figures for the hospitalization rate of men and women in the different age groups range within broad limits. The proportion of all those hospitalized for nervous diseases in the total number of admissions for the same diseases is 10.2%. For various age groups of diseases the following percentages were hospitalized:

Cerebral arteriosclerosis and other vascular lesions of the brain, with the exception of hypertension with cerebral hemorrhage	7.7%
Epilepsy	33.3%
Hereditary, familial and other CNS diseases	26.9%
Lumbosacral radiculitis, neuritis and sciatica	12.3%
Other nerve diseases	6.6%
Neuroses	6.4%

Table 121

AVERAGE INTENSIVE AGE INDEXES OF HOSPITALIZATION OF THE POPULATION ACCORDING TO THE DATA OF FIVE CITIES (No. of cases hospitalized per 1,000 population of the corresponding age and sex)

Name of disease	Age groups									total
	under 4 years	5–6 years	7–13 years	14–19 years	20–29 years	30–39 years	40–49 years	50–59 years	60 years and over	
Both sexes										
Nervous diseases	0.7	1.2	0.7	2.6	4.5	9.1	12.3	10.6	6.4	5.8
Arteriosclerosis	—	—	—	—	0.1	0.1	0.5	1.8	2.2	0.4
Epilepsy	0.1	0.4	—	0.3	0.3	0.3	0.8	0.1	—	0.3
Hereditary, familial and other CNS diseases	0.3	0.4	0.3	0.8	0.5	1.3	0.9	0.5	1.3	0.7
Lumbosacral radiculitis, neuritis and sciatica	—	—	—	0.3	1.9	5.1	6.4	5.5	2.0	2.7
Other nerve diseases	—	—	0.2	0.5	0.5	0.6	1.3	1.4	0.7	0.5
Neuroses and psycho- neuroses	0.2	0.4	0.3	0.7	1.2	1.7	2.4	1.3	0.3	1.1
Men										
Nervous diseases	0.8	1.6	0.8	2.7	5.0	14.1	16.6	15.3	11.3	7.6
Arteriosclerosis	—	—	—	—	—	0.1	0.4	2.6	3.9	0.5
Epilepsy	0.2	0.7	—	0.1	0.2	0.5	1.0	—	—	0.3
Hereditary, familial and other CNS diseases	0.6	0.4	0.4	0.9	0.7	1.4	1.1	0.8	2.6	1.0
Lumbosacral radiculitis, neuritis and sciatica	—	—	—	0.2	2.8	9.0	10.3	9.1	3.8	4.1
Other nerve diseases	—	—	0.2	0.5	0.2	0.9	1.8	1.4	0.7	0.6
Neuroses and psycho- neuroses	—	0.5	0.2	1.0	1.1	2.2	1.9	1.3	0.2	1.1
Women										
Nervous diseases	0.6	0.7	0.7	2.4	4.0	5.5	10.3	7.7	3.8	4.5
Arteriosclerosis	—	—	0.02	—	0.16	0.08	0.5	1.4	1.3	0.36
Epilepsy	0.05	0.05	0.02	0.6	0.6	0.3	0.9	0.15	—	0.40
Hereditary, familial and other CNS diseases	—	0.4	0.2	0.8	0.4	1.2	0.7	0.3	0.5	0.6
Lumbosacral radiculitis, neuritis and sciatica	—	—	—	0.3	1.16	2.2	3.7	3.1	1.1	1.5
Other nerve diseases	0.1	—	0.2	0.5	0.8	0.4	1.0	1.4	0.6	0.6
Neuroses and psycho- neuroses	0.5	0.3	0.3	0.4	1.1	1.4	2.8	1.4	0.36	1.1

It should be pointed out that the highest proportion in the total number of cases hospitalized for nervous diseases is from lumbosacral radiculitis.

Attendance at Outpatient-Polyclinic Institutions by the Urban Population for Nervous Diseases

In determining the number of visits for nervous diseases we took into account, in addition to the visits for the class of nervous diseases, the large group of patients who need treatment by specialists in the various fields and at the same time require obligatory (at least once) consultation with the neuropathologists.

The attendance at outpatient-polyclinic institutions for purposes of treatment is determined by the rate and distribution of the total morbidity. The work volume of neuropathologists in prophylactic care of the population depends chiefly on the tenets and directives of the Ministry of Health of the USSR, as well as on work experience of neurological institutions accumulated in regular examination of various population groups (examinations of students, industrial workers, workers in the trade and food industry, etc.). The attendance rate is shown in Table 122.

Table 122

AVERAGE FIGURES FOR ATTENDANCE AT OUTPATIENT POLYCLINIC INSTITUTIONS FOR TREATMENT PURPOSES FOR NERVOUS DISEASES IN FIVE CITIES (No. of visits per 1,000 population)

Visits	To physicians of all specialties				Including those to neuropathologists			
	actually made	added by the experts	total	average number of visits for treatment per case	actually made	added by the experts	total	average number of visits for treatment per case
Nervous diseases (total)	165.1	54.26	220.86	3.9	73.4	33.72	107.12	1.9
These include:								
Cerebral arteriosclerosis and other vascluar lesions, with the exception of hypertension with cerebral hemorrhage	12.5	4.86	17.68	3.4	3.7	2.09	5.79	1.1
Epilepsy	2.3	1.38	3.68	4.1	1.8	0.18	1.98	2.2
Hereditary, familial and other CNS diseases	10.5	1.29	11.79	4.5	6.0	0.49	6.49	2.5
Lumbosacral radiculitis, neuritis and sciatica	84.6	15.64	100.24	4.6	39.8	12.34	52.14	2.4
Other nerve diseases	22.3	11.45	33.75	3.7	9.9	7.66	17.56	1.9
Neuroses and psycho-neuroses	32.9	19.64	54.04	3.1	12.2	10.96	23.16	1.3
In addition, visits for other diseases					29.6	50.1	79.7	—
Total					103.0	83.8	186.82	

As is evident from Table 122, the total number of visits for treatment actually made for nervous diseases is 165.1 per 1,000 population, including 73.4 to neuropathologists.

The great majority of visits for nervous diseases is for lumbosacral radiculitis, neuritis and sciatica, 84.6 per 1,000 population or 50%. In second place with respect to visitation rate is the group of neuroses and psychoneuroses, 32.9 per 1,000 population. The visitation rate for other diseases of the central nervous system is 10.5 per 1,000 inhabitants; 12.5 per 1,000 for cerebral arteriosclerosis; 2.3 for epilepsy, and 22.3 for other nervous diseases.

Above we pointed out that for the purpose of determining the number of visits needed for outpatient treatment of patients an expert analysis was made of each patient on the basis of the initial medical records. The clinical picture of disease in each patient and the treatment measures taken at the current level of our knowledge were used as a basis, and other factors were also taken into account.

The expertise made it possible to determine the number of visits needed for treatment of each patient with a certain nervous disease. After introducing the corrections made by the experts the incidence of nervous diseases in the population rose to 220.86, i. e., by 1.3 times. As is evident from the table, the total number of visits to neuropathologists actually made plus those added by the experts is 107.12.

Of great importance for determining the population's requirement of neurological care is a record of all visits to neuropathologists made not only for nervous diseases but also for other diseases, which for the most part are treated by physicians in other specialties by way of medical consultations. The number of visits to neuropathologists for medical consultations is 79.7. Therefore the total number of visits to neuropathologists for various nervous diseases is 186.82 per 1,000 population.

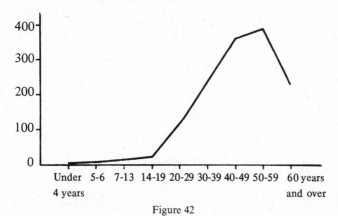

Figure 42

Average age indexes of visitation rate of the population for nervous diseases (No. of visits per 1,000 population of the corresponding age).

The age indexes of the visitation rate for nervous diseases are shown in Figure 42 and Table 123. As is evident from Table 123, the visitation rate figures for nervous diseases in children under 4 are low; they rise with age. However, the visitation rate for various diseases is different in the different age groups. While in the early ages there is a predominance of hereditary and congenital nervous diseases, in the middle age groups lumbosacral radiculitis, neuroses, and other nerve diseases predominate; at the later ages we have also the highest number of visits for arteriosclerosis.

There are certain characteristic features in the visitation rate distribution according to age in men and women. In all age groups the visitation rate for lumbosacral radiculitis is higher in men than in women. The highest number of visits for this condition in men is seen at the ages of 50-59 years, in women at 40-49 years.

It should be noted that in the majority of the other CNS disease groups the visitation rates for men are also higher than for women, with the exception of the neuroses, in which the visitation is almost twice as high for women (42.1) as for men (20.8). In the other nerve diseases the visitation rate among women is also somewhat higher.

Along with the visits for purposes of treatment it is exceedingly important also to take into consideration visits for prophylactic purposes. Among the prophylactic visits we included regular house calls to children under the age of one, dispensary care of children entering school (up to the age of 7), examinations of preschool child-

Table 123

AVERAGE INTENSIVE INDEXES OF THERAPEUTIC OUTPATIENT-POLYCLINC VISITS FOR NERVOUS DISEASES IN FIVE CITIES (No. of visits per 1,000 population of the corresponding sex and age)

Name of disease and distribution of visits according to sex	Total	Age groups								
		under 4 years	5–6 years	7–13 years	14–19 years	20–29 years	30–39 years	40–49 years	50–59 years	60 years and over
Cerebral arteriosclerosis and other vascular lesions of the brain, with the exception of hypertension with cerebral hemorrhage:										
both sexes	12.5	—	—	—	0.6	1.3	3.5	6.8	38.6	96.2
men	12.5	—	—	—	1.2	0.8	2.9	3.7	56.3	114.5
women	12.5	—	—	—	0.2	1.6	4.0	9.0	27.1	83.8
Epilepsy:										
both sexes	2.3	—	2.0	2.0	1.5	2.3	3.7	4.0	0.1	0.5
men	3.1	—	3.6	3.1	—	2.7	5.5	8.2	—	1.7
women	1.6	—	0.4	0.8	3.1	2.1	2.9	1.1	0.2	—
Hereditary, familial and other CNS diseases:										
both sexes	10.5	0.5	2.5	1.5	2.7	12.6	14.3	19.8	12.3	12.8
men	11.4	0.9	2.9	1.9	3.2	15.5	13.0	24.5	17.6	13.6
women	9.9	—	2.0	1.0	2.3	11.2	14.9	16.8	8.6	12.4
Lumbosacral radiculitis, neuritis and sciatica:										
both sexes	84.6	0.2	1.1	1.6	5.9	47.7	110.6	198.1	232.8	76.2
men	109.1	0.3	—	2.5	8.4	73.2	157.4	258.4	345.6	104.8
women	65.6	—	2.2	0.7	3.5	28.6	78.2	159.5	156.5	59.7
Other nerve diseases:										
both sexes	22.3	1.6	1.5	3.0	5.0	18.6	32.8	44.9	40.9	26.0
men	20.9	1.3	1.3	3.5	4.4	22.0	32.7	42.9	31.8	41.6
women	23.6	3.0	1.8	2.5	5.6	16.5	33.2	46.5	46.8	20.0
Neuroses and psycho-neuroses:										
both sexes	32.9	2.6	2.5	4.9	6.5	30.6	58.6	66.8	46.1	9.1
men	20.8	2.3	2.8	4.5	4.1	28.4	40.1	39.5	20.1	2.7
women	42.1	3.0	2.2	3.8	9.1	32.5	72.9	84.5	63.9	12.0

ren, prophylactic examinations of schoolchildren and adolescent workers, examinations of pregnant women and of workers in the public dining room system, children's institutions and municipal enterprises, visits for the purpose of obtaining various kinds of certificates, checkups during the dispensary care of patients, and other prophylactic visits. The data of prophylactic visits are shown in Table 124.

Table 124
FREQUENCY OF PROPHYLACTIC VISITS TO
NEUROPATHOLOGISTS

Type of prophylactic visits	No. of visits per 1,000 population
Regular visits for treatment of children under 1 year of age	0.04
Examinations of preschool children	0.13
Dispensary care of children entering school (7-year-old children)	0.27
Examinations of schoolchildren	0.67
Prophylactic examinations of workers	9.98
Examinations of adolescent workers	0.18
Examinations of pregnant women	0.04
Examinations of workers in public dining rooms, municipal enterprises	0.22
Issuance of various certificates	0.22
Checkups during dispensary care of patients	0.76
Other prophylactic visits	24.90
Total	41.17

As is evident from the table, the number of prophylactic visits to neuropathologists is 41.17 per 1,000 population. The amount of prophylactic work in nervous diseases in Stupino is low. Therefore, in determining the need for neurological care these data should be modified in accordance with the existing instructions, principles and directives of the Ministry of Health of the USSR. Consideration of all the visits (therapeutic and prophylactic) is the basis for working out the standards of neurological care of the population. The expertise permits us to introduce corrections into the number of visits actually made for the various conditions.

Standards of Outpatient-Polyclinic Care of the Urban Population

A comparison of the figures for the sickness rate and the frequency with which chronic cases are detected during complete medical checkups is given in Table 125.

From Table 125 it is evident that during the course of the medical checkups a considerable number of chronic cases was detected, for which the population had not come for medical care. However, the newly detected chronic cases in the entire population examined cannot be mechanically added to the number of cases found from sickness rate, because in the next few years not all of the population will be given examinations. Apparently it is necessary to take into account only the cases found in the population groups that are already being examined regularly by physicians.

In calculating the population's requirement of visits to outpatient-polyclinic institutions for the next few years (1965-1970), we used as a basis the fact that all persons with arteriosclerosis and other vascular lesions of the brain (with the exception of hypertension with cerebral hemorrhage) need therapeutic care to the extent found according to sickness rate (taking into consideration the corrections made by the experts). The number of cases of these diseases is 5.8 per 1,000 population (of these 5.2 were previously known from sickness rate, 0.6 newly found in the population examined) (Table 126). The number of visits, according to sickness rate obtained by physicians of all specialties for these diseases is 17.36 per 1,000 population; the number of additional treatment visits for the newly found cases was 2.0. Therefore the total number of visits to physicians in all specialties needed will be 19.36 per 1,000 population per year, or 3.3 visits for treatment per case.

In epilepsy the number of cases per 1,000 population is 1.2, including 0.9 actual admissions and 0.3 newly detected. The number of visits, according to sickness rate data, is 3.68 per 1,000 population. The number of additional visits on account of newly detected diseases is 1.2.

The total number of indispensable visits due to epilepsy is 4.88 per 1,000 population. The number of visits for treatment per case is 4.1.

Table 125

PREVALENCE OF NERVOUS DISEASES AMONG THE URBAN POPULATION, ACCORDING TO THE SICKNESS RATE DATA AND THE MATERIAL OF COMPLETE MEDICAL CHECKUPS

Name of disease	Per 1,000 population	
	average intensive indexes of population sickness rate of five cities	No. of previously unknown chronic cases detected on medical checkups
Cerebral arteriosclerosis and other vascular lesions of the brain, with the exception of hypertension with cerebral hemorrhage	5.2	7.5
Epilepsy	0.9	0.8
Hereditary, familial and other CNS diseases	2.6	5.4
Lumbosacral radiculitis, neuritis and sciatica	21.8	13.7
Other nerve diseases	9.1	5.7
Neuroses and psychoneuroses	17.2	25.2
Total	56.8	58.3

The rate of hereditary, familial and other CNS diseases is 5.8 per 1,000 population, including 2.6 according to sickness rate data and 3.2 detected on complete medical checkups of the chronic cases. The rate of visits for treatment actually made, according to sickness rate data, is 11.79 per 1,000 population, and 14.4 additional visits for the newly detected cases. The total number of visits for treatment in these conditions is 29.19. There will be an average of 4.5 visits per case.

Lumbosacral radiculitis, neuritis, and sciatica make up the largest group in the nervous diseases. Their incidence is 23.7 per 1,000 population, including 21.8 according to sickness rate data and 1.9 additionally detected during medical examinations.

The number of visits for treatment of lumbosacral radiculitis, neuritis, and sciatica, according to the sickness rate data, is 100.24 per 1,000 population. For the newly detected cases 8.7 visits were added. The total of visits for these conditions was 108.94 per 1,000 population. This is 4.6 visits per case for treatment purposes.

The number of miscellaneous nerve diseases comes to 9.9 per 1,000 population, including 9.1 according to sickness rate and 0.8 added from the medical examinations per 1,000 population.

The number of visits for the miscellaneous nerve diseases was 33.75 per 1,000 population, according to sickness rate data. For the newly detected cases 3 visits were added. The total number of visits for these conditions there is 36.75 per thousand. There are 3.7 visits for treatment per case.

The incidence of neuroses and psychoneuroses is 20.5, including 17.2 according to sickness rate data and 3.3 per 1,000 population added from the medical examinations.

The frequency of visits for treatment of the neuroses and psychoneuroses is 54.04 per 1,000 population according to sickness rate. For newly detected cases 10.2 visits were added. The total number of visits for these conditions will be 64.24 per 1,000 population. This is 3.1 visits per case.

On the basis of the calculations given we can compute the total number of visits for treatment to physicians of all specialties for nervous diseases, which will amount to 260.36 per 1,000 population; this includes 126.92 visits to neuropathologists.

In addition, consideration should be given to visits to neuropathologists for a number of diseases which are treated essentially by physicians in other specialties. The total number of visits for treatment to neuropathologists for these conditions is 79.7 per 1,000 population, according to the data of five cities.

Now we may proceed with a determination of the work volume in the dispensary care of patients and in prophylactic examinations of the urban population by neuropathologists. At present we are not posing the problem of complete coverage of all patients by dispensary observation.

At present patients with chronic diseases of the peripheral nervous system, lumbosacral radiculitis, and sequelae of cerebral circulatory disorders, are subject to dispensary care by neuropathologists.

In calculations of the need for dispensary visits by patients with lumbosacral radiculitis we used as a basis the data of a number of authors in the literature. In the opinion of the majority (E. E. Golofastova, S. Ya. Freidlin, P. M. Al'perovich), patients with lumbosacral radiculitis need dispensary visits once every two months; they require physiotherapy and drug treatment.

In stubborn, chronic cases some of the patients (about 25%) need hospital treatment. The number with chronic lumbosacral radiculitis who need dispensary care, according to our figures, is 13.8 per 1,000 population. In addition, the newly detected diseases, for which the patients did not go to the physician, amounted to 1.9. Essentially these are the initial and mild forms of disease. In these cases the patients did not need dispensary care, as a rule.

For the purpose of getting a stable remission in chronic lumbosacral radiculitis about six visits are needed.

Therefore, the total number of visits for treatment for the given condition will be 82.8 per 1,000 population.

The number of visits needed for the dispensary care of patients with cerebral circulatory disorders (1.2 cases per 1,000 population) will be 7.2 per 1,000 population, given the present actual number of six.

In these calculations we used as a basis the need for giving dehydration and symptomatic treatment as well as active physiotherapeutic exercises throughout the year, for which observation by neuropathologists is needed.

The total number of visits by way of dispensary care of patients is, therefore, 93.6 per 1,000 population.

In determining the population requirement of prophylactic visits we used the directives of the Ministry of Health of the USSR, as well as instructions on methods and instructions for the care of the various healthy population groups doing the same kind of work or under the same physiological conditions.

According to Directive No. 136-m of the Ministry of Health of the USSR dated September 7, 1957, concerning prophylactic checkups of workers in the various branches of industry, and other directives, neuropathologists should examine 49.7 of each 1,000 workers.

On mass examinations of schoolchildren and adolescent workers, according to the existing directives of the Ministry of Health of the USSR, neuropathologists should examine 69 persons per 1,000 population and, in addition, 19.7 per 1,000 population in the group of those entering school (preschool children).

According to Directive No. 707 of the Ministry of Health of the USSR dated August 24, 1950, persons admitted to occupational and technical schools should be examined; 6.8 examinations per 1,000 population are needed.

The total number of prophylactic examinations of the population by neuropathologists, taking into account the calculations given, will be 145.2 per 1,000 population.

Therefore complete outpatient-polyclinic care of the urban population by neuro-

Table 126
STANDARDS OF OUTPATIENT-POLYCLINIC CARE FOR 1966–1970 (per 1,000 population)

Name of disease	Morbidity as judged from sickness rate	No. of visits for treatment		No. of cases newly detected among the population groups subject to examinations	No. of additional visits for treatment		Total cases (as judged from sickness rate plus those newly detected on medical examinations)	Total number of visits for treatment		No. of visits for treatment during dispensary care	Prophylactic medical examinations of healthy persons					No. of outpatient visits	
		total	including those to neuro-pathologists		total	including those to neuro-pathologists		total	including those to neuro-pathologists		total	examinations of adolescents	examinations of preschool children	examinations of workers	other examinations	total	to neuro-pathologists
Cerebral arteriosclerosis and other vascular lesions of the brain, with the exception of hypertension with cerebral hemorrhage	5.2	17.36	5.79	0.6	2.0	0.7	5.8	19.36	6.49	7.2	—	—	—	—	—	—	—
Epilepsy	0.9	3.68	1.98	0.3	1.2	0.7	1.2	4.88	2.68	—	—	—	—	—	—	—	—
Hereditary, familial and other CNS diseases	2.6	11.79	6.49	3.2	14.4	8.0	5.8	26.19	14.49	—	—	—	—	—	—	—	—
Lumbosacral radiculitis, neuritis and sciatica	21.8	100.24	52.14	1.9	8.7	4.6	23.7	108.94	56.74	82.8	—	—	—	—	—	—	—
Other nerve diseases	9.1	33.75	17.56	0.8	3.0	1.5	9.9	36.75	19.06	3.6	—	—	—	—	—	—	—
Neuroses and psycho-neuroses	17.2	54.04	23.16	3.3	10.2	4.3	20.5	64.24	27.46	—	—	—	—	—	—	—	—
Total	56.8	220.86	107.12	10.1	39.5	19.8	66.9	260.36	126.92	93.6	—	—	—	—	—	—	—
In addition, visits to the neuropathologist for consultations	—		79.7	—	—	—	—		79.7	—							
Total	56.8	220.86	186.82	10.1	39.5	19.8	66.9	260.36	206.62	93.6	145.2	69.0	19.7	49.7	6.8	499.16	445.42

pathologists can be provided with 445.42 visits per year per 1,000 population, including 206.62 treatment visits, 145.2 prophylactic and 93.6 dispensary visits. Most of the numerical data presented has been given in Table 126.

Standards of Hospital Care in Neuropathology

The data for the total morbidity as judged by sickness rate of the population are basic also for determining the standards of the population's requirement of hospital care (Table 127). The complete medical examinations made it possible to detect an additional number of persons needing hospital care from the group of those with previously unknown chronic diseases. The number of cases hospitalized in the neurological department was 5.8 per 1,000 population in the group admitted.

Table 127

STANDARDS OF HOSPITAL CARE OF THE URBAN POPULATION IN THE FIELD OF NEUROPATHOLOGY

Name of disease	Per 1,000 population					
	No. of cases (according to sickness rate and medical examination data)	No. of cases hospitalized		No. of cases hospitalized among the newly detected cases	total	average length of treatment
		actual	added by experts			
Cerebral arteriosclerosis and other vascular lesions of the brain, with the exception of hypertension with cerebral hemorrhage	5.8	0.4	0.1	—	0.5	21.0
Epilepsy	1.2	0.3	0.2	—	0.5	9.8
Hereditary, familial and other CNS diseases	5.8	0.7	—	0.36	1.06	19.4
Lumbosacral radiculitis, neuritis and sciatica	23.7	2.7	0.1	0.04	2.84	13.9
Other nerve diseases	9.9	0.6	—	0.04	0.64	17.4
Neuroses and psychoneuroses	20.5	1.1	0.2	0.04	1.34	13.9
Total	66.9	5.8	0.6	0.48	6.88	

In the group of newly detected cases hospitalization is needed in 0.48 case per 1,000 population.

Therefore, the total number hospitalized in the neurological department is 6.88 per 1,000 population, with consideration of all the corrections and additions.

The average length of treatment in the neurological departments is 20 days. We consider it possible to accept these figures for calculations for the next few years (1966–1970).

Standards of Therapeutic-Prophylactic Care of the Urban Population in the Field of Psychiatry

The method of obtaining data on the prevalence of neuropsychiatric conditions among the urban population was substantially different from that used by physicians in all other specialties.

This difference is brought about by the fact that some mental patients (especially with schizophrenia) sometimes avoid encounters with the psychiatrist. Other patients, for example, those who have had a psychotic break in the past, those with epilepsy with few seizures, and those with chronic alcoholism, are embarrassed by their conditions and attempt to conceal them on examination. A certain number of the patients are not treated at the polyclinic for their area but rather seek aid at the nearest inter-district or regional neuropsychiatric dispensary; therefore there may be no polyclinic information on them.

The majority of the most seriously ill patients may be in mental hospitals, nursing homes for patients with chronic mental diseases or boarding houses for mentally retarded children for a long time when the dispensary records are made and, therefore, are not among the patients detected.

In addition, the characteristics of psychiatric diagnosis, the importance of obtaining such information as the year of onset of the disease, the nature of its course, the stage, degree of clinical and social compensation, and so forth, with respect to mental patients, make it necessary to fill out a comparatively detailed medical record card on each patient detected.

The work of psychiatrists in dispensary care of the population of the experimental districts of Stupino was to a considerable degree facilitated by the presence of a dynamic statistical record of patients with neuropsychiatric diseases kept in the Central [Moscow] Region Card-File, in which there were cards on all patients on

259

record in the district and city neuropsychiatric dispensaries, the neuropsychiatric clinics of the district polyclinics, and those in mental hospitals, nursing homes for mental patients with chronic courses of their disease, and boarding houses for mentally retarded children.

Therefore, before the investigation of the Stupino population began, there was already complete information about patients with neuropsychiatric diseases, living in the corresponding districts, at the disposal of the psychiatrists.

A special examination by psychiatrists was made of the population of 22,049 persons in the experimental districts of Stupino.

This examination was made by concurrent house-to-house surveys in which medical record cards were filled out on all patients with detected neuropsychiatric diseases. Then these patients underwent consultation.

For the purpose of assuring complete coverage of the entire population, a record card indicating the surname, first name, and patronymic, year of birth, and address was first made out for each inhabitant of the experimental districts. These cards were grouped according to apartments, houses, and streets. The cards on patients with neuropsychiatric conditions who lived in the experimental districts of Stupino, which had been obtained from the Central [Moscow] Region Card-File, were distributed similarly according to groups.

Seven physicians and seven assistants made the psychiatric examinations of the population of the experimental districts for three months (from December 6, 1962, through March 12, 1963).

Patients living in the experimental districts who were in psychiatric hospitals during the time of the examination were studied by groups of physicians in these hospitals.

In addition, abstracts from the hospital case histories were made for all patients with detected schizophrenia and epilepsy who had previously been treated in mental hospitals, as well as for the majority of other patients previously hospitalized for neuropsychiatric diseases.

In the first half of 1964 a group of psychiatrists made up of the same members reexamined (by means of house-to-house surveys) the population of one of the four experimental districts, as well as all the patients with neuropsychiatric diseases in whom there was any doubt about the diagnosis.

Prevalence of Neuropsychiatric Diseases in the Urban Population

In the study of 22,049 inhabitants of Stupino, 740 patients with neuropsychiatric conditions were detected. Of this group 657 were to be treated by psychiatrists and 83 by neuropathologists. Some of them with the so-called borderline states as well as all those with chronic alcoholism, were referred to psychiatrists.

The prevalence of the various conditions in the Stupino population of different sexes is shown in Table 128.

In Table 129, for purposes of comparison, the intensive indexes of the prevalence of neuropsychiatric diseases for Stupino are given according to the data of examination as well as the figures obtained on the basis of dispensary records of patients with neuropsychiatric diseases in the cities of Elektrostal', Ramenskoe, Noginsk, and Kolomna.

As is evident from Table 129, the prevalence of the mental diseases proper for the various cities shows only slight variations. Differences are seen in the figures for the borderline state and chronic alcoholism, as well as traumatic and organic diseases of the brain. The differences among the figures for the five cities are explained not only by the fact that data of examination of the population were used in Stupino and material from dispensary records were utilized in the other cities, but also by the fact that in these cities patients with borderline states, chronic alcoholism, traumatic and organic diseases of the brain, with no manifest psychotic symptoms or gross intellectual disorders, were recorded variously.

Turning now to the data of examination of the population in Stupino, it should be pointed out that, aside from the 740 patients detected, 298 patients were examined who had been kept on the records of the neuropsychiatric clinic with diagnoses of borderline states (neurasthenia, astheno-depressive syndrome, astheno-hypochon-

Table 128

PREVALENCE OF VARIOUS NEUROPSYCHIATRIC CONDITIONS IN THE STUPINO POPULATION EXAMINED (per 1,000 persons of the corresponding sex)

Neuropsychiatric disease	both sexes	men	women	Needing treatment by psychiatrists			Needing treatment by neuropathologists		
				men	women	both sexes	men	women	both sexes
Schizophrenia	4.0	3.7	4.3	3.7	4.3	4.0	—	—	—
Epilepsy	3.1	4.2	2.1	3.5	1.8	2.6	0.7	0.3	0.5
Manic-depressive psychosis	0.045	—	0.085	—	0.085	0.045	—	—	—
Cerebral arteriosclerosis and other vascular lesions of the brain	2.1	1.2	2.8	0.9	2.5	1.8	0.3	0.3	0.3
Presenile psychoses	0.3	0.1	0.5	0.1	0.5	0.3	—	—	—
Senile psychoses	0.3	—	0.5	—	0.5	0.3	—	—	—
Cerebral syphilis	0.045	0.098	—	0.098	—	0.045	—	—	—
Chronic alcoholism	4.9	9.9	0.5	9.9	0.5	4.9	—	—	—
Mental disorders from cerebral trauma	6.3	8.9	4.1	7.9	3.7	5.7	1.0	0.4	0.6
Organic lesions of the CNS	3.4	3.6	3.2	3.3	2.9	3.1	0.3	0.3	0.3
Oligophrenia	1.2	2.0	0.6	2.0	0.6	1.2	—	—	—
Pathological development of the personality (psychopathy)	1.5	1.6	1.5	1.6	1.5	1.5	—	—	—
Neuroses and reactive states	6.2	3.1	8.9	2.1	6.1	4.3	1.0	2.8	1.9
Total	33.4	33.3	29.2	35.0	25.1	29.7	3.3	4.1	3.6

driacal syndrome, neuroses, and others). All these patients have some somatic disease (essential hypertension, hypotension, endocrine disorders, peptic ulcer, etc.). The neurotic symptomatology detected in them is secondary, included in the symptom-complex of the main somatic condition. This group of patients should be kept under the observation of internists, endocrinologists, and other specialists. These patients need psychiatric consultations only from time to time (no more than once or twice a year) and should not be put on the records of psychiatric institutions.

Thus in Stupino 29.5 cases needing psychiatric help to a greater or lesser degree were found per 1,000 population (see Table 130).

If we exclude those with so-called borderline states (neuroses, reactive states and psychopathy) and those with chronic alcoholism from the total number of patients detected, the intensive index will drop to 19 per 1,000 population. If, in addition to those with borderline states and those with chronic alcoholism, we exclude also the patients with cerebral arteriosclerosis, traumatic and organic cerebral diseases (without psychotic symptoms or gross intellectual impairment), the intensive index will be 12.6 per 1,000 inhabitants. Finally, if we exclude from this group the patients with epilepsy who have no psychotic symptoms or gross intellectual impairment, leaving in it only those with psychoses and other manifest mental disorders (including oligophrenia), the intensive index for the incidence of mental diseases proper will be 11.2 per 1,000 population.

Study of the neuropsychiatric morbidity in Stupino was made on the basis of data on 657 patients needing psychiatric help. Patients with oligophrenia, for which various persons do not need medical care by virtue of social compensation, were included in this group.

Data characterizing only the prevalence of neuropsychiatric diseases are inadequate to determine the population's requirement of psychiatric care.

It is also necessary to have data on the nature of the course of the disease, the frequency of remissions in the patients outside the hospitals, the degree of expression of the defect, i.e., the degree of social and clinical compensation, and the loss of work fitness associated with it.

In the data which we obtained through examination of the population of Stupino all the types listed are present. We are presenting them textually for the most common nosologic entities.

The prevalence of schizophrenia, its duration, severity and complexity of treatment, the need for regular active observation of the patients, and their comparatively great need of hospitalization largely determine the amount of hospital and outpatient neuropsychiatric care of the population.

The information about the prevalence of schizophrenia, that is, about the number of patients with schizophrenia per 1,000 population according to the data in the literature, are contradictory. It is customarily considered that two patients with schizophrenia are found per 1,000 population. This figure is reduced by various

Table 129

PREVALENCE OF NEUROPSYCHIATRIC CASES AMONG THE POPULATION OF
DIFFERENT CITIES (No. of patients per 1,000 population)

Neuropsychiatric disease	City				
	Stupino	Elektrostal'	Ramenskoe	Noginsk	Kolomna
Schizophrenia	4.0	5.3	5.0	4.2	3.9
Epilepsy	3.1	2.1	2.1	3.2	2.4
Manic-depressive psychosis	0.045	0.05	0.08	0.05	0.04
Cerebral arteriosclerosis and other vascular lesions of the brain	2.1	1.5	0.7	2.6	2.3
Presenile psychoses	0.3	0.6	0.6	1.1	0.3
Senile psychoses	0.3	0.2	0.2	0.4	0.3
Cerebral syphilis	0.045	0.16	0.06	0.08	0.2
General paresis	—	—	0.04	0.05	0.01
Psychoses from intoxications	—	0.04	0.12	0.2	—
Psychoses from infectious and virus diseases	—	0.1	0.6	1.8	0.3
Alcoholic psychosis and chronic alcoholism	4.9	7.1	8.1	8.4	8.6
Mental disorders from diseases of the internal organs, vitamin deficiency, metabolic and endocrine disorders	—	0.6	0.02	0.4	0.6
Mental disorders from cerebral trauma	6.3	3.2	1.3	4.4	3.3
Organic lesions of the CNS	3.4	3.0	1.3	4.9	2.8
Oligophrenia	1.2	4.1	3.6	4.7	2.4
Pathological development of the personality (psychopathy)	1.5	2.8	0.7	1.4	0.6
Neuroses and reactive states	6.2	3.3	3.4	9.7	5.7
Other neuropsychiatric and undiagnosed cases	—	0.02	—	0.02	—
Total	33.4	34.1	27.9	47.6	33.8

authors to 0.5 (A. L. Leshchinskii) or 1.34 (G. V. Zenevich), or increased to 2.9
(M. Ya. Koltunova, M. I. Rybal'skii), 5.14 (G. V. Zenevich), or 6 (V. V. Borinevich).

According to data in the foreign press, as A. V. Snezhnevskii reports it, the number
of patients with schizophrenia per 1,000 inhabitants is 3 per thousand in Denmark,
5 in England, 8 in the Federal Republic of Germany. On examination of inhabitants
of the experimental districts of Stupino, an average of 4 patients per 1,000 population
was found.

The reliability of the diagnosis of schizophrenia in all the patients detected in
Stupino is confirmed not only by the carefulness of the examination, but also by the
fact that in the majority of cases (89.9%) the diagnosis of schizophrenia was made
in the hospital.

Table 130

PREVALENCE OF NEUROPSYCHIATRIC DISEASES NEEDING TREATMENT BY PSYCHIATRISTS AMONG THE POPULATION OF BOTH SEXES AND DIFFERENT AGE (No. of patients per 1,000 population of the corresponding age and sex)

Disease	Sex	Age groups											Total
		under 1 year	1–2 years	3–6 years	7–12 years	13–15 years	16–19 years	20–29 years	30–39 years	40–49 years	50–59 years	60 years and over	
Schizophrenia	Male	—	—	—	—	—	4.9	6.0	6.9	6.8	3.1	—	3.7
	Female	—	—	—	—	—	2.5	6.7	4.3	8.7	8.2	1.0	4.3
Epilepsy	Male	—	—	2.9	5.9	5.0	2.4	2.0	1.4	9.1	—	4.2	3.5
	Female	—	—	1.4	2.9	1.6	2.5	1.0	2.6	1.2	3.0	—	1.8
Manic-depressive psychosis	Male	—	—	—	—	—	—	—	—	—	—	—	—
	Female	—	—	—	—	—	—	—	0.4	—	—	—	0.09
Cerebral arteriosclerosis and other vascular lesions of the brain	Male	—	—	—	—	—	—	—	—	1.5	5.1	4.2	0.9
	Female	—	—	—	—	—	—	—	—	4.0	10.4	9.0	2.5
Presenile psychoses	Male	—	—	—	—	—	—	—	—	—	1.0	1.0	0.1
	Female	—	—	—	—	—	—	—	—	3.0	0.7	—	0.5
Senile psychoses	Male	—	—	—	—	—	—	—	—	—	—	6.0	0.5
	Female	—	—	—	—	—	—	—	—	—	—	6.0	0.1
Cerebral syphilis	Male	—	—	—	—	—	—	—	0.5	—	—	—	—
	Female	—	—	—	—	—	—	—	—	—	—	—	—
Chronic alcoholism	Male	—	—	—	—	—	—	4.7	24.0	22.6	9.2	6.3	9.9
	Female	—	—	—	—	—	—	—	0.9	0.6	1.5	1.0	0.5
Mental disorders	Male	—	—	—	4.6	3.8	—	2.7	9.7	19.6	16.3	8.4	7.9
	Female	—	—	1.4	0.7	1.6	2.5	1.0	4.7	9.3	7.4	1.0	3.7
Organic lesions of the CNS	Male	—	3.2	2.9	7.2	7.6	4.9	4.0	—	2.3	2.0	—	3.2
	Female	—	—	1.4	3.6	8.1	4.9	2.6	3.0	2.3	2.2	2.0	2.9
Oligophrenia	Male	—	3.2	1.4	5.9	1.3	4.9	2.7	0.5	0.8	—	—	2.0
	Female	—	—	—	1.5	3.3	4.9	—	—	—	—	0.7	0.6
Pathological development of the personality (psychopathy)	Male	—	—	1.4	3.9	2.5	—	0.6	1.8	0.8	1.0	—	1.6
	Female	—	—	—	0.7	—	—	1.0	3.0	2.9	2.2	—	1.5
Neuroses and reactive states	Male	—	—	2.9	4.6	2.5	—	—	1.8	5.3	—	—	2.1
	Female	—	—	—	2.2	—	2.5	0.5	9.4	18.5	9.6	—	6.1
Total													29.5

Of the total number of patients with schizophrenia undergoing hospital examination, 65.2% had been in mental hospitals two or more times during their life. Information on the number of admissions to mental hospitals by patients with schizophrenia in Stupino is given in Table 131.

Table 131
DISTRIBUTION OF PATIENTS WITH SCHIZOPHRENIA
ACCORDING TO NUMBERS OF ADMISSIONS TO
MENTAL HOSPITALS (in percent of the total)

No. of admissions for hospital treatment	Men	Women	Both sexes
Not admitted to mental hospitals	7.9	11.6	10.1
Admitted to mental hospitals	92.1	88.4	89.9
This includes:			
once	28.9	21.7	24.7
twice	23.8	19.6	21.4
3 times	10.5	15.7	13.5
4 times	10.5	7.8	8.9
5 times	5.3	5.9	5.6
6 times	2.6	5.9	4.5
7 times	5.3	2.0	3.4
8 times	—	2.0	1.1
9 times	2.6	3.9	3.4
10 times or more	2.6	3.9	3.4
Total	100	100	100

The total number of patients with schizophrenia in Stupino includes not only those who had been hospitalized previously, but also those who had first been detected on examination of the population by psychiatrists. Over half of the patients with schizophrenia who had never been in the hospital were those with a slow-moving course of the neurotic or psychopathic-type symptoms, as well as those with relatively compensated defects after having had a single attack in the past.

The absence of a government neuropsychiatric service outside hospitals and of dispensary care and records of patients in the capitalist countries forces psychiatrists there to determine the numbers of patients with schizophrenia mainly from hospital data. Therefore, the intensive indexes for prevalence and morbidity derived by investigators outside the USSR require corrections which would take into account patients who have not been hospitalized for mental disease.

The reduction in the severity of the course of schizophrenia may to some degree be judged on the basis of data on the loss of work fitness (Table 132).

As shown by Table 132, of the total number of those with schizophrenia 71.9% are incapable of working (including first- and second-category invalids and unemployed), while 11.2% show an impaired work fitness (third-group invalids), i.e.,

Table 132
DISTRIBUTION OF PATIENTS WITH SCHIZOPHRENIA
ACCORDING TO DEGREE OF LOSS OF WORK FITNESS
(in percent of the total)

Work fitness	Men	Women	Total
First category invalidism	7.9	5.9	6.7
Second category invalidism	50	56.8	53.9
Third category invalidism	15.8	7.8	11.2
No invalidism—not working	5.3	15.8	11.3
No invalidism—working	21.0	15.7	16.9
Total	100	100	100

Table 133
INCIDENCE OF CASES OF SCHIZOPHRENIA AMONG THE POPULATION OF
DIFFERENT AGE AND BOTH SEXES (No. of patients per 1,000 population of the
corresponding age and sex)

	Age groups						Total
	16–19 years	20–29 years	30–39 years	40–49 years	50–59 years	60 years and over	
Men	4.9	6.0	6.9	6.8	3.1	—	3.7
Women	2.5	6.7	4.3	8.7	8.2	1.0	4.3
Both sexes	3.7	6.4	5.5	7.9	6.0	0.7	4.0

an overt schizophrenic defect with clinical and social decompensation or partial compensation is noted in 83.1% of the patients; 16.9% of schizophrenics are not considered invalids and they work.

These data to a certain degree characterize the amount of psychiatric care which schizophrenic patients need and, therefore, should be used for determining the standards of psychiatric care (Table 133).

Among patients with schizophrenia there is a predominance of younger and middle-aged persons.

Data on the distribution of schizophrenic patients, according to the year of onset of the condition, are very interesting (Table 134).

The average figure for the annual incidence of schizophrenia is 0.25 per 1,000 population. However, considering the inadequately complete data for 1962 and the earlier years (before 1956), the average annual incidence is best determined for the period from 1957 through 1961; for this period it proves to be equal to 0.28 per 1,000 population.

Table 134
ANNUAL INCIDENCE OF
SCHIZOPHRENIA AMONG MEN
AND WOMEN IN STUPINO FROM
1953 THROUGH 1962 (No. of new
cases in the given year per 1,000
population of the corresponding sex)

Year	Men	Women	Both sexes
1962	0.19	0.17	0.18
1961	0.19	0.34	0.27
1960	0.19	0.34	0.27
1959	0.29	0.34	0.31
1958	0.29	0.34	0.31
1957	0.29	0.25	0.27
1956	0.48	0.08	0.27
1955	0.19	0.25	0.22
1954	0.29	0.08	0.18
1953	0.10	0.25	0.18
Average for the year	0.25	0.24	0.25

In connection with the fact that the incidence of schizophrenia in children under 14 is comparatively low, according to data in the literature, and since in Stupino there are no children under 16 who have schizophrenia, we deemed it practical to calculate the intensive indexes of the annual incidence of the adult population only (Table 135).

Therefore, the average annual incidence of schizophrenia in the population over 15 years in 1953–1962 was equal to 0.33 per 1,000 adults.

Epilepsy and other diseases in which the epileptiform syndrome is predominant were combined in the same group, with the epileptiform symptom complex in its clinical picture. Such a grouping, although arbitrary and disputable, is still expedient for practical purposes, because it facilitates the calculation of the need for psychiatric care by a large group of patients whose treatment and hospital maintenance is complicated by their epileptiform seizures.

A clinical-statistical study of the data on the prevalence of epilepsy was made by many psychiatrists, but to date there is no agreement (on record) on the number of patients with epilepsy living among the population or admitted to mental hospitals and already in them. This is connected with the fact that patients with epilepsy are treated and maintained on the records of physicians in different specialties (neuro-pathologists, psychiatrists, internists, or pediatricians), in accordance with the form and nature of the course of the disease; not uncommonly they are not put on record at all, are not treated, and are hospitalized comparatively rarely. Therefore the inten-

Table 135
ANNUAL INCIDENCE OF
SCHIZOPHRENIA IN MEN AND
WOMEN OVER 15 FROM 1953
THROUGH 1962 (No. of new cases
per 1,000 population of the
corresponding sex and age)

Year	Men	Women	Both sexes
1962	0.27	0.27	0.24
1961	0.27	0.44	0.36
1960	0.27	0.44	0.36
1959	0.41	0.44	0.42
1958	0.41	0.44	0.42
1957	0.41	0.33	0.36
1956	0.69	0.11	0.36
1955	0.27	0.33	0.30
1954	0.41	0.11	0.24
1953	0.13	0.38	0.24

sive indexes of the incidence of epilepsy, according to the data of the various authors, vary within limits of 1.5 and 2.5 per 1,000 population.

Epilepsy and organic diseases of the brain with an epileptiform syndrome predominate in the young population. For epilepsy the highest figures were found in the population of both sexes and age groups from 7 to 12 (3.5 per thousand), and 13–15 (3.6 per thousand); in the group of patients with organic cerebral diseases with epileptiform syndrome the figures were 1.4 per thousand in the age group 13–15, 1.2 per thousand from 16 to 19, and 1.5 per thousand from 20 to 29.

In traumatic epilepsy the highest figures were noted between 40 and 49 years, particularly in men.

Usually persons in the older age groups (50–59, 60 and over) had traumatic disease of the brain with epileptiform syndrome.

In conclusion, the very important question must be dealt with of the relationship of patients with overt psychotic symptoms or gross intellectual impairment and those without psychotic symptoms or gross intellectual impairment.

These relationships should be kept in mind in determining the requirement for various types of psychiatric care.

According to our data, over half of all patients included in the groups with epilepsy and other epileptiform conditions were made up of those with psychotic symptoms or gross intellectual impairment (2.2 per thousand out of the total of 4.3 per thousand).

Therefore 28% of all patients with detected neuropsychiatric diseases are those with schizophrenia, epilepsy, or organic and traumatic diseases of the brain with an epileptiform syndrome. The other forms of neuropsychiatric disease, including the borderline states (19.5 %), occur in much lower proportion in the total number of patients found.

All forms of oligophrenia (including Down's disease), as well as cases of retarded mental development from organic brain diseases in infancy, have been included in the group of diseases characterized by congenital or infancy-acquired mental retardation. Grouping these two conditions together is explained by the following factors: first of all, in a number of cases it is difficult in practice to differentiate congenital mental deficiency from mental retardation caused by cerebral diseases in infancy; secondly, many authors, speaking about the prevalence of oligophrenia, do not distinguish the congenital from the infancy-acquired mental retardation. According to various authors, the number of cases of oligophrenia per 1,000 inhabitants ranges from 1 to 2.7.

In the study of the population of Stupino, 1.2 patients with congenital mental deficiency (oligophrenia) were found per 1,000 population. If we also consider the patients with mental retardation from organic cerebral diseases in infancy, this figure rises to 2.2 per 1,000 persons. Among those with oligophrenia, children with mongolism (Down's disease) constitute 0.09 per 1,000 of the whole population.

It should be noted that in the group under analysis we did not include those with mental retardation from organic cerebral diseases and epileptiform syndrome suffered in infancy, because they have been included in the large group of patients in whom the disease has an epileptiform syndrome.

The great majority of those with oligophrenia are mental defectives.

In combining patients with oligophrenia and patients with organic cerebral diseases and mental retardation in the same group, we should note that the need for medical care by these patients shows substantial differences: patients with mental retardation from organic diseases of the brain suffered in infancy need both treatment and pedagogical and social correction in most instances; whereas those with oligophrenia need chiefly pedagogical and social correction. Some of them are in a state of adequate social compensation and do not need any help at all.

Completely to overlook patients who have oligophrenia with only mild defectiveness would not be perfectly correct, because while clinical and particularly social compensation occurs with age, still this is a compensation which may be dynamic. Therefore, in calculations of the standards for requirement of neuropsychiatric care, patients with oligophrenia with mild defectiveness and adequate clinical and social compensation should be put into the category of those who need regular consultations with the psychiatrist for the rest of their lives.

The group of traumatic and organic (with different etiologies) cerebral diseases (with the exception of cases with an epileptiform syndrome and mental retardation from early childhood) was arbitrarily divided into two sub-groups, patients with overt psychotic manifestations or gross intellectual impairment and patients without permanent overt psychotic symptomatology or gross intellectual impairment but who need treatment by psychiatrists rather than neuropathologists.

In the group being analyzed we did not include patients with traumatic and organic cerebral diseases who need treatment by neuropathologists (Table 136).

Table 136
PREVALENCE OF TRAUMATIC AND ORGANIC DISEASES OF THE
BRAIN IN THE POPULATION OF BOTH SEXES (No. of cases per 1,000
population of the corresponding sex)

Nosologic group	Total	With pronounced psychotic symptoms or gross intellectual impairment	Without pronounced psychotic symptoms or gross intellectual impairment
Traumatic cerebral diseases			
men	6.2	1.8	4.4
women	3.2	0.7	2.5
both sexes	.6	1.2	3.4
Organic cerebral diseases			
men	1.4	0.4	1.0
women	1.4	0.5	0.9
both sexes	1.4	0.5	0.9

As seen from Table 136, among those suffering from traumatic cerebral diseases the minority have pronounced psychotic problems or gross intellectual impairment.

In calculating standards of psychoneurological care, which is lacking for patients suffering from traumatic and organic cerebral diseases, data on their invalidity are very important, since the occurrence of these diseases is to a considerable extent a consequence of the war, epidemics of viral influenza, etc.

The group of patients with neuropsychiatric disease at an older age included patients who had cerebral arteriosclerosis with overt psychotic symptoms or gross intellectual impairment and those with cerebral arteriosclerosis without overt psychotic symptoms or gross intellectual impairment who still need treatment by psychiatrists (Table 137).

In the group of those with mental disease in the older age group, the marked predominance of women is noteworthy; this coincides with data in the literature.

In the group over 60, cases of cerebral arteriosclerosis with overt psychotic symptoms or gross intellectual impairment (4 per 1,000 population) constitute over half of the cases of cerebral arteriosclerosis (7.4 per 1,000 population).

Of the whole group of patients in the older age group with neuropsychiatric conditions chiefly those with presenile and senile psychoses, and psychoses of a cerebral arteriosclerotic nature, need hospital and outpatient neuropsychiatric care. At the same time, all these conditions and especially cerebral arteriosclerosis require considerable prophylactic work of a psychiatric nature, which should be

Table 137

PREVALENCE OF NEUROPSYCHIATRIC DISEASES OF THE OLDER AGE GROUP AMONG THE POPULATION OF BOTH SEXES AND DIFFERENT AGES (per 1,000 population of the corresponding sex and age)

Disease	Whole population	Age groups		
		40–49 years	50–59 years	60 years and over
Cerebral arteriosclerosis				
men	0.9	1.5	5.1	4.2
women	2.5	4.0	10.4	9.0
both sexes	1.8	2.9	8.2	7.4
This includes:				
cerebral arteriosclerosis with pronounced psychotic symptoms or gross intellectual impairment				
men	0.2	—	1.0	2.1
women	0.9	—	4.5	5.0
both sexes	0.6	—	3.0	4.0
cerebral arteriosclerosis without pronounced psychotic symptoms or gross intellectual impairment				
men	0.7	1.5	4.1	2.1
women	1.6	4.0	5.9	4.0
both sexes	1.2	2.9	5.2	3.4
Presenile psychosis				
men	0.1	—	1.0	—
women	0.5	3.0	0.7	1.0
both sexes	0.3	1.3	0.9	0.7
Senile psychosis				
men	—	—	—	—
women	0.5	—	—	6.0
both sexes	0.3	—	—	4.1

Table 138

PREVALENCE OF THE SO-CALLED BORDERLINE STATES AMONG THE POPULATION OF DIFFERENT AGES AND BOTH SEXES (number of cases per 1,000 population of the corresponding age and sex)

Nosologic group	Under 2 years	3–6 years	7–12 years	13–15 years	16–19 years	20–29 years	30–39 years	40–49 years	50–59 years	60–69 years	Whole popu-lation
Psychopathy											
men	—	1.4	3.9	2.5	—	0.7	0.5	1.8	1.0	—	1.6
women	—	—	0.7	—	—	1.0	3.0	2.9	2.2	—	1.5
both sexes	—	0.7	2.4	1.4	—	0.9	2.4	2.0	1.7	—	1.5
Neuroses, reactive states											
men	—	2.9	4.6	2.5	—	—	1.8	5.3	—	—	2.1
women	—	—	2.2	—	2.5	0.5	9.4	18.5	9.6	—	6.1
both sexes	—	1.4	3.5	1.4	1.2	0.3	5.8	12.8	5.6	—	4.3

taken into account in determining the standards for their therapeutic-prophylactic care.

The group of diseases with the so-called borderline states includes cases of psychopathy, neuroses, and reactive states requiring psychiatric treatment. Those in whom the neurotic symptoms are included in the symptoms of some basic somatic or neurological disease and who, therefore, need treatment by neuropathologists, internists, endocrinologists, and others have been excluded from this group.

According to examination data for the population of Stupino, the number of cases of psychopathy proved to be 1.5; of neuroses and reactive states, 4.3; and the total figure, 5.8 per 1,000 population.

As is evident from Table 138, there are no essential differences in the figures for psychopathy in men and women, whereas the incidence of neuroses and reactive states in women was three times as great as in men.

The statistical and clinical-statistical data presented above on the incidence of neuropsychiatric diseases detected on examination of the population of the experimental districts of Stupino permit proceeding with determination of the standards for the urban population requirement of various types of neuropsychiatric care. However, such calculations are hard to make without considerable additional general information on the entire group of patients with neuropsychiatric diseases.

This information deals primarily with the degree of loss of work fitness, the amount of hospitalization, and the number of new patients with mental diseases during the year. For the purpose of determining the amount of outpatient and hospital psychiatric care needed by all patients with neuropsychiatric diseases detected on examination, it is also necessary to take into consideration the severity of the condition of these patients at present, to determine the duration of their illness, the frequency of hospitalization in the past, and, finally, the number of new patients during

To a certain extent, information about the degree of loss of work fitness can serve as the criterion of the severity of the neuropsychiatric diseases detected in the inhabitants of Stupino (Table 139).

As is evident from this table, of the total number of persons who need treatment by psychiatrists, 24% are incapable of working (including first- and second-category invalids, those who are not invalids and are not working, and children incapable of studying). This percentage should be considered very large if we take into account the fact that the total number of patients who must be treated by psychiatrists includes those with the so-called borderline states as well as persons who suffer from chronic alcoholism.

If from the total number of patients we exclude patients with borderline states and those with chronic alcoholism, the patients who have lost the ability to work mentioned above will come to 32.7%.

Of special interest is the degree of loss of work fitness in the groups of patients with mental diseases who constitute the greatest proportion of the whole neuro-

Table 139

DISTRIBUTION OF PATIENTS WITH NEUROPSYCHIATRIC DISEASES IN STUPINO ACCORDING TO THE DEGREE OF LOSS OF WORK FITNESS (in percent of the total)

Form of neuropsychiatric disease	Total	With invalidism			Groups without invalidism		Those receiving old-age pensions	Studying	Not studying	Preschool children
		first category	second category	third category	not working	working				
I. Schizophrenia	100.0	6.8	53.9	11.2	11.2	16.9	—	—	—	—
II. Group of epileptic and epileptiform diseases										
epilepsy	100.0	1.1	18.9	16.8	5.3	30.4	1.1	11.6	9.5	5.3
traumatic epilepsy	100.0	2.8	22.2	2.8	2.8	27.8	—	19.4	13.9	8.3
organic disease of the brain with epileptiform syndrome	100.0	—	19.0	9.5	9.5	38.1	4.8	4.8	9.5	4.8
III. Group of diseases characterized by mental retardation	100.0	—	13.3	20.0	6.7	20.0	—	20.0	13.3	6.7
oligophrenia	100.0	—	4.2	6.1	6.1	10.2	—	36.8	20.4	12.2
organic disease of the brain with mental retardation	100.0	—	7.4	7.4	3.7	18.5	—	29.7	22.2	11.1
IV. Traumatic and organic diseases	100.0	—	9.1	4.5	9.1	—	—	45.5	18.2	13.6
traumatic diseases of the brain*	100.0	—	8.8	20.6	2.9	52.0	4.9	9.8	—	1.6
organic diseases of the brain**	100.0	3.3	20.0	10.0	10.0	30.0	—	23.4	—	3.3
V. Psychoses from diseases in older ages										
cerebral arteriosclerosis	100.0	—	7.7	7.7	15.4	43.6	25.6	—	—	—
presenile psychosis	100.0	—	14.3	—	28.6	57.1	—	—	—	—
senile psychosis	100.0	—	—	16.7	50.0	33.3	—	—	—	—
VI. Manic-depressive psychosis	100.0	—	—	—	—	100.0	—	—	—	—
cerebral syphilis	100.0	—	—	—	—	100.0	—	—	—	—
VII. Chronic alcoholism	100.0	—	0.9	0.9	1.9	93.5	2.8	—	—	—
VIII. Borderline states	100.0	—	—	—	3.1	80.5	1.6	12.5	—	2.3
psychopathy	100.0	—	—	—	8.8	58.9	2.9	26.5	—	2.9
neuroses and reactive states	100.0	—	—	—	1.0	88.3	1.0	7.4	—	2.1
Total	100.0	1.2	13.9	8.9	6.2	51.9	3.2	9.4	2.9	2.4

* Not including patients with epileptiform syndrome.
** Not including patients with epileptiform syndrome and mental retardation since infancy.

psychiatric morbidity. Thus, among the patients with schizophrenia the number who are completely incapable of working proves to be 71.9% (with 11.2% third-category invalids); among patients with epilepsy and epileptiform diseases, the number is 34.8% (including 16.8% third-category invalids and 1.1% old-age pensioners).

Information about the hospitalization rate during the entire disease period (Table 140) represents a certain addition to the data on the degree of loss of work fitness characterizing the distribution of patients with neuropsychiatric diseases.

As is evident from Table 140, in such diseases as schizophrenia, epilepsy and others,

Table 140

DISTRIBUTION OF PATIENTS DETECTED IN STUPINO ACCORDING TO THE HOSPITALIZATION RATE DURING THE ENTIRE DISEASE PERIOD IN MENTAL HOSPITALS (in % of the total)

Neuropsychiatric diseases	All	Including mental hospitals		Group of patients treated in mental hospitals— number of times hospitalized				
		never hospitalized during lifetime	hospitalized some time during life	once	twice	3 times	4 times	5 times or more
I. Schizophrenia*	100	10.1	89.9	27.5	23.8	15.0	9.9	23.8
II. Group of epileptic and epileptiform diseases	100	78.9	21.1	35.0	35.0	10.0	5.0	15.0
epilepsy	100	77.8	22.2	37.5	25.0	12.5	12.5	12.5
traumatic epilepsy	100	71.4	28.6	33.3	50.0	—	—	16.7
traumatic disease of the brain with epileptiform syndrome	100	73.9	26.1	33.3	33.3	16.7	—	16.7
organic disease of the brain with epileptiform syndrome	100	100	—	—	—	—	—	—
III. Group of diseases characterized by mental retardation	100	100	—	—	—	—	—	—
oligophrenia	100	100	—	—	—	—	—	—
organic disease of the brain with mental retardation	100	100	—	—	—	—	—	—
IV. Traumatic and organic diseases traumatic and organic diseases of the brain**	100	91.2	8.8	66.7	11.1	11.1	—	11.1
organic diseases of the brain†	100	90.0	10.0	100.0	—	—	—	—
V. Mental diseases of the older age group cerebral arteriosclerosis	100	97.4	2.6	100.0	—	—	—	—
presenile psychoses	100	28.6	71.4	40.0	40.0	20.0	—	—
senile psychoses	100	83.3	16.7	—	100.0	—	—	—
VI. Manic-depressive psychosis	100	—	100.0	100.0	—	—	—	—
cerebral syphilis	100	—	100.0	100.0	—	—	—	—
VII. Chronic alcoholism	100	57.0	43.0	58.7	30.4	2.2	2.2	6.5
VIII. Borderline states	100	93.8	6.2	100.0	—	—	—	—
psychopathy	100	94.1	5.9	100.0	—	—	—	—
neuroses and reactive states	100	93.6	6.4	100.0	—	—	—	—

* Information on the number of admissions to mental hospitals for patients with schizophrenia is given with respect to the number hospitalized rather than the total number of patients.

** Not including patients with epileptiform syndrome.

† Not including patients with epileptiform syndrome and mental retardation since infancy.

not only is the total number of patients hospitalized during the whole disease period high (for example, for schizophrenia, 89.9%) but also the number of repeat cases of hospitalization.

Aside from information about the number of hospitalized cases, Table 140 gives us an idea of the relative number of cases in which the diagnosis of a neuropsychiatric disease was established on an outpatient basis or confirmed in the hospital (third and fourth columns).

Thus, confirmation of the diagnosis as the result of investigation in a psychiatric

Table 141

AVERAGE ANNUAL FIGURES OF INCIDENCE OF NEUROPSYCHIATRIC DISEASES AMONG THE POPULATION OF STUPINO IN THE FIVE-YEAR PERIOD 1956–1960 (No. of cases per 1,000 population per year)

Disease	Average annual incidence of neuropsychiatric cases
I. Schizophrenia	0.29
II. Group of diseases with epileptiform syndrome	0.25
epilepsy	0.14
traumatic epilepsy	0.05
traumatic disease of the brain with epileptiform syndrome	0.04
organic cerebral disease with epileptiform syndrome	0.02
III. Group of cases characterized by mental retardation	0.05
oligophrenia	0.01
organic cerebral disease with mental retardation	0.04
IV. Traumatic and organic diseases of the brain	
traumatic diseases of the brain*	0.23
organic diseases of the brain**	0.09
V. Mental diseases of older age	
cerebral arteriosclerosis	0.18
presenile psychoses	0.03
senile psychoses	0.01
VI. Manic-depressive psychosis	—
cerebral syphilis	0.01
VII. Chronic alcoholism	0.22
VIII. Borderline states	0.44
psychopathy	0.10
neuroses, reactive states	0.34
Total	1.8

* Not including patients with epileptiform syndrome.
** Not including patients with epileptiform syndrome and mental retardation.

hospital occurred in 89.9% of the cases of schizophrenia, 71.4% of presenile psychoses, and 22.2% of epilepsy.

For determination of the average annual index of the incidence of neuropsychiatric diseases, information for 1956–1960 is most suitable (Table 141).

Thus, during the five-year period (1956–1960), each year an average of 1.8 persons per 1,000 population became ill, for all the neuropsychiatric diseases.

In conclusion we should dwell on data concerning the hospitalization rate of patients detected in Stupino in 1961. However, it should be emphasized that this information gives us an idea only of the actual hospitalization occurring during the year (Table 142). In 1961 not all the patients were hospitalized but only those who needed it particularly, because there were not enough beds available in mental hospitals in 1961 for all those needing hospital treatment (Table 142).

Table 142

NUMBER OF PATIENTS WITH NEUROPSYCHIATRIC DISEASES HOSPITALIZED IN 1961 AND THE PATIENT'S AVERAGE LENGTH OF STAY IN BED DURING THE YEAR

Neuropsychiatric diseases	No. of hospitalized patients (absolute figures)	Average length of stay in bed (in days) during the year
Schizophrenia	36	150.5
Epilepsy	2	60.0
Presenile psychoses	3	64.7
Chronic alcoholism	21	34.4
Mental disorders from cerebral trauma	1	30.0
Neuroses and reactive states	2	32.5
Total	65	98.3

Therefore, of the population group of the experimental districts in Stupino 68 patients were hospitalized in 1961; they spent a total of 6,684 bed-days in the mental hospitals (neuropsychiatric hospitals). In other words, during 1961, 18.3 beds, or 0.83 bed per 1,000 population, were continuously occupied with neuropsychiatric patients detected among the population group of 22,049 persons.

Standards of Neuropsychiatric Care of the Urban Population

Neuropsychiatric care needed by the population is composed of two main types, outpatient and hospital. ·

Outpatient neuropsychiatric care in turn includes the following work divisions:
a) mental hygiene and prophylactic work (health education, etc.);
b) investigation of the population made with the aim of detecting mental patients

and those with borderline forms of neuropsychiatric illness (neuroses, psychopathy, etc.);

c) dispensary care of patients with neuropsychiatric disease;

d) outpatient treatment of patients (including maintenance therapy with neuroleptic agents and work therapy);

e) social prophylactic work, including housing and working arrangements for mental patients;

f) expertise (work, military, and forensic psychiatric expertise).

All these divisions of the activity of the neuropsychiatric dispensary are united by a single concept, dispensary neuropsychiatric care of the population.

Hospital psychiatric care includes organization of treatment and the maintenance of patients with neuropsychiatric disease in the mental hospitals, in neuropsychiatric and somatic nervous disease sanatoria, and in nursing homes for mental patients with chronic courses of disease.

In the organization of the outpatient and hospital neuropsychiatric care, a division of all institutions into those for adults and those for children and adolescents is needed.

Standards of Outpatient Neuropsychiatric Care

In the investigation of the population of Stupino, of the total number of patients detected (29.8 per 1,000 population) 74.2% (22.11 per 1,000 population) needed outpatient care (Table 143).

Noteworthy is the fact that over half of those with schizophrenia, about three-fourths of those with epileptiform syndromes, and the majority of patients with traumatic cerebral diseases and borderline states needed outpatient therapy in the neuropsychiatric dispensary at the time of the investigation.

The average number of visits per year per patient is being given here according to the data of the neuropsychiatric dispensary of Elektrostal', a city very similar to Stupino in the nature of work and life of the population and its age and sex distribution. In this city dispensary care of patients with neuropsychiatric diseases is well organized.

It should be noted that the data on the number of visits by patients with such forms of disease as schizophrenia and epilepsy are very similar in Elektrostal' to the findings in Ramenskoe also.

In our calculations the number of annual visits per patient with schizophrenia or epilepsy is somewhat increased, because the introduction of free treatment of these patients since 1965 entails a considerable increase in their attendance at therapeutic-prophylactic institutions. Moreover, it should be taken into consideration that patients with epilepsy should be treated regularly throughout life. Here we are usually dealing only with a change in dosages of drugs and the replacement of certain

Table 143

AMOUNT OF OUTPATIENT-POLYCLINIC CARE IN THE FIELD OF PSYCHIATRY

Neuropsychiatric diseases	No. of patients needing outpatient care (per 1,000 population)	Average No. of visits per patient per year	Total number of visits (per 1,000 population)
I. Schizophrenia	2.4	15	36.00
II. Group of epilepsy and other diseases with epileptiform syndrome			
epilepsy	1.27	12	15.24
traumatic epilepsy	0.59	12	7.08
traumatic disease of the brain with epileptiform syndrome	0.86	12	10.32
organic disease of the brain with epileptiform syndrome	0.50	12	6.00
III. Group of cases characterized by mental retardation			
oligophrenia	0.05	1.8	0.09
organic brain diseases with mental retardation	0.41	1.8	7.738
IV. Traumatic and organic diseases			
traumatic diseases of the brain	4.27	3.2	13.664
organic diseases of the brain -	1.18	2.8	3.304
V. Mental diseases of the older age group			
cerebral arteriosclerosis presenile psychoses	1.77	2.6	4.602
senile psychoses	0.09	2.1	0.105
VI. Manic-depressive psychosis	0.05	2.4	0.12
cerebral syphilis	0.05	1.5	0.075
VII. Chronic alcoholism	2.99	2.8	8.372
VIII. Borderline states			
psychopathy	1.32	1.9	2.508
neuroses, reactive states	4.26	3.3	14.058
Total	22.06		129.3

drugs with others. In connection with this, the patients need long medical observation even in those cases where the convulsive seizures and other epileptiform manifestations have already disappeared, because the slightest disruption of the routine and of the medical treatment prescribed inevitably leads to a marked exacerbation of the course of the epilepsy and to social and work decompensation of the patients.

In schizophrenia maintenance therapy with neuroleptics in combination with other psychopharmacologic drugs should be given for years also. Of particularly great importance for increasing the efficacy of the maintenance therapy is social and work reconstruction of the patients with schizophrenia, carried out in therapeutic workshops and day hospitals organized at the neuropsychiatric dispensaries. While the number of visits amounts to 12 per year per patient with epilepsy and other diseases with an epileptiform syndrome, patients with schizophrenia who need to have maintenance therapy (36%) visit the dispensary 24 times a year.

The average number of visits per patient with schizophrenia will come to 15 per year.

The total number of visits by patients with all forms of neuropsychiatric diseases detected on examination of the Stupino population was 122.4 per 1,000 population.

In addition, the visits of patients with neuropsychiatric diseases not found at the time of examination of the population of the four experimental districts of Stupino should be taken into consideration.

Among these diseases are psychoses from infectious and virus diseases, intoxications, diseases of the internal organs, vitamin deficiency diseases, metabolic and endocrine disorders with mental disorders.

The number of visits by patients with the forms of neuropsychiatric diseases listed was deduced from the data of the Elektrostal' dispensary and was found to be 3.74 per 1,000 population.

In accordance with the calculations, the total number of medical consultation visits will amount to 126.1 per 1,000 population; prophylactic visits to 39.3, and the total to 165.4 visits per year per 1,000 population.

In calculations of standards for the requirement of neuropsychiatric care we should not overlook the clinic-type institutions included in the neuropsychiatric dispensary. In the dispensary of a city (or city district) servicing 250,000–300,000 population, an integrated combination of medical-reconstructive institutions is needed in the form of therapeutic workshops, a special shop on the premises, a day hospital and a night prophylactorium.

Standards of Hospital Neuropsychiatric Care

At the present time, the maintenance of the following types of psychiatric and neuropsychiatric hospitals is sufficiently well substantiated.

1. Mental hospitals (departments) for acutely ill patients and those with an ordinary attack (or recurrence) of the disease.

2. Mental hospitals (departments) for patients with chronic courses of the disease (chronic patients).

3. Nursing homes for mental patients with chronic courses (including nursing homes for imbeciles and idiots).

4. Neuropsychiatric sanatoria (sanatorium departments, for neuropsychiatric patients, convalescents, and those who are in a state of remission).

5. Somatic nervous disease sanatoria for those with neuroses.

6. Neuropsychiatric hospitals of the public health agencies for those with chronic alcoholism.

For all the types of hospitals listed the calculations of the requirement are given simultaneously for all age groups with further divisions in accordance with the following age intervals: for children (0–14 years), adolescents (15–16 years), and adults (17 years and over).

Calculation of the requirement of hospital beds per 1,000 of the whole population was made according to the generally accepted method but with consideration of the number of repeat hospitalizations for the various nosologic entities.

In calculation of the number of beds required for acutely ill patients, not only the data on the need for hospital care by patients on record, but also data on those needing hospitalization in the group of patients detected for the first time, were used in the calculation.

The average annual occupancy of a single bed is assumed to be the following: in hospitals (or departments) of all categories, 340 days per year, and in nursing homes and colonies for drug addicts, 350 days.

Mental Hospitals (or Departments) for Patients with Acute Illness who have Recently Become Sick and Those with a New Attack (Recurrence) of the Disease

All newly detected cases, as well as patients in whom a second attack has occurred after remission (recurrence) of the disease (Table 144), are admitted to hospitals for acute cases of recent onset.

In addition, hospitalization is needed for patients with brief psychoses terminating in complete recovery (0.46 per 1,000 population). With an average duration of their stay in the hospital of 60 days, an additional 27.6 bed-days are needed per 1,000 population. The number of those included in the psychiatric work expertise for every 1,000 persons should be about 0.2, which, with an average length of stay of 25 days, requires an additional 5 bed-days.

Therefore, for a single admission (116.9 + 27.6 + 5) 149.5 bed-days should be allotted for all patients with acute disease.

With an average bed occupancy of 340 days 0.44 bed per 1,000 population will be needed.

Taking into consideration the repeated admissions in the same year (repetition factor of 1.1) the number of beds needed for acute patients per 1,000 population will be 0.48, including 0.06 bed for children and adolescents.

Mental Hospitals (or Departments) for Patients with Chronic Diseases with Protracted Courses

The bed requirement in hospitals of this type is determined by data on the prevalence of neuropsychiatric disease in the population. The annual increase in the number of chronic patients needing hospitalization is not considered, because the natural reduction in the number of these patients partly compensates for the "accumulation";

Table 144

HOSPITALIZATION RATE OF PATIENTS WITH ACUTE DISEASES, AVERAGE LENGTH
OF TREATMENT PER PATIENT AND TOTAL NUMBER OF BED-DAYS NEEDED

Neuropsychiatric diseases	No. of patients acutely in need of hospitalization per 1,000 population			Average length of stay of one patient in the hospital	Total number of bed-days (per 1,000 population)
	number previously put on record	number sick for the first time	total		
I. Schizophrenia	0.27	0.29	0.56	75	42.0
II. Group of epilepsy and epilepti-form diseases					
epilepsy	0.14	0.012	0.152	45	6.8
traumatic epilepsy	0.09	0.005	0.095	60	5.7
traumatic diseases of the brain with epileptiform syndrome	0.05	0.002	0.052	60	3.1
III. Group of cases characterized by mental retardation					
organic disease of the brain with mental retardation	0.05	0.001	0.051	60	3.1
IV. Traumatic and organic diseases of the brain					
traumatic disease of the brain	0.18	0.009	0.189	45	8.5
organic disease of the brain	0.14	0.009	0.149	60	8.9
V. Mental diseases of the older age group					
cerebral arteriosclerosis	0.18	0.09	0.27	60	16.2
presenile psychoses	0.27	0.03	0.30	50	15.0
senile psychoses	0.05	0.01	0.04	150	6.0
VI. Borderline states					
psychopathy	0.05	0.003	0.053	30	1.6
Total					116.9

therefore during the next 8–10 years the bed requirement will not change substantially.

Therefore the total number of bed-days needed for this patient group is 384.9 per 1,000 population, which, with a repetition factor of 1.3 and a duration of bed occupancy of 340 days per year, requires 1.47 beds per 1,000 population, including 0.15 for children and adolescents (see Table 145).

Nursing Homes for Mental Patients with Chronic Diseases

The bed requirement in nursing homes for chronic mental patients has been determined here separately for adults (Table 146), and for children (including imbeciles and idiots) (Table 147).

Table 145
HOSPITALIZATION RATE OF CHRONIC PATIENTS, AVERAGE LENGTH OF
TREATMENT OF A SINGLE PATIENT AND TOTAL NUMBER OF BED-DAYS NEEDED

Neuropsychiatric diseases	No. of cases needing hospitalization (per 1,000 population)	Average length of stay of a patient in bed	Total number of bed-days needed (per 1,000 population)
I. Schizophrenia	1.37	150	205.5
II. Group of epilepsy and epileptic diseases			
epilepsy	0.18	300	54.0
traumatic epilepsy	0.27	120	32.4
traumatic diseases of the brain with epileptiform syndrome	0.09	90	8.1
organic cerebral disease with epileptiform syndrome	0.09	250	22.5
III. Group of cases characterized by mental retardation			
oligophrenia	0.09	90	8.1
organic cerebral disease with mental retardation	0.5	150	7.5
IV. Traumatic and organic cerebral disease			
traumatic cerebral disease	0.09	90	8.1
organic cerebral disease	0.09	150	13.5
V. Senile psychoses	0.09	280	25.2
Total			384.9

The total number of patients needing to be placed in nursing homes is 0.52 per 1,000 population, which, with a length of a single patient's bed stay of 368 days and 350 days of bed operation per year, will be 0.54 bed per 1,000 population (Table 146).

The total number of sick children and adolescents needing to be placed in nursing homes is 0.32 per 1,000 population, which requires 0.33 bed per 1,000 population (average length of treatment of one patient 365 days, duration of bed operation per year 350 days).

Sanatoria (Sanatorium Departments) for Neuropsychiatric Patients—Convalescents and Patients who are in a State of Remission

Specialized neuropsychiatric sanatoria and sanatorium departments of mental hospitals are designed for mental patients, convalescents who are in a state of remission, or the most seriously ill patients with neuroses and reactive states (Table 148).

Thus, the total number of patients requiring treatment in neuropsychiatric sanatoria (sanatorium departments) is 2.3 per 1,000 population; with an average length of treatment of 30 days and 340 days of bed operation per year, the bed requirement is 0.2 per 1,000 population (including 0.04 for children and adolescents).

Table 146
HOSPITALIZATION RATE OF CHRONIC PATIENTS WITH NEUROPSYCHIATRIC DISEASES IN NURSING HOME

Neuropsychiatric diseases	No. of patients needing to stay in nursing homes (per 1,000 population)
I. Group of epilepsy and epileptiform diseases	
epilepsy	0.05
traumatic epilepsy	—
traumatic disease of the brain with epileptiform syndrome	0.05
organic disease of the brain with epileptiform syndrome	0.18
II. Traumatic and organic diseases of the brain	
traumatic diseases of the brain	0.05
organic diseases of the brain	0.05
III. Mental diseases of the older age group	
cerebral arteriosclerosis with pronounced dementia	—
senile dementia	0.14
Total	0.52

Table 147
HOSPITALIZATION RATE OF SICK CHILDREN AND ADOLESCENTS IN NURSING HOME FOR MENTAL PATIENTS WITH A CHRONIC COURSE

Neuropsychiatric diseases	No. of patients needing to be in nursing homes (per 1,000 population)
Oligophrenia to the extent of imbecility and idiocy	0.23
Other neuropsychiatric diseases, chiefly organic and traumatic with dementia	0.09
Total	0.32

Somatic Nervous Disease Sanatoria for Patients with Neuroses

Neurosis patients requiring sanatorium treatment comprised 2.8 per 1,000 population; with a treatment duration of 24 days and 340 days of bed operation per year, the bed requirement is 0.2 per 1,000 population (including 0.003 for children and 0.03 for adolescents).

Table 148
FREQUENCY OF HOSPITALIZATION CASES
AND SPECIALIZED NEUROPSYCHIATRIC
SANATORIA (DEPARTMENTS)

Neuropsychiatric diseases	No. of patients needing sanatorium treatment (per 1,000 population)
Schizophrenia	0.45
Epilepsy	0.31
Traumatic cerebral disease	0.73
Organic cerebral disease	0.36
Cerebral arteriosclerosis	0.23
Manic-depressive psychosis	0.045
Compulsive-obsessive neurosis	0.18
Total	2.3

Neuropsychiatric Hospitals of the Public Health Services for Persons Suffering from Chronic Alcoholism

Patients with second-stage chronic alcoholism needing hospital treatment were detected to the extent of 2.08 per 1,000 population. For their treatment 0.13 bed per 1,000 population is needed (treatment time, 21 days; duration of bed operation, 340 days).

Therefore, per 1,000 urban population the bed requirement will be:

1) 0.48 (including 0.06 for children and adolescents) in mental hospitals for patients with acute diseases;

2) 1.47 (including 0.15 for children) in mental hospitals for patients with longer-lasting courses and chronic patients;

3) 0.2 (including 0.04 for children) in neuropsychiatric hospitals (departments) of the sanatorium category;

4) 0.13 in neuropsychiatric hospitals for persons with chronic alcoholism.

Total in mental and neuropsychiatric institutions of the Ministry of Health of the RSFSR 2.28 (including children and adolescents 0.025);

5) in nursing homes for mental patients with chronic courses, 0.54;

6) in nursing homes for child mental patients with chronic courses, 0.33;

Total in neuropsychiatric institutions who are within the domain of social security agencies, 0.87;

7) in somatic nervous disease sanatoria of the All-Union Central Trade Union Council, 0.20 (including 0.03 for children and adolescents).

Provision has also been made for a substantial increase in the number of beds in mental hospitals with the aim of complete coverage of all patients found to have mental diseases and requiring hospitalization.

Provision is also being made for beds for patients with logoneuroses.

Standards of Therapeutic-Prophylactic Care of the Urban Population in the Field of Tuberculosis

In working out the standards of tuberculosis control in the population we used the following material:

a) data of the detailed study of morbidity, sickness rate, hospitalization rate and outpatient attendance, collected in five cities located in different climato-geographic areas of the country;

b) data of complete medical checkups of the population of the Stupino experimental districts.

The investigation showed that most often the population sought medical care for pulmonary tuberculosis.

For men the incidence of pulmonary tuberculosis was 40.3% higher than in women; for extrapulmonary tuberculosis, 16.2% higher.

It is important to note that in studying the sickness rate according to data of the five cities consideration was given not only to patients with active but also those with inactive tuberculosis, in other words, groups III and IV on the dispensary records. This is confirmed by the fact that the incidence of pulmonary tuberculosis (groups I, II and III on the dispensary records) as well as tuberculosis of the other organs (groups Va and Vb) is, on the average for the RSFSR, not much different from the figures for its incidence in the five cities.

The admission rate for pulmonary tuberculosis in children increases with age. The lowest incidence of pulmonary tuberculosis is in children under 4 years; the highest, from 7–13. In adolescents (age group 14–19) a reduction in the incidence is noted.

Beginning with the age of 20 the sickness rate for pulmonary tuberculosis increases, reaching a maximum at 40–49. At 50–59 the sickness rate remains quite high, while at the age of 60 and over a reduction is noted.

Therefore it may be considered that the highest sickness rate of pulmonary tuberculosis in both sexes occurs at 40–49 and 50–59. Approximately the same patterns are noted in the sickness rate for tuberculosis of other organs.

In comparing the age indexes of the sickness rate for pulmonary tuberculosis in men and women under 30, we observed no particular differences in these figures. In subsequent age groups the sickness rate in men is much higher than in women. At the ages of 30–39 the sickness rate in men is 1.6 times as high as in women; at 40–49, 2.5 times; at 50–59, three times; at 60 and over, four times, which is noted also in the records for the RSFSR.

Men and women are almost equally afflicted with the other forms of tuberculosis, among which extrapulmonary tuberculosis accounts for a considerable fraction.

In determining the standards of care in the field of tuberculosis, data on the seasonality of the sickness rate in the population are interesting. Most often the admissions for tuberculosis were in January, March, and May; least often, in August and December. This confirms the rule established by practicing physicians that the tuberculous process is exacerbated most often in the spring and to a lesser degree in the autumn.

The considerable increase in sickness rate in the spring is probably connected largely with the occurrence of vitamin deficiency, which in turn depends on the fact that prophylactic courses of chemotherapy are given to patients with active tuberculosis in the spring and autumn.

Incidence of Tuberculosis in the Urban Population According to the Data of Complete Medical Examinations

Calculating the optimum standards of therapeutic-prophylactic care in treatment of tuberculosis from the incidence of tuberculosis in the population is difficult because it is well known that pulmonary or other organ changes often fail to produce the corresponding clinical symptoms that would cause the patient to go to the physician at the opportune time. Particularly great changes in the clinical course of tuberculosis and an increase in the number of patients with an unnoticed course of the disease have occurred because of the extensive practical use of antibiotics and chemotherapeutic agents in the past 10–15 years. Mass medical examinations of the population with the aim of early detection of tuberculosis assume tremendous importance. At present much attention is being given to this matter. Data of mass examinations in combination with sickness rate data of the population permit the determination of the true morbidity of the population and by the same token the determination of the optimum need for therapeutic-prophylactic treatment of the population.

Table 149

INCIDENCE OF NEWLY DETECTED CASES OF TUBERCULOSIS (for which there had been no admissions in previous years) IN COMPLETE MEDICAL EXAMINATIONS IN STUPINO

(No. of cases per 1,000 population)

Name of disease	Age groups								
	both sexes	men	women	both sexes	men	women	both sexes	men	women
	under 1 year			1–2 years			3–6 years		
Pulmonary tuberculosis	—	—	—	—	—	—	3.1	6.7	—
Extrapulmonary tuberculosis	—	—	—	8.1	15.4	—	9.4	10.0	8.8
	7–12 years			13–15 years			16–19 years		
Pulmonary tuberculosis	3.9	4.6	2.3	—	—	—	2.1	—	4.3
Extrapulmonary tuberculosis	3.1	1.5	4.7	—	—	—	—	—	—
	20–29 years			30–39 years			40–49 years		
Pulmonary tuberculosis	7.6	13.0	3.9	8.4	8.0	8.6	7.8	6.1	8.9
Extrapulmonary tuberculosis	2.3	1.8	2.6	2.9	3.4	2.6	1.8	1.5	2.0
	50–59 years			60 years and over			total		
Pulmonary tuberculosis	12.7	17.4	9.4	3.2	5.4	2.3	6.3	7.3	5.7
Extrapulmonary tuberculosis	—	—	—	1.6	—	2.3	2.5	2.5	2.5

Table 149 shows data of medical checkups of the Stupino population.

As seen in Table 149, patients with pulmonary tuberculosis are detected almost $2\frac{1}{2}$ times as often as those with extrapulmonary tuberculosis. In men pulmonary tuberculosis is detected almost $1\frac{1}{2}$ times as often as in women (7.3 and 5.7), whereas the detection rate of tuberculosis of the other organs is the same for men and women (2.5 and 2.5). This once again confirms the principle that men contract pulmonary tuberculosis more than women, in contrast to extrapulmonary tuberculosis, in which the incidence is about the same for both.

Pulmonary tuberculosis is detected most often in the 50–59 age group in both men and women. Here there are certain differences from the figures obtained in the study of the sickness rate. This fact gives rise to the need for increasing therapeutic-prophylactic work in tuberculosis among older persons.

Attendance at Tuberculosis Institutions by the Urban Population for Pulmonary and Extrapulmonary Tuberculosis

As is well known, the attendance at tuberculosis institutions for treatment purposes is determined primarily by the total incidence of tuberculosis.

Table 150

ATTENDANCE FOR TREATMENT OF PULMONARY AND EXTRAPULMONARY TUBERCULOSIS (No. of visits per 1,000 population)*

Name of disease	Women			Men			Both sexes		
	actually made	added by experts	total	actually made	added by experts	total	actually made	added by experts	total
Pulmonary tuberculosis	61.0	4.84	65.84	126.2	8.94	135.14	89.3	6.7	96.0
Extrapulmonary tuberculosis	10.8	1.21	12.01	11.4	1.99	13.39	11.1	1.6	12.7
Total	71.8	6.05	77.85	137.6	10.93	148.53	100.4	8.3	108.7

* The table shows information on visits not only to phthisiologists but also to other specialists. At the same time, it should be kept in mind that phthisiologists visited patients for other, nontuberculous diseases.

The figures for outpatient attendance of the population of three cities (Dneprodzerzhinsk, Rubezhnoe and Stupino) are shown in Table 150.

From Table 150 it is evident that the number of visits for tuberculosis of the respiratory organs is 89.3 per 1,000 population, which is almost 8 times as high as the number for extrapulmonary tuberculosis (11.1). The attendance of men for pulmonary tuberculosis is twice as high as that of women (126.2 per 1,000 men and 61 per 1,000 women).

The attendance of men with extrapulmonary tuberculosis is not much different from that of women (11.4 for men and 10.8 for women).

From Table 151 it is seen that the attendance for pulmonary tuberculosis is relatively low in the age groups under 4 and from 5 to 6. Beginning with the age of 7 an increase is seen in the figure, which reaches a maximum at 20–29 and 30–39. Beginning with the age of 40 the number of visits per 1,000 population appreciably decreases, reaching a minimum at the age of 60 and over.

The attendance rate of patients with other forms of tuberculosis increases with age in children, reaching a maximum in the 7–13 age group (29.8 per 1,000 population).

In the age groups 14–19, 20–29 and 30–39 a relative stabilization of the figure is noted (11.5, 7.4 and 10.0), with a subsequent rise at 40–49 years (15.1). Beginning with the age of 50 the number of visits decreases, reaching a minimum at the age of 60 and over (1.8 visits per 1,000).

The attendance figures for men in almost all age groups (except 7–13) are higher than for women. The difference becomes particularly great beginning with the age of 30, at which time the attendance of men is $4\frac{1}{2}$ times as great as that of women, and in the 60 and over age group, when it is six times as great. The data given show tendencies similar to the age changes in the sickness rate figures.

As has been pointed out above, for determining the standards of the number of visits during outpatient treatment of patients an expertise was given on the basis of

Table 151
AVERAGE AGE INDEXES OF ATTENDANCE OF THE POPULATION OF BOTH SEXES
FOR PULMONARY AND EXTRAPULMONARY TUBERCULOSIS (No. of visits for treatment
per 1,000 population of the corresponding age and sex)

Name of disease	Age groups								
	men	women	both sexes	men	women	both sexes	men	women	both sexes
	under 4 years			5–6 years			7–13 years		
Pulmonary tuberculosis	8.9	5.4	7.2	9.3	5.0	7.1	26.8	39.0	32.8
Extrapulmonary tuberculosis	8.4	4.5	6.5	14.5	8.83	11.6	31.8	28.0	29.8
	14–19 years			20–29 years			30–39 years		
Pulmonary tuberculosis	56.2	51.4	53.8	178.1	106.4	136.2	225.0	68.0	131.7
Extrapulmonary tuberculosis	11.5	11.4	11.5	10.9	5.1	7.4	6.0	13.0	10.0
	40–49 years			50–59 years			60 years and over		
Pulmonary tuberculosis	185.2	82.5	122.0	178.0	38.0	95.0	79.5	1.07	33.1
Extrapulmonary tuberculosis	13.0	16.5	15.1	6.2	7.6	7.0	1.3	2.0	1.3

the initial medical records of each patient. Usually the clinical picture of the course of each patient's disease in the dispensary record group was used as a basis. Table 152 shows the figures on the number of visits added by the experts according to data on the study of the initial records in Stupino. We believe that if an expertise had been given in other cities studied, the number of visits added by the experts for each disease would have been the same as for Stupino.

After the correction made by the experts the attendance figures for patients with pulmonary tuberculosis in Stupino rose from 38.6 to 45.3 per 1,000 population (6.7 visits added by experts per 1,000 population).

Prior to evaluation by the experts the attendance for extrapulmonary tuberculosis in Stupino was 9.2 per 1,000 population. After introduction of the experts' corrective factor (1.6) this rate rose to 10.8 per 1,000 population.

As is evident from Table 152, the total of visits actually made and those added by the experts for pulmonary tuberculosis was 96 per 1,000 population; for extrapulmonary tuberculosis, 12.7.

Of great importance for determination of the population requirement of care in the field of tuberculosis is the correct recording of visits to the phthisiologist not only for the main condition, tuberculosis, but also for other diseases by way of

Table 152

DISTRIBUTION OF VISITS FOR TREATMENT OF TUBERCULOSIS AMONG PHYSICIANS OF DIFFERENT SPECIALTIES

Per 1,000 population

Name of disease	average number of visits for treatment for 3 cities	added by the experts	total	this includes: internal medicine	surgery	ENT	ophthal-mology	tuber-culosis	neurology	psychiatry	stomatology	dermato-venereology	obstetrics and gynecology	pediatrics	speech training	oncology
Pulmonary tuberculosis	89.3	6.7	96.0	4.9	0.1	0.1	—	90.5	—	—	0.1	—	0.2	0.1	—	—
Extrapulmonary tuberculosis	11.1	1.6	12.7	1.1	0.8	0.1	0.4	6.7	0.2	—	—	0.1	2.1	1.2	—	—
Total	100.4	8.3	108.7	6.0	0.9	0.2	0.4	97.2	0.2	—	0.1	0.1	2.3	1.3	—	—

Table 153

HOSPITALIZATION RATE OF URBAN POPULATION FOR PULMONARY AND EXTRAPULMONARY TUBERCULOSIS

(No. of cases per 1,000 population)

Name of disease	Actual			Added by the experts			Chronic cases of tuber-culosis newly detected on examination, needing hospitalization			No. of cases actually hospitalized plus those added by the experts plus chronic cases newly detected, needing hospital treatment		
	men	women	both sexes	men	women	both sexes	men	women	both sexes	men	women	both sexes
Pulmonary tuberculosis	6.1	2.4	4.1	0.2	—	0.1	0.7	0.7	0.7	7.0	3.1	4.9
Extrapulmonary tuberculosis	0.9	0.9	0.9	—	0.1	0.05	—	—	—	0.9	1.0	0.95

medical consultations and a record of the number of visits to physicians in other specialties made by tuberculosis patients. The distribution of visits for treatment (actual and added by the experts) according to the medical specialties is shown in Table 152. The number of visits by patients with pulmonary tuberculosis was highest to the phthisiologist (90.5 visits per 1,000 population). Among the visits made by patients with pulmonary tuberculosis to physicians in other specialties the highest rate was to the internist (4.9 per 1,000 population). The visits by patients with pulmonary tuberculosis to physicians in other specialties ranged from 0.1 to 0.2 per 1,000 population.

Visits to phthisiologists by patients with extrapulmonary tuberculosis comprised only half of the total (6.7 out of 12.7 per 1,000 population). The other visits (4.2 per 1,000 population) to the phthisiologist were for other diseases. Most often the patients with extrapulmonary tuberculosis visited obstetrician-gynecologists (2.1 per 1,000 population); then, pediatricians (1.2 per 1,000 population) and internists (1.1 per 1,000 population); least often, ENT specialists and dermatovenereologists (0.1 per 1,000 population). In all, the number of visits to the phthisiologist by patients with pulmonary and extrapulmonary tuberculosis was 97.2 per 1,000 population. The total number of visits to physicians in the various specialties (including the phthisiologist) for the three cities was 108.7 visits per 1,000 population.

The highest number of medical consultation visits needed to phthisiologists was for respiratory and infectious diseases (for common colds, 2.56 visits; for respiratory diseases, 2.15 per 1,000 population, etc.).

Hospitalization of the Urban Population for Tuberculosis

Data on hospitalization for pulmonary and extrapulmonary tuberculosis for five cities (Dneprodzerzhinsk, Rubezhnoe, Kopeisk, Chelyabinsk, and Stupino) are given in Table 153.

As seen from Table 153, the hospitalization rate of the population of both sexes for pulmonary tuberculosis is 4.1 per thousand. In men it is 6.1 per thousand, in women 2.4. The hospitalization rate for extrapulmonary tuberculosis in men and women is the same and comes to 0.9 per thousand. Therefore, the main and most frequent cause of hospitalization is pulmonary tuberculosis. Men are more often hospitalized than women. Standardization did not change the actual hospitalization rate figures practically.

As has already been pointed out, the data of sickness rate, hospitalization rate, and attendance were subjected to expert analysis so as to determine the population requirement of outpatient and hospital treatment. At the same time, the data of medical examinations of the population were of importance, permitting determination of the additional number of admissions, visits, and hospitalization required.

In Table 153 we see data on the number of cases actually hospitalized, the corrective factors introduced by the experts, and the data on hospitalization rate of patients newly detected on examination.

From the table it is evident that *in toto* the number of cases actually hospitalized, plus the number added by experts, plus the number of cases hospitalized among the patients newly detected by examinations who need hospital treatment for pulmonary tuberculosis amounted to 4.9 per 1,000 population, whereas the figure for extrapulmonary tuberculosis was 0.95 per 1,000 population. The age indexes for hospitalization rate (average for five cities) are given in Table 154.

As is evident from Table 154, in the children's and young adolescents' groups the hospitalization rates for pulmonary tuberculosis are about the same and vary from 2.4 to 2.5 per 1,000 population, with the exception of the age groups from 5 to 6 years, in which the hospitalization rate was 1.6 per 1,000 children of this age. Beginning with the age of 20, an increase in hospitalization rate is noted, which reaches a maximum

Table 154

AGE INDEXES OF HOSPITALIZATION RATE OF THE POPULATION OF FIVE CITIES (No. of cases hospitalized per 1,000 population of the corresponding age and sex)

Name of disease	Age groups					
	men	women	both sexes	men	women	both sexes
	under 4 years			5–6 years		
Pulmonary tuberculosis	3.0	1.8	2.4	1.5	1.8	1.6
Extrapulmonary tuberculosis	1.3	3.5	2.2	0.8	0.16	0.4
	7–13 years			14–19 years		
Pulmonary tuberculosis	1.7	3.2	2.5	1.9	2.8	2.4
Extrapulmonary tuberculosis	0.6	0.6	0.6	1.2	0.7	0.9
	20–29 years			30–39 years		
Pulmonary tuberculosis	6.1	3.6	4.7	0.7	2.4	6.8
Extrapulmonary tuberculosis	1.1	0.8	0.8	0.7	0.8	0.7
	40–49 years			50–59 years		
Pulmonary tuberculosis	9.7	2.1	5.1	8.6	1.9	4.4
Extrapulmonary tuberculosis	1.6	0.8	1.0	0.6	0.5	0.5
	60 years and over			total		
Pulmonary tuberculosis	5.2	0.2	1.7	6.1	2.4	4.1
Extrapulmonary tuberculosis	0.4	0.3	0.3	0.9	0.9	0.8

at 30–39 and 40–49 (6.8 and 5.1, respectively, per 1,000 population). At the age of 50 and over a reduction in hospitalization rate is noted.

In patients with extrapulmonary tuberculosis the highest hospitalization rate is seen under the age of 4 (2.2 per 1,000 population), the lowest in the age group 60 and over (0.3 per 1,000 population).

Table 155

DISTRIBUTION OF HOSPITALIZED PATIENTS IN THE VARIOUS HOSPITAL DEPARTMENTS (per 1,000 population)

Name of disease	Total cases hospitalized	Distributed among the following departments			
		internal medicine	tuberculosis	infectious-disease (for adults)	other
Pulmonary tuberculosis	4.2	0.1	4.0	0.1	—
Extrapulmonary tuberculosis	0.95	—	—	—	0.95
Total	5.15	0.1	4.0	0.1	0.95

An analysis of data on the distribution of patients with tuberculosis in the various departments of the hospital showed that patients with pulmonary tuberculosis were hospitalized largely in the tuberculosis department (hospitalization rate in these departments was 4 per 1,000 population with a total average hospitalization rate for the five cities of 4.2 per 1,000 population). The remaining 0.2 case hospitalized was in the department of internal medicine (0.1 case per 1,000 population) and infectious-disease department (0.1 case per 1,000 population). At the same time, patients with extrapulmonary tuberculosis were usually hospitalized in the various somatic-disease departments of the hospital (Table 155).

Standards of Therapeutic-Prophylactic Care of the Urban Population in the Field of Tuberculosis

We analyzed the standards of therapeutic-prophylactic care of the urban population in the field of tuberculosis for the next few years, with calculation of the optimum provision for tuberculosis patients with all types of medical care.

As has been pointed out above, calculation of the standards of care in the field of tuberculosis from the sickness rate data of the population alone is impossible without the data of complete medical examinations, to assist in the detection of tuberculosis in those who have not sought medical care.

According to Directive No. 529 of the Ministry of Health of the RSFSR dated November 4, 1960, and Directive No. 426 dated November 6, 1960, 50% of the urban population should be examined every year with the aim of detecting tuberculosis.

Considering the fact that every year the number of patients examined for tuberculosis and correspondingly the number of newly detected cases will increase through expansion of mass prophylactic checkups, as well as in view of the improvement in diagnosis and improvement of the quality of work in early detection of tuberculosis prior to the development of its focal forms, some increase in the number of groups of patients with tuberculosis is to be expected for the next few years.

It may be supposed that in the next few years (1966–1970), despite the increase in total incidence because of the examinations, progressively fewer acute forms of tuberculosis will be encountered in its distribution and, correspondingly, the number of patients with the chronic forms will increase. This is explained not only by an increase in the longevity of the population generally and of patients with chronic tuberculosis in particular, but also by the fact that, because of the considerable expansion of prophylactic examinations of the nonorganized population for tuberculosis, there will be more patients with the chronic forms of the disease, not found in previous years, among the newly detected cases.

The data given above, however, concern both the active and inactive forms of tuberculosis and require a differentiated approach. For the purpose of dividing the group of patients with tuberculosis into active and inactive forms, we used the record data on the relationship between patients with active and inactive tuberculosis in 1963 (58.8% of the patients had active and 41.2% inactive pulmonary tuberculosis, 41.3% had active and 58.7% inactive extrapulmonary tuberculosis).

Standards for Outpatient-Polyclinic Care in the Field of Tuberculosis

As has been pointed out above, in determining the outpatient attendance for tuberculosis we used as a basis the data of detailed study in three cities (Dneprodzerzhinsk, Rubezhnoe, and Stupino) and the corrections made by the experts in Stupino. On the basis of these data the estimated attendance of patients who would be additionally detected as the result of prophylactic examinations of the population was determined. Some increase in the number of persons in the groups of patients with tuberculosis in the next few years naturally will entail an increase in the number of visits to phthisiologists by the tuberculosis patients.

Along with data on the number of visits to phthisiologists by patients in the first, second, and third dispensary record groups as well as by those visiting phthisiologists for follow-up examinations, visits of healthy persons seen because of contacts with tuberculosis patients (group IV on the dispensary records), whose attendance should come to 38.5 per 1,000 population, should be taken into account. Calculation of the attendance rate by persons in contact with tuberculosis patients was made in the following way. Persons in contact with those excreting bacilli should have visited the tuberculosis-control institutions four times. In addition, according to a letter on methods of drug prophylaxis of tuberculosis in children, for adolescents and adults under the age of 30 who are in constant contact with patients with the open form of tuberculosis, drug prophylaxis should be conducted. They should also visit the tuberculosis-control institutions four times a year.

In the calculation per 1,000 population the number of visits by persons in contact with tuberculosis patients will be 38.5. The overall attendance by persons of dispensary record groups I, II, and III for patients with pulmonary tuberculosis as well as those sent in for follow-up examinations will be 231.6 per 1,000 population (89.3 + 6.7 + 53.3 + 38.5 + 43.8).

As for patients with extrapulmonary tuberculosis, the total number of visits (actual plus expert corrections plus additional visits for patients newly detected at prophylactic examinations) will be 24.9 per 1,000 population (11.1 + 1.6 + 12.2). Data obtained from the calculations are shown in Table 156.

Table 156
STANDARDS OF OUTPATIENT CARE OF THE POPULATION IN THE FIELD OF TUBERCULOSIS

	Pulmonary tuberculosis	Extrapulmonary tuberculosis	Total
No. of actual visits (per 1,000 population)	89.3	11.1	100.4
No. of visits added by experts (per 1,000 prophylactic)	6.7	1.6	8.3
No. of additional visits of patients newly detected by medical examinations (per 1,000 population)	53.3	12.2	65.5
No. of persons sent in for follow-up to phthisiologists, using fluorography (per 1,000 population)	43.8		43.8
No. of visits by persons kept on records in dispensary record group IV (per 1,000 prophylactic)	38.5	–	38.5
Total visits (per 1,000 population)	231.6	24.9	256.5
Total number of visits per admission for tuberculosis	13.3	6.0	—

It should be noted that the number of visits to phthisiologists, according to record data in 1963, was 0.3 per inhabitant per year, which is somewhat less than our figures (0.26 per inhabitant per year), but approaches those of I. D. Bogatyrev (1959) and A.P. Zhuk (1960) and others.

Table 157 shows the attendance of patients with active and inactive tuberculosis and those with tuberculous intoxication in the outpatient tuberculosis institutions.

As is evident from Table 157, the number of visits per admission for patients with active tuberculosis of the lungs is almost three times as high as the number of visits

Table 157
OUTPATIENT ATTENDANCE FOR TUBERCULOSIS OF DIFFERENT FORMS

	Pulmonary tuberculosis	Extrapulmonary tuberculosis
Actual number of visits per 1,000 population plus those added by experts	96.0	12.7
Of these		
for patients with active tuberculosis	56.5	4.6
for patients with inactive tuberculosis	39.5	6.1
for patients with tuberculous intoxication	—	2.0
No. of additional visits for patients newly detected at medical examinations	53.3	12.2
Of these		
for patients with active tuberculosis	31.4	4.4
for patients with inactive tuberculosis	21.9	5.9
for patients with tuberculous intoxication	—	1.9
Total visits for patients with active tuberculosis	61.4	12.0
Total visits for patients with tuberculous intoxication	—	3.9
No. of visits per admission for patients with active tuberculosis	11.6	3.6
No. of visits per admission for patients with inactive tuberculosis	63	6.7
No. of visits per admission for patients with tuberculous intoxication	—	6.5

per admission in the case of patients with active extrapulmonary tuberculosis (11.6 and 3.6 per 1,000 population), whereas the number of visits per admission in patients with inactive pulmonary tuberculosis is almost the same as that per admission for patients with inactive extrapulmonary tuberculosis. Patients with active pulmonary tuberculosis visit tuberculosis institutions almost twice as often as those with inactive pulmonary tuberculosis, while the attendance per admission in the case of those with active extrapulmonary tuberculosis is a little more than half of that for patients with inactive extrapulmonary tuberculosis.

Age indexes of the outpatient attendance of the population for tuberculosis are interesting (Table 158).

From the table it is evident that the highest attendance for pulmonary tuberculosis is in the age groups from 40 to 49 and 50 to 59, while the lowest is in the group of 60 years and over. The highest attendance for extrapulmonary tuberculosis is in young adults.

The amount of hospital care depends both on the sickness rate and on the result of examinations. The complete standards for hospital care in the field of tuberculosis are given in Table 159.

Table 158
AGE INDEXES OF VISITATION RATE OF THE ADULT POPULATION TO PHYSICIANS IN OTHER SPECIALTIES FOR TUBERCULOSIS IN THE NEXT FEW YEARS (per 1,000 population)

Age groups	Pulmonary tuberculosis	Extrapulmonary tuberculosis
20—29 years		
visits actually made	42.98	5.71
added by experts	4.9	2.18
additional visits for cases detected at phrophylactic examinations	84.8	7.73
total	132.68	15.62
30—39 years		
visits actually made	51.24	13.09
added by experts	9.76	1.33
additional visits for cases detected at prophylactic examinations	68.2	13.2
total	129.2	27.62
40—49 years		
visits actually made	80.88	17.76
added by experts	12.05	1.59
additional visits for cases detected at prophylactic examinations	46.6	8.8
total	139.53	28.15
50—59 years		
visits actually made	59.22	1.44
added by experts	9.63	—
additional visits for cases detected at prophylactic examinations	68.1	—
total	136.95	1.44
60 years and over		
visits actually made	34.58	0.69
added by experts	13.14	0.69
additional visits for cases detected at prophylactic examinations	13.1	1.92
total	60.82	3.30

Table 159
STANDARDS OF HOSPITAL CARE OF THE POPULATION IN THE FIELD OF TUBERCULOSIS

Name of disease	No. of cases actually hospitalized			No. added by experts			New cases detected at medical examinations requiring hospital treatment			Total number of cases		
	men	women	both sexes	men	women	both sexes	men	women	both sexes	men	women	both sexes
Pulmonary tuberculosis	6.1	2.4	4.2	0.2	—	0.1	0.7	0.7	0.7	7.0	3.1	4.9
Extrapulmonary tuberculosis	0.9	0.9	0.9	—	0.1	0.05	—	—	—	0.9	1.0	0.95
Total	7.0	3.3	5.0	0.2	0.1	0.15	0.7	0.7	0.7	7.9	4.1	5.9

Standards of Therapeutic-Prophylactic Care of the Urban Population in the Field of Dermatovenereology

Total Morbidity of the Urban Population (according to sickness rate at the therapeutic-prophylactic institutions)

The average intensive indexes of total incidence of skin and venereal diseases in the population of five cities (as judged by sickness rate) are shown in Table 160.

The standardized indexes (composition of the urban population according to the 1959 census is taken as the standard) are not substantially different from the actual morbidity figures, which speaks for the absence of essential differences in age and sex composition of these cities compared with the data for the USSR as a whole.

Table 160
AVERAGE INCIDENCE OF DISEASES LARGELY UNDER THE CARE OF DERMATOVENEREOLOGISTS IN THE POPULATION OF FIVE CITIES

Disease	Per 1,000 population					
	No. of cases (admissions)			standardized figures		
	men	women	both sexes	men	women	both sexes
Skin diseases	60.7	47.4	53.3	60.8	45.5	52.2
These include:						
pyoderma	20.6	12.8	16.4	21.2	12.8	16.7
eczema	5.3	5.2	5.2	5.3	5.1	5.2
other skin diseases	34.8	29.4	31.7	34.3	27.6	30.3
Mycoses and other diseases	10.2	6.7	8.3	10.1	5.9	7.6

Table 161

AVERAGE AGE INDEXES FOR INCIDENCE (according to sickness rate) OF SKIN DISEASES,
FUNGUS DISEASES AND OTHER DISEASES IN THE POPULATION OF FIVE CITIES

(No. of admissions per 1,000 population of the corresponding age and sex)

Disease	Age groups								
	under 4 years			5–6 years			7–13 years		
	men	women	both sexes	men	women	both sexes	men	women	both sexes
Skin diseases	54.1	54.4	54.3	38.5	44.2	41.2	28.6	34.1	31.1
These include:									
pyoderma	26.2	23.7	24.9	17.3	18.7	18.0	11.2	13.6	12.4
eczema	4.0	2.6	3.4	2.1	1.9	2.1	1.0	1.4	1.2
other skin diseases	23.8	28.1	26.0	19.1	23.6	21.2	16.3	19.1	17.7
Mycoses and other diseases	6.2	5.4	4.9	7.1	4.4	5.8	6.8	4.4	5.6

Disease	Age groups								
	14–19 years			20–29 years			30–39 years		
	men	women	both sexes	men	women	both sexes	men	women	both sexes
Skin diseases	61.2	52.0	56.6	77.1	51.5	62.7	67.8	45.9	55.3
These include:									
pyoderma	23.8	14.7	19.4	24.9	14.9	20.0	24.5	11.5	17.4
eczema	2.3	2.9	2.5	5.1	5.4	5.2	7.2	6.7	6.9
other skin diseases	35.1	34.4	34.7	47.1	31.2	37.6	36.1	27.7	31.0
Mycoses and other diseases	5.4	4.8	5.2	28.8	8.3	13.0	11.9	8.5	10.1

Disease	Age groups								
	40–49 years			50–59 years			60 years and over		
	men	women	both sexes	men	women	both sexes	men	women	both sexes
Skin diseases	71.1	44.7	55.3	70.3	43.5	54.0	51.3	35.4	40.1
These include:									
pyoderma	2x.9	10.6	15.3	19.1	8.4	12.3	10.4	4.3	6.0
eczema	8.0	5.9	6.7	10.0	7.9	8.7	10.4	7.2	8.1
other skin diseases	41.2	28.2	33.3	41.2	27.1	33.0	30.6	23.9	26.0
Mycoses and other diseases	7.5	5.7	6.5	8.1	4.2	5.8	4.2	2.3	2.9

The highest number of admissions to dermatovenereological institutions occurs in the case of skin diseases. The average figure as a whole for the class of skin diseases is 53.3 per thousand. Among men this figure is higher (60.7 per thousand) than for women (47.4 per thousand).

Of the class of "Skin diseases," pyoderma and eczema were distinguished separately for study, because they are the cause of a considerable number of outpatient visits, and patients with eczema are comparatively frequently hospitalized.

The average figure for the incidence of pyoderma is 16.4 per thousand. In analysis a higher incidence in men than in women is noted (20.6 and 12.8 per thousand, respectively).

The average incidence of eczema is 5.2 per thousand; it is nearly the same for both sexes.

The admission rate for other skin diseases is 31.7 per 1,000 population (for men 34.8, for women 29.4 per thousand).

The age indexes for the population morbidity in the cities studied are shown in Table 161.

The total incidence of skin diseases in the under-4 age group is quite high (54.3 per thousand) and is nearly the same in boys and girls. At 13 years it drops, and then gradually rises again, reaching a maximum at 20–29 years, and drops considerably only in the 60 and over group.

The incidence of skin diseases in men, beginning with 20–29 and over, is $1\frac{1}{2}$ times higher than in women.

The incidence of pyoderma is highest under the age of 4 (24.9 per thousand); at the age of 60 and over it is least (6.0 per thousand). Under 13 years there is no essential difference between the incidence of pyoderma in boys and girls. Beginning with the age of 14, the incidence in men is $1\frac{1}{2}$–2 times higher than in women.

The incidence of eczema in children under the age of 4 is much higher ($1\frac{1}{2}$–2 times) than the incidence in older children (5–13 years). Beginning with the 20–29 age group, the incidence increases, reaching a maximum at 50–59 years (8.7 per thousand). In the age group 40–49 and over the incidence in men is higher than in women.

The incidence of other skin diseases is highest in the age group 20–29 years (37.6 per thousand). Beginning with this age, the incidence in men is higher than in women.

In Stupino, data of the population's sickness rate have been worked out for skin diseases as seen by physicians in various specialties. The proportion of diagnoses made by dermatovenereologists is very high (Table 162).

In the analysis of data on seasonality of the sickness rate of the population for various skin and venereal diseases, note should be taken of the increase in admissions for epidermophytosis and pyoderma during the autumn-winter season. As for eczema, the highest number of admissions occur during the winter months. For the other nosologic entities no particular variations connected with seasonality were noted.

Table 162
PROPORTION OF FIRST ADMISSIONS TO
DERMATOVENEREOLOGISTS FOR CERTAIN
SKIN DISEASES (in percent of total number of
admissions for these diseases)

Disease	% of admissions to dermato-venereologists
Trichophytosis	66.67
Microsporidiosis	100.0
Epidermophytosis	85.96
Miscellaneous fungus diseases	36.84
Pyoderma	51.41
Eczema	88.23
Neurodermatitis	61.11
Psoriasis	92.0
Lupus erythematosis	66.67
Scleroderma	66.66
Other skin diseases	75.37

Morbidity of the Urban Population According to Data of Complete Medical Examinations

Complete medical examinations of the population permit supplementing the total morbidity data (according to sickness rate) with data on the chronic diseases, for which the population did not seek medical care at all (although it was needed) or did not seek it in the year when the sickness rate was studied.

By complete medical examinations a large number of cases of fungus diseases were found (54.7 per 1,000 examined); of these the great majority were fungus diseases of the feet (55.7 per thousand population). In the examinations 34.3 per 1,000 were found to have skin diseases; of these 1.7 had pyoderma; 7.6, eczema; 25.0 per thousand, other skin diseases.

Among the newly detected cases an important place is occupied by patients with chronic diseases who need treatment (Table 163).

Patients with mycoses of the feet are constant sources of dissemination of the infection, and the incidence of epidermophytosis and rubrophytosis remains at a high level from year to year because of the impossiblility of taking the full routine therapeutic-prophylactic measures.

For successful control of fungus diseases of the feet timely detection and treatment of patients are needed, including the initial and abortive forms, and broad prophylactic measures need to be taken.

According to medical examination data of the population of Stupino, fungus

Table 163
PREVALENCE OF NEWLY DETECTED SKIN DISEASES IN COMPLETE EXAMINATIONS

Disease	Per thousand examined	
	No. of cases detected by medical examinations	total number of chronic cases needing medical care
Mycoses	54.7	52.0
Skin diseases	34.3	12.9
Pyoderma	1.7	0.1
Eczema	7.6	6.0
Miscellaneous skin diseases	25.0	6.8

diseases of the feet affect 5.2% of the population, because only the clinically manifest forms of these diseases were put on record. Therefore we included almost all cases of fungus diseases of the feet in the group of chronic cases.

In addition, of the group of skin diseases newly detected at examinations (34.3 per 1,000 examined) only 12.9 per thousand were included in the group of chronic cases requiring medical care (pyoderma, 0.1 per thousand; eczema, 6 per thousand; miscellaneous skin diseases, 6.8 per thousand).

Attendance of the Urban Population at Outpatient-Polyclinic Institutions for Therapeutic and Prophylactic Purposes

The rate and distribution of the total morbidity are determined chiefly by the attendance at outpatient-polyclinic institutions for therapeutic purposes. In addition, dermatovenereologists are doing considerable prophylactic work in investigating members of the families and persons in contact with patients with venereal and fungus diseases, investigating and bringing in for treatment persons who are sources of infection of patients who have interrupted treatment or declined it, observing patients with venereal and fungus diseases until they are cured, putting patients with disseminated skin disease under observation, offering consultations for persons sent by physicians in other specialties, etc. The entire work is conducted in accordance with the tenets, instructions and directives of the Ministry of Health.

The rate and distribution of the attendance at dermatovenereological institutions in the various cities are given for these cities in Table 164.

The number of admissions for skin diseases is 111.3 per 1,000 population, for mycoses and other diseases 27.2. Men visit dermatovenereologists more often. It should also be taken into account that visits for a number of other diseases are included in the group visiting dermatovenereologists only. The total number of visits to dermatovenereologists for all skin diseases is 63.1%; to internists, 6.15%; to

Table 164
ATTENDANCE OF THE URBAN POPULATION AT OUTPATIENT-POLYCLINIC
INSTITUTIONS FOR TREATMENT BY PHYSICIANS IN ALL SPECIALTIES
(per 1,000 population)

Disease	Visits actually made			Added by experts			Total		
	men	women	both sexes	men	women	both sexes	men	women	both sexes
Skin diseases	111.3	138.0	91.2	32.07	34.87	28.72	143.37	172.87	119.92
These include:									
pyoderma	13.2	16.2	10.9	8.82	10.53	7.43	22.02	26.73	18.33
eczema	14.5	15.5	13.8	5.7	4.77	5.49	20.5	20.27	19.29
miscellaneous skin diseases	83.6	106.3	66.4	17.55	19.57	15.8	101.15	125.87	82.2
Mycoses and other diseases	27.2	35.5	20.7	5.97	4.72	6.70	33.17	40.58	27.40
Total	138.5	173.5	111.9	38.04	39.95	35.42	176.54	213.45	147.32
This includes: visits to dermato-venereo-logists	108.2	—	—	37.3	—	—	145.5	—	—

surgeons, 14%; to ENT specialists, 1.3%; to ophthalmologists, 0.05%; to phthisiologists, 0.1%; to neuropathologists, 0.8%; to obstetrician-gynecologists, 0.2%; to pediatricians, 8.1%; to oncologists, 0.2%.

For the purpose of determining the number of visits needed in the outpatient treatment of patients, an expert analysis was made on the basis of the medical records for each disease. The clinical experts rendered their conclusions, taking into consideration the clinical picture of the disease, the therapeutic measures taken, their efficacy, etc., with the aim of determining the number of visits needed for complete care of the patient. Table 164 also shows the data on the number of visits actually made for treatment for each disease and the number added by the experts. As is evident from Table 164, the total number of visits actually made was 138.5 per 1,000 population. The number of visits added by the experts is 38.04 per thousand, while the total actually made and added by the experts is 176.54 per thousand.

The age indexes of attendance of the population for medical consultation purposes are shown in Table 166.

For the purpose of determining the population requirement of dermatovenereological care it is necessary to take into account also medical consultations that are rendered by dermatovenereologists to patients largely under the care of physicians in related specialties, as well as determination of the fraction of visits to other specialists made by patients with skin and venereal diseases.

Table 165
PROPORTION OF OUTPATIENT VISITS TO
DERMATOVENEREOLOGISTS FOR SKIN
DISEASES (in percent of total number of visits actually
made for these diseases)

Disease	% of outpatient visits to dermato-venereologists
Mycoses	83.0
Pyoderma	57.5
Eczema	92.1
Miscellaneous skin diseases	74.0

The number of visits for medical consultations to dermatovenereologists for other diseases is 17.27 per 1,000 population (on the average for five cities).

According to the data of the dermatovenereological dispensaries of Moscow, the minimum number of visits for rubrophytosis is 15; for epidermophytosis, 6; for trichomycosis, 10. For the calculations the relationships of the percentages of the various nosologic entities of mycoses in Stupino were used (mycoses of the feet, 67%; trichomycoses, 10.5%; other mycoses, 22.3%). The incidence of trichomycosis per 1,000 population is 0.68; for mycosis of the feet, 4.29, of which rubrophytosis comprises 40% (according to the figures of Professor Arievich, 50%; according to Moscow dispensary data, 30%; according to the Dermatovenereological Dispensary of the Lithuanian Republic, 48.9%; to the Dermatovenereological Dispensary of the Chelyabinsk Region, 79% (i.e., 1.7 per 1,000 population)): epidermophytosis, 60%, i.e., 2.59 per 1,000 population; miscellaneous mycoses, 1.43 per 1,000 population.

The total visits for trichomycosis is 6.8 (10×0.68); for epidermophytosis, 15.54 (6×2.59); for rubrophytosis, 25.5 (15×1.7). We took the average number of visits for the other mycoses from the calculations derived for the five cities (2.3) The total visits for the other mycoses was 3.29 (2.3×1.43). The total visits for all mycoses should amount to 51.13 ($6.8 + 15.54 + 25.5 + 3.29$).

The average number of visits per case of mycosis was 7.99 (or 8). According to the Stupino data, the attendance for pyoderma is 32.3 per thousand, while the morbidity is 14.2 per thousand, or 2.3 visits per case. The average number of visits per case of eczema is 3.57; for other skin diseases, 2.3.

In a similar manner the number of visits needed for the treatment of venereal disease was determined.

Aside from the visits for treatment, consideration should also be given to visits to dermatovenereologists for prophylactic purposes. Among these visits are examinations of schoolchildren, dispensary care of children admitted to school, prophylactic examinations of workers, examinations of adolescent workers, examinations of

Table 166

AGE INDEXES OF POPULATION ATTENDANCE FOR MEDICAL CONSULTATIONS
(No. of medical consultation visits per 1,000 population of the corresponding age and sex)

Disease	Age groups								
	under 4 years			5–6 years			7–13 years		
	men	women	both sexes	men	women	both sexes	men	women	both sexes
Skin diseases	73.5	85.9	79.5	34.5	63.5	47.8	31.3	48.9	37.5
These include:									
pyoderma	33.4	28.4	30.9	9.1	17.1	12.9	6.3	8.3	7.2
eczema	3.8	1.7	4.3	1.2	4.2	2.6	0.7	2.5	1.6
other skin diseases	36.4	55.8	44.2	24.1	42.2	32.4	24.3	33.2	28.7
Mycoses and other diseases	6.6	5.8	6.2	9.9	7.3	8.8	6.2	7.1	6.7

Disease	Age groups								
	14–19 years			20–29 years			30–39 years		
	men	women	both sexes	men	women	both sexes	men	women	both sexes
Skin diseases	125.6	105.6	116.2	211.3	102.7	147.3	148.5	107.2	123.9
These include									
pyoderma	12.4	7.2	9.9	21.5	12.7	16.5	20.2	11.4	15.3
eczema	10.2	7.8	9.2	14.2	13.4	13.6	20.6	24.8	22.3
other skin diseases	103.0	50.6	97.0	175.6	76.5	117.3	108.4	72.6	86.3
Mycoses and other diseases	9.8	17.2	13.6	104.5	48.0	72.9	36.9	17.7	25.2

Disease	Age groups								
	40–49 years			50–59 years			60 years and over		
	men	women	both sexes	men	women	both sexes	men	women	both sexes
Skin diseases	182.6	103.2	133.6	188.2	83.2	126.0	114.8	70.4	85.0
These include:									
pyoderma	13.4	10.6	11.7	20.7	12.5	16.7	8.8	2.1	4.0
eczema	24.1	20.0	21.5	36.8	13.2	22.4	24.1	11.9	15.7
other skin diseases	145.2	72.6	100.3	130.7	37.6	87.5	81.9	56.4	65.3
Mycoses and other diseases	16.8	17.0	16.8	18.0	13.4	15.2	3.8	2.9	3.2

public dining room workers, workers in children's institutions and municipal enterprises, examinations at the time of issuance of various certificates, checkups during the dispensary care of patients, and other prophylactic visits. Data on the frequency of prophylactic visits to dermatovenereologists are shown in Table 167.

In all, prophylactic visits to dermatovenereologists amounted to 59.97 per thousand population.

Table 167
VISITS TO DERMATOVENEREOLOGISTS OF
OUTPATIENT POLYCLINIC INSTITUTIONS FOR
PROPHYLACTIC PURPOSES (No. of visits per 1,000
population)

Type of prophylactic visit	No. of visits
Regular house calls to children under 1 year of age	—
Examinations of preschool children	0.4
Dispensary care of children entering school (7-year-olds)	1.38
Examinations of schoolchildren	18.76
Prophylactic examinations of workers	6.06
Examinations of adolescent workers	0.09
Examinations of pregnant women	—
Examinations of public dining room workers, workers in children's institutions and municipal enterprises	29.0
Issuance of various certificates	1.92
Checkups of patients during dispensary care	0.04
Other prophylactic visits	2.32
Total	59.97

Hospitalization of the Urban Population for Venereal, Fungus and Skin Diseases

Data on the hospitalization of the population of various cities in the dermatovenereological institutions are shown in Table 168.

From Table 168 it is evident that 2.5 per thousand population were actually hospitalized, including 3.7 per thousand men and 1.96 per thousand women. The most common cause of hospitalization is skin disease, 1.7 per 1,000 population. For all diseases men are hospitalized 1–2 times as often as women.

Table 169 reflects the average age indexes of hospitalization of the population of five cities.

Children under 4 years of age (2.2 per thousand) are most often hospitalized for all skin diseases. At the ages of 5–13 this figure drops by half, and beginning with 14

Table 168

HOSPITALIZATION RATE OF THE URBAN POPULATION IN DERMATOVENEREO-
LOGICAL DEPARTMENTS (No. of cases hospitalized per 1,000 population)

Disease	No. of cases actually hospitalized			No. added by experts			No. of cases actually hospitalized plus those added by experts		
	men	women	both sexes	men	women	both sexes	men	women	both sexes
Skin diseases	2.3	1.2	1.7	0.6	0.8	0.3	2.9	1.28	2.0
These include:									
pyoderma	0.7	0.4	0.4	0.1	—	0.04	0.8	0.4	0.44
eczema	0.6	0.3	0.4	0.4	0.08	0.22	1.0	0.38	0.72
other skin diseases	1.1	0.7	0.9	0.1	—	0.04	1.2	0.7	0.94
Mycoses and other diseases	1.4	0.21	0.9	0.1	0.08	0.08	1.5	0.83	0.98
Total	3.7	1.96	2.5	0.7	0.16	0.38	4.4	2.11	2.98

and continuing until 50–59 years it remains at almost the same level (2.1–1.9 per thousand).

Higher hospitalization rate figures for pyoderma are noted in children under 4 years of age (0.9 per thousand), which is connected with the comparatively high incidence of pyoderma at this age. In the age groups 5–6 and 7–13 the hospitalization rate drops to 0.1–0.2 per thousand and again rises to 0.7 per thousand at the age of 14–19. In subsequent groups it drops and remains at the 0.4–0.5 per thousand level, and at the age of 60 and over it amounts to 0.2 per thousand.

For a more correct idea of the population hospitalization requirement of dermato-venereological institutions, an expert analysis was made of the initial records. Table 168 shows the figures for the actual average hospitalization rate for the five cities, the additions made by the experts and sum of these (number of cases per 1,000 population).

The length of confinement to bed for skin and venereal diseases differs. Thus, on the average, patients were treated for 20.1 days for venereal diseases, 26.5 for mycoses, and 17.8 days for skin conditions. The average number of days spent in bed as a whole for the specialty is 21.4.

Standards of Therapeutic-Prophylactic Care of the Urban Population in the Field of Dermatovenereology

Aside from the sickness rate data, attendance and hospitalization rate data were also utilized on the cases detected in medical examinations in Stupino.

However, complete medical examinations of the whole population will evidently not be accomplished in the near future, and therefore in working out the standards

Table 169

AGE INDEXES OF HOSPITALIZATION IN THE DERMATOVENEREOLOGICAL DISEASE DEPARTMENT

(No. of cases hospitalized per 1,000 population of the corresponding age and sex)

Age groups

Disease	under 4 years			5–6 years			7–13 years			14–19 years			20–29 years		
	men	women	both sexes	men	women	both sexes	men	women	both sexes	men	women	both sexes	men	women	both sexes
Skin diseases	2.5	1.7	2.2	0.4	1.4	0.9	1.2	0.9	1.0	2.9	1.3	2.1	2.4	1.4	1.9
These include:															
pyoderma	1.4	1.3	0.9	0.1	0.1	0.1	0.3	0.2	0.2	1.4	0.6	0.7	0.7	0.5	0.4
eczema	0.9	0.05	0.5	0.4	0.07	0.3	0.1	0.1	0.1	—	0.1	—	0.6	0.3	0.6
other skin diseases	0.6	0.9	0.8	—	1.3	0.6	0.8	0.6	0.7	1.7	1.9	1.3	1.2	0.9	0.9
Mycoses and other diseases	0.6	0.25	0.4	1.1	0.3	1.0	1.3	0.9	2.0	0.6	0.55	0.5	2.4	1.15	1.5

Age groups

Disease	30–39 years			40–49 years			50–59 years			60 years and over			total		
	men	women	both sexes	men	women	both sexes	men	women	both sexes	men	women	both sexes	men	women	both sexes
Skin diseases	3.1	1.1	1.9	2.8	1.4	2.0	3.6	0.9	1.9	1.5	1.6	1.5	2.3	1.2	1.7
These include:															
pyoderma	0.7	0.4	0.4	1.0	0.5	0.5	1.5	0.2	0.5	0.8	0.17	0.2	0.7	0.4	0.4
eczema	0.7	0.5	0.6	1.0	0.4	0.6	1.3	0.3	0.6	0.9	0.7	0.9	0.6	0.3	0.4
other skin diseases	1.9	0.4	1.0	1.2	0.8	1.0	1.4	0.5	0.8	0.2	0.7	0.5	1.1	0.7	0.9
Mycoses and other diseases	1.3	0.92	0.9	0.9	0.7	0.7	2.1	0.08	0.7	1.9	0.1	0.4	1.4	0.7	0.9

we gave only partial consideration to the data on cases detected by medical examinations.

By taking advantage of the morbidity figures per 1,000 population for the five cities and the average number of visits per case, determined with consideration of the corrective factors based on data for the USSR, we derived the number of therapeutic visits to dermatovenereologists per 1,000 urban population.

The number of all visits for therapeutic purposes for the cases under the care of dermatovenereologists was 231.27 per 1,000 population (Table 170).

For every patient with venereal disease seeking medical care there are contacts among which the dermatovenereologists must detect the source of infection and those who may be infected through contact with the patient. At the time of the visit to the physician those who have been in contact with the patients and members of their families are investigated, and some of them receive preventive treatment.

According to the data of concurrent surveys of the activity of some of the dermatovenereological institutions for 1963, there are 3.3 persons in contact with every patient with syphilis who has been put on record for the first time in the current year. Of these, 50% receive two courses of preventive treatment (according to the treatment routines for syphilis); i.e., there are 30 visits to physicians for each person. The remaining persons in contact with him must visit the physician for examination 8 times on the average.

On the average there are 1.5 persons who have been in contact with the gonorrhea patient. Of these, 20% will have preventive treatment. These are mainly women with the clinical picture of chronic gonorrhea but in whom the gonococcus is not detected. They are treated like patients with chronic gonorrhea, and each of them makes an average of 20 visits. The others who have been in contact with the gonorrhea patients visit the physician merely for investigation (six visits, on the average).

For each patient with mycosis an obligatory investigation is made of the members of their family. On the average, the family consists of 3.5 persons (All-Union Population Census of 1959). Therefore, if we consider that each of the family contacts will, according to instructions, be examined three times, the total of such visits per 1,000 population will be 67.3 ($3.5 \times 6.4 \times 3$).

According to data for Stupino, 0.3 per 1,000 population is put on dispensary care for mycosis, 2.7 for eczema. In accordance with the instructions on methods of the Ministry of Health of the USSR dated September 9, 1961, there must be four dispensary visits per year, on the average, per patient. Therefore, there should be 1.2 visits for mycosis and 10.8 visits per 1,000 population for eczema.

According to the same instructions, patients with all forms of psoriasis and lupus erythematosus and the majority with neurodermatitis should be on dispensary care. Therefore we made calculations of the amount of work involved in the dispensary care of all patients with these diseases, the number of which was established on the basis of the Stupino morbidity data. Among the miscellaneous skin diseases in

Table 170

STANDARDS FOR THE URBAN POPULATION REQUIREMENT OF OUTPATIENT-POLYCLINIC CARE IN THE FIELD OF DERMATOVENEREOLOGY

Disease	Average morbidity figures for 5 cities	No. of visits for treatment per 1,000 population to the various specialists			Average number of visits to dermatovenereologists per case (with corrective factors)	No. of visits for treatment to dermatovenereologists for skin diseases per 1,000 population (with corrective factors)	No. of visits by contacts for examination and preventive treatment per 1,000 population	No. of dispensary visits	No. of prophylactic visits	No. of visits to dermatovenereologists for other diseases	Total visits to dermatovenereologists per 1,000 population
		actual	added by the expert	total							
Skin diseases	53.3	111.3	32.07	143.37							
These include:											
pyoderma	16.4	13.2	8.82	22.02	2.3	37.72		10.8			
eczema	5.2	14.5	5.7	20.2	3.57	18.6		16.72			
other skin diseases	31.7	83.6	17.55	101.15	2.3	72.91					
Mycoses and other diseases	8.3	27.2	5.97	51.17	69.8	112.04		1.2			
Total						231.27	88.7	28.7	59.97	17.27	425.9

Stupino the proportion of psoriasis, neurodermatitis, and lupus erythematosus is 13.2 per thousand. On the average for five cities there are 31.7 visits per 1,000 population for miscellaneous skin diseases, and 13.2% of this group corresponds to 4.18 per 1,000 population. The number of dispensary visits needed for these diseases will be 16.72. Therefore the total number of dispensary visits for mycosis and skin diseases together will come to 28.72 per 1,000 population.

The total number of prophylactic visits is 59.97 per 1,000 population, and the number of visits for other diseases is 17.27 per thousand. Therefore the total number of therapeutic-prophylactic visits to dermatovenereologists should amount to 425.9 per 1,000 population (Table 170).

In determining standards for the population requirement of hospital care, chiefly morbidity data were used according to the population's visits to dermatovenereological institutions for the five cities with corrections added by the experts. In all, 5.05 per 1,000 population need hospital treatment for skin and venereal diseases.

The average treatment period in the venereal disease department of the hospital is 20.1 bed-days, in the mycology department 26.5, and in the skin disease department 17.8. On the average, the patient spends 21.4 days in the dermatovenereological institution (Table 171).

Table 171

STANDARDS FOR HOSPITAL CARE OF THE URBAN POPULATION
IN THE FIELD OF DERMATOVENEREOLOGY

Disease	Morbidity judged by sickness rate (per 1,000 population)	Hospitalization rate (after the additional expert analysis) per 1,000 population
Skin diseases	53.3	2.6
These include:		
pyoderma	16.4	0.4
eczema	5.2	1.3
other diseases	31.7	0.9
Mycoses and other diseases	8.3	2.45
Total	51.6	5.05

Standards of Therapeutic-Prophylactic Care of the Urban Population in the Field of Logopedics

Total Prevalence of Speech Pathology According to Medical Examination Data

Data of the population sickness rate gathered on the basis of the initial medical records cannot be used in the study of speech pathology, because at present speech therapy in the medical institutions is not very satisfactory, and the population avails itself of it only for very serious speech disorders. The basic data used in making up the standards for the requirement of speech therapy can be only the material of mass examinations of the population.

We made medical examinations in conjunction with a group of other specialists. In the performance of the examinations the following problems were posed:

1) detection of all speech disorders found.

2) determination of the population's requirement of various types of speech therapy.

3) distinction of the forms of speech pathology requiring treatment by the logopedist only from those needing consultation with and medical care by a physician.

The examination was preceded by a population census of the districts under investigation on the basis of the house records of the housing offices. This afforded the opportunity to obtain some idea of the number of persons needing speech therapy per 1,000 population. For the examination two experimental districts of Stupino in the Moscow Region with a total population of 10,054 persons were used; a medical examination card was filled out for each person examined, and in the column "Logopedist's examination" all the speech pathology detected was entered. In the examination we took into account the following: 1) various types of dyslalia; 2) aphasia; 3) alalia; 4) various types of stammering; 5) speech of those who have

313

lost hearing later in life; 6) speech of deaf-mutes; 7) speech of the feeble-minded; 8) cluttering.

On completion of the examinations all the medical record cards were subjected to a careful analysis by experts. Consideration was given to the need for outpatient and hospital treatment. Separate consideration was given to the requirement of dispensary observation.

The medical examinations showed that for every thousand inhabitants there were 54.4 cases of different types of speech disorders (Table 172).

Most often encountered were simple dyslalia (25.8 per 1,000 persons examined), stammering (15.5), and complicated dyslalia (8.8). Less frequent were such speech disorders as cluttering, speech of the hard of hearing, alalia, aphasia and other speech disorders (respectively, 0.8, 0.7, 0.4, 0.3 and 1.3 cases per thousand). In planning logopedic care special attention should be given to the organization of care for stammering and the various types of dyslalia.

From Table 172 it is seen that the figures for the prevalence of speech disorders are substantially different in the different age and sex groups of the population. These types of speech disorders are most often seen in children of preschool, elementary and secondary school ages.

The number of cases of simple dyslalia per 1,000 children examined were: 134.6 from 5 to 6 years; 72.4 from 7 to 13; 24.4 from 14 to 19. In the older age groups the frequency of dyslalia falls considerably.

The number of cases of stammering per 1,000 children examined was: 11.0 from 5 to 6 years; 30.4 from 7 to 13; 22.6 from 14 to 19.

In the subsequent age groups the prevalence of stammering also falls appreciably. Most often it is seen at ages 7 to 13. This is explained apparently by the fact that during this period children enter school, where they have the opportunity to come into contact with a large group of their peers and respond during class sessions.

The data we obtained are in agreement with those of Yu. A. Florenskaya, *"Sovetskaya Nevropatologiya, Psikhiatriya i Psikhogigiena" (Soviet Neuropathology, Psychiatry and Mental Hygiene)*, Vol. 4, No. 2, pp. 160–167, 1935, who has also demonstrated that stammering and dyslalia are most often present at the preschool school ages. In her opinion, the "ascending growth curve of stammering crosses the descending curve of declining dyslalia."

Reduction of all speech disorders occurs at the ages of 30–39 but some speech disorders (of the aphasia type) are found more often after age 50, because aphasia occurs most often as a complication of internal diseases (hemorrhages, thrombosis of cerebral vessels, etc.).

The examination showed that men usually suffer more often from speech disorders than women. For example, the number of cases of stammering per 1,000 persons examined was 25.3 in men and 8 in women; the number of cases of complicated dyslalia was 12 in men and 6.2 in women.

Table 172

AGE INDEXES OF THE PREVALENCE OF SPEECH DISORDERS, ACCORDING TO THE DATA OF MEDICAL EXAMINATIONS OF THE POPULATION OF STUPINO (No. of cases per 1,000 population)

Age groups

Name of disease	under 4 years			5-6 years			5-13 years			14-19 years			30-29 years		
	both sexes	men	women	both sexes	men	women	both sexes	men	women	both sexes	men	women	both sexes	men	women
Stammering	3.3	6.3	—	11.0	13.5	8.8	30.4	44.5	15.8	22.6	28.9	15.4	19.8	37.0	7.8
Simple dyslalia	6.6	12.6	—	134.6	143.8	126.5	72.4	81.2	63.2	24.4	28.9	19.3	12.3	16.6	9.1
Complicated dyslalia	—	—	—	72.0	83.6	61.8	14.0	21.4	6.3	11.7	12.0	11.5	3.8	5.6	2.6
Aphasia	—	—	—	4.7	6.8	2.9	0.8	1.5	—	—	—	—	—	—	—
Alalia	—	—	—	—	—	—	—	—	—	—	—	—	3.8	5.6	2.6
Other speech disorders	—	—	—	—	—	—	1.6	3.1	—	—	—	—	—	—	—
Speech of those who become deaf late	—	—	—	—	—	—	—	—	—	—	—	—	2.3	1.9	2.6
Speech of deaf-mutes	—	—	—	—	—	—	1.5	—	—	—	—	—	0.8	1.9	—
Speech of the feeble-minded	—	—	—	—	—	—	—	—	—	—	—	—	—	—	—
Cluttering	—	—	—	—	—	1.6	0.8	—	1.5	—	—	—	0.8	—	1.3
Total	9.5	19.0	—	223.7	251.0	141.0	122.3	153.3	88.5	64.2	73.2	54.0	43.6	68.5	26.1

Name of disease	30-39 years			40-49 years			50-59 years			60 years and over			total		
	both sexes	men	women	both sexes	men	women	both sexes	men	women	both sexes	men	women	both sexes	men	women
Stammering	6.2	25.2	9.5	8.4	13.6	4.9	8.2	15.2	3.1	4.7	16.1	—	15.5	25.3	8.0
Simple dyslalia	8.4	6.9	9.5	6.6	9.1	5.0	3.6	2.2	4.7	6.4	10.8	4.6	25.8	31.3	21.5
Complicated dyslalia	1.5	2.3	0.9	—	—	—	0.9	2.2	—	—	—	—	8.8	12.0	6.2
Aphasia	—	—	—	—	—	—	—	—	—	—	—	—	0.3	0.2	0.4
Alalia	—	—	—	—	—	—	—	—	—	4.8	5.4	4.6	0.4	0.7	0.2
Other speech disorders	—	—	—	2.4	4.6	1.0	—	—	—	—	—	—	1.5	1.6	1.4
Speech of those who become deaf late	0.5	1.1	—	—	—	—	0.9	—	1.6	1.6	—	2.3	0.7	0.9	0.5
Speech of deaf-mutes	1.0	1.1	0.9	—	—	—	—	—	—	—	—	—	0.3	0.5	0.2
Speech of the feeble-minded	—	—	—	—	—	—	—	—	—	—	—	—	0.4	0.5	0.4
Cluttering	—	—	—	1.8	3.0	1.0	0.9	—	1.6	—	—	—	0.8	0.9	0.7
Total	28.5	37.8	21.6	19.3	30.4	12.0	14.6	19.6	22.0	17.6	32.2	11.4	54.5	73.6	39.3

The figures obtained are in agreement with the data given in the literature. For example, R. A. Khersonskaya (*Sotsial'nye problemy zaikaniya u detei (Social Problems of Stammering in Children)*. Medgiz. 1930) notes that stammering in boys is found about four times as often as in girls.

In describing in such detail the prevalence of speech pathology among the population, we used as a basis the fact that the work along these lines is being conducted for the first time. However, in comparing the standards for the need of logopedic care only those cases of speech pathology were used where special treatment was necessary.

Evaluation made by experts of the examination data, as well as the participation in the present examination of the population by various specialists, permitted evaluation of the speech pathology as secondary, the result of the basic disease. In a number of cases, for example, aphasia appeared in persons who had had cerebral hemorrhages, thromboses, emboli or skull injury, and speech disorders in those with manifest deafness, secondary stammering (after wartime injury), in those of middle or older age groups, etc.

In these cases we considered the speech pathology as a disease, but in calculating the standards we did not plan the full volume of logopedic care for patients, but considered it possible to limit ourselves to a single consultation by the speech therapist for this category of patients solving the problem of subsequent sessions with the logopedist.

Nor did we plan visits for treatment to the speech therapist for simple dyslalia in younger children, under the age of six, nor in persons over 60.

In determining the amount of logopedic care for patients with cluttering, we took into account only cases of possible transition of cluttering into stammering. No logopedic care was planned for complicated dyslalia in those over 40. For speech disorders of deaf-mutes we did not recommend either outpatient or hospital treatment by the logopedists, because patients with such pathology are sent to special institutions, where work is done to restore their speech function over several years. Speech therapy for the feeble-minded in the outpatient departments was recommended only in several cases where mental defectiveness was demonstrated (the diagnosis of the latter was made in cooperation with the psychiatrist).

Based on everything stated above, we showed that various types of outpatient logopedic care are needed in 38.8 cases out of 1,000 persons examined (55.7 in men and 21.2 in women). All the data on the need for outpatient treatment for the various types of speech pathology obtained in medical examinations of the Stupino population are given in Table 173.

Most common in the distribution of speech pathology requiring treatment is simple dyslalia (39.2); then comes stammering (37.1%), then complicated dyslalia (21.6%). The remaining forms of speech pathology (aphasia, alalia, speech of those who become deaf late, speech of the feeble-minded, cluttering) constitute 2.1% in total. The incidence of speech disorders needing various types of treatment varies in the different age and sex groups of the population. These differences are particularly noticeable for stammering and dyslalia. In both forms of pathology the greatest need of treatment is seen in children under 15 years. The need at this age in the case of dyslalia comes to 39.3 per 1,000 population examined; for stammering, 20.7 per 1,000 examined. Similar figures from 16 to 60 are, respectively, 10.1 and 5.6 per 1,000 population examined. For the other forms of speech pathology the highest requirement of treatment is also noted under the age of 15.

Table 173

PREVALENCE OF SPEECH DISORDERS REQUIRING OUTPATIENT TREATMENT (per 1,000 population)

Name of disease	Children under 15			From 16 to 60			Total		
	both sexes	men	women	both sexes	men	women	both sexes	men	women
Stammering	20.7	29.6	11.4	10.1	19.5	6.3	14.4	23.1	7.6
Simple dyslalia	39.3	44.1	34.2	5.6	7.0	4.7	15.2	19.2	12.0
Complicated dyslalia	25.6	30.3	20.7	1.6	2.3	1.1	8.4	12.0	6.0
Aphasia	—	—	—	0.1	0.2	—	0.1	0.2	—
Alalia	0.3	0.6	—	—	—	—	0.1	0.2	—
Speech of those who become deaf late	0.7	1.3	—	—	—	—	0.2	0.4	—
Speech of the feeble-minded	0.7	0.6	1.4	—	—	—	0.2	0.2	0.3
Cluttering	0.3	1.3	0.7	0.8	—	0.2	0.2	0.4	0.3
Total	87.6	107.8	68.4	18.8	29.0	12.3	38.8	55.7	21.2

In all age groups and in all the nosologic entities the treatment requirement is much higher for men than for women. The total need of outpatient treatment for men is 55.7 per 1,000 population examined; for women 21.2.

In the case of stammering the treatment requirement for men is 23.1 per 1,000 persons examined; for women, 7.6. In the case of dyslalia the analogous figures are, respectively, 19.2 for men and 12 for women.

The predominance of speech pathology in men also occurs in all other nosologic entities of speech pathology. These are the main patterns of the prevalence of speech pathology in the various age and sex groups of the population; they were taken into account in determining the need for outpatient-polyclinic care and hospitalization for the various forms of speech pathology.

Attendance at Outpatient-Polyclinic Institutions for Various Forms of Speech Pathology

In determining the need for outpatient attendance for the various forms of speech pathology, we used as a basis the data of the morbidity yielded upon examination and the frequency of the necessary visits for the various speech disorders. Having at our disposal the information on the need for outpatient treatment per 1,000 population for the various forms of speech disorders and knowing the best times for this treatment by the physician and the speech therapist, we determined the size of the premises needed for the outpatient-polyclinic institutions of the urban population for various speech disorders.

In determining the attendance we used the average and the optimum number of visits to the physician and logopedist in the various forms of speech pathology.

	Visits to the physician	Visits to the logopedist
Stammering	3	60
Simple syslalia	1	20
Complicated dyslalia	1	30
Aphasia	—	30
Alalia	2	30
Speech of those who become deaf late	1	30
Speech of the feeble-minded	—	30
Cluttering	1	30

Since, at present, care for patients with speech disorders is given by physicians and speech therapists, we considered it practical to represent the visitation rate to physicians who usually make the diagnosis, examine the patients, prescribe drug therapy and supervise the course of treatment, and to the logopedists who carry out the routine sessions of speech correction.

In planning three visits to physicians for stammering, we used as a basis the fact that the first visit is necessary for making the diagnosis, prescribing drug treatment and for sessions with the logopedist; the second, for observation of the course of treatment; and the third, for checking on the treatment given.

Based on our work experience we determined that 60 visits to the logopedist are needed, because the treatment of stammering requires long sessions.

We believe that this number of visits is best and is possible at the present time. For the various forms of dyslalia, aphasia, and cluttering only one visit to the physician is being planned.

When there is further need for observation by a physician, a consultation with the physician may be recommended.

For alalia two visits to physicians are needed, in view of the fact that children who need careful observation of their general state of health most often have this disorder.

Visits to physicians for speech of the feeble-minded (mental defectives) are not being planned at all, because such patients are usually examined and observed by the psychiatrist.

On the basis of the data we determined the required volume of outpatient-polyclinic care for the various speech disorders (Table 174).

Table 174

AVERAGE AGE INDEXES FOR THE REQUIREMENT OF VISITS TO THE SPEECH THERAPIST AND THE LOGOPEDIST IN THE OUTPATIENT-POLYCLINIC INSTITUTIONS FOR SPEECH DISORDERS (per 1,000 of the population examined)

Name of disease	Age groups												Total visits					
	under 15						from 16 to 60						to physician			to logopedist		
	visits to physician			visits to logopedist			visits to physician			visits to logopedist								
	both sexes	men	women	both sexes	men	women	both sexes	men	women	both sexes	men	women	both sexes	men	women	both sexes	men	women
Stammering	62.1	88.8	34.2	1242.0	1796.0	684.0	30.5	58.5	18.9	804.0	1398.0	408.0	43.2	63.9	22.8	864.0	1386.0	456.0
Simple dyslalia	39.3	44.1	34.2	786.0	882.0	684.0	5.6	7.0	4.7	112.0	140.0	94.0	15.2	19.2	12.0	304.0	384.0	240.0
Complicated dyslalia	25.6	30.3	20.7	768.0	909.0	621.0	1.6	2.3	1.1	48.0	69.0	33.0	8.4	12.0	6.0	252.0	360.0	180.0
Aphasia	—	—	—	—	—	—	—	—	—	—	—	—	—	—	—	—	—	—
Alalia	0.6	1.2	—	18.0	36.0	—	—	—	—	3.0	6.0	—	0.2	0.4	—	2.7	6.0	—
Speech of those who become deaf late	0.7	0.7	—	21.0	21.0	—	—	—	—	—	—	—	0.4	0.8	—	8.0	16.0	—
Speech of the feeble-minded	—	—	—	21.0	21.0	—	—	—	—	—	—	—	0.4	0.8	—	6.0	6.0	9.0
Cluttering	0.3	1.3	0.7	9.0	39.0	21.0	0.8	—	0.2	24.0	—	6.0	0.2	0.4	0.3	6.0	12.0	9.0
Total	128.6	166.5	89.8	2865.0	3701.0	2052.0	38.3	67.8	24.9	991.0	1624.0	541.0	67.6	102.5	41.1	1445.7	2176.0	894.0

As is evident from Table 174, with the existing level of speech pathology, 67.6 visits to the physician and 1,445.7 visits to the logopedist are necessary per 1,000 of the urban population.

The highest number of visits for therapeutic purposes is for stammering, 43.2 per 1,000 to the physicians and 864 per 1,000 to the logopedist; for simple dyslalia, 15.2 and 304, respectively.

The number of visits for complicated dyslalia is considerable: 8.4 per 1,000 to the physician and 252 to the logopedist.

The lowest number of visits is noted for speech pathology of the alalia type, for speech of those who become deaf later in life, and for cluttering (the number of visits are, respectively, 0.2, 0.4 and 0.2 per 1,000 population to the physician and 2.7, 8 and 6 per 1,000 to the logopedist).

In the various age and sex groups of the population there is an essential difference in the attendance at outpatient-polyclinic institutions for therapeutic purposes. The table shows that the highest number of visits for therapeutic purposes is noted in children from 0 to 15 years of age. Visits to the physician by children of this age amount to 128.6 per 1,000 population examined; to the logopedist, 2,865. At ages 16 to 60 this figure drops considerably: 38.3 to the physician and 991 to the logopedist.

In all age groups the rate of visitation by men is greater than by women. In children from 0 to 15 years of age the rate of visits to the physician by boys is 166.5 per 1,000 children examined and by girls 89.8; visits to the logopedist by boys 3,701 and by girls 2,052. Approximately the same relationship exists in persons from 16 to 60 years of age.

The attendance for various forms of speech pathology is substantially different in the various age groups. The highest number of visits for stammering in both boys and girls is noted from 0 to 15 years of age (88.8 and 34.2 visits, respectively, per 1,000 population to the physician and 1,796 and 684 visits to the logopedist).

In the older age groups, from 16 to 60, this figure drops and amounts to 58.5 and 18.9 visits to the physician per 1,000 population and 1,398 and 408, respectively, to the logopedist.

For simple dyslalia a higher attendance is also noted from 0 to 15 years of age. The number of visits to the physician for simple dyslalia is 44.1 per 1,000 examined in boys and 34.2 in girls. From 16 to 60 the figures are, respectively, 7 in boys and 4.7 in girls.

For complicated dyslalia, from 0 to 15 years of age the number of visits to the physician is 30.3 per 1,000 boys examined and 20.7 for girls. These figures are considerably lower from 16 to 60 years of age, being, respectively, 2.3 visits to the physician by men and 1.1 by women.

In all the other forms of speech pathology a predominance of visits by children from 0 to 15 years of age is also noted at the outpatient-polyclinic institutions. All this once again convinces us of the need for a more careful prevention and treatment of speech disorders in preschool and schoolchildren.

Need for Hospitalization in the Various Forms of Speech Pathology

In examinations of the Stupino population we showed the need for hospitalization for speech pathology. Of the group of chronic cases newly detected (Table 175), we used only two nosologic entities of diseases, stammering and alalia, for which hospital treatment was recommended. For all the other forms of speech pathology we advise outpatient treatment.

Table 175

STANDARDS FOR THE URBAN POPULATION REQUIREMENT OF HOSPITALIZATION

Name of disease	Age groups						Total		
	from 0 to 15			from 16 to 60					
	both sexes	men	women	both sexes	men	women	both sexes	men	women
Stammering	2.1	3.4	0.7	—	—	—	0.5	1.1	0.1
Alalia	1.0	2.0	—	—	—	—	0.3	0.6	—
Total	3.1	5.4	0.7	—	—	—	0.8	1.7	0.1

The total hospitalization requirement for speech pathology is 0.8 per 1,000 population examined. In the distribution of patients hospitalized for speech pathology, the highest proportion is shown by those with stammering (0.5 per 1,000 population). The hospitalization requirement is higher among men than among women. The hospitalization figures per 1,000 persons of the corresponding sex are 1.7 and 0.1.

There is an essential difference in the hospitalization rate of the population of both sexes in the other diseases also. Thus, for stammering men need more hospital treatment (1.1 per 1,000 population). The hospitalization rate of women for this condition is much lower (0.1 per 1,000 population).

The hospitalization rate differs in the various age groups. Taking into consideration the fact that among those with speech pathology there are more children and adolescents under the age of 15, we considered it practical to divide the hospitalization requirement into that for children and adolescents from 0 to 15 and that for adults from 16 to 60. According to our data, the adult population (from 16 to 60) does not need hospitalization, for the most part. The total hospitalization requirement for stammering in the case of children and adolescents from 0 to 15 years of age is 2.1 per 1,000 population.

The hospitalization requirement for alalia applies only to children and is 1 per 1,000 population.

It is assumed that in the future, when regular dispensary observation of preschool children is organized and when there is smooth operation of a system of children's day hospitals, the figures for those needing hospitalization for speech pathology will drop even further through elimination of speech disorders in early childhood. These factors must be taken into account in making up the standards for the logopedic care requirement in general outlines for the future.

Standards of Therapeutic-Prophylactic Care of the Urban Population in the Field of Logopedics

An analysis of the cases of speech pathology demonstrated by examinations makes it possible to approach working out the standards for the population requirement of outpatient-polyclinic and hospital care for the next few years and may serve as the basis for long-range planning of public health.

Considering the fact that the data for the incidence of speech pathology cannot be basic for working out standards, we shall use as a basis essentially the medical examination data. All cases of speech pathology demonstrated by medical examinations and requiring various types of specialized care are presented in Table 176.

Table 176

REQUIREMENT OF VARIOUS TYPES OF SPECIALIZED MEDICAL CARE FOR 1965–1970 (per 1,000 population)

Name of disease	No. of cases of speech disorders	Of these		No. of visits to physician required
		those needing outpatient therapy	those needing hospital treatment	
Stammering	15.5	14.4	0.5	43.2
Simple dyslalia	25.8	15.2	—	15.2
Complicated dyslalia	8.8	8.4	—	8.4
Aphasia	0.3	0.1	—	—
Alalia	0.4	0.1	0.3	0.1
Speech of those who become deaf late	0.7	0.2	—	0.4
Learned speech in deaf-mutes	0.3	—	—	—
Speech of the feeble-minded	0.4	0.2	—	—
Cluttering	0.8	0.2	—	0.3
Total	54.5	38.8	0.8	67.6

In calculating the population requirement of therapeutic care for stammering we took as a basis the fact that almost all cases of stammering need various types of care (with the exception of a very small number, 0.6 per 1,000). We included persons over 50 in the latter group; in them stammering appeared as the result of wartime injury and they adapted themselves, for the most part, to their speech defect. This category of persons is under the observation of neuropathologists and does not need special logopedic treatment.

We included all children with various speech disorders (incorrect pronunciation of vowels and consonants, various types of lisping—nondental, labiodental, lateral fricative, and nasal) in the group with simple dyslalia.

Considering the fact that the time needed for formulating the sounds by these patients ranges from two to four weeks, we used one visit to the physician and 20 to the logopedist as the number to be used for this condition.

Children with considerable speech disorders, in whom the pronunciation of syllables and words was distorted to the point of complete or partial incomprehensibility, were included in the same group.

The number of visits for this type of speech pathology was determined from the calculation of one visit to the physician and 30 to the logopedist; this, comes, respectively, to 8.4 visits per 1,000 population to the physician and 232 visits per 1,000 to the logopedist.

In our investigations aphasia was encountered only in elderly persons (aged 60 and over). Usually all these patients were observed by neuropathologists and internists; therefore, they did not need visits to the speech therapist but they all had to visit the logopedist, because it is well known that logopedic work with patients of this age is very effective and assists in the rapid and complete restoration of speech function. The total number of visits to the logopedist in examinations of the population is 3.0 per 1,000.

The number of outpatient visits to the physician for alalia is 0.2 and to the logopedist, 7.0 per 1,000 population.

In the group "Speech of those who become deaf late" we included cases of hearing loss in persons in whom speech had already been developed. The speech of such patients frequently becomes ungrammatical and needs appropriate observation and treatment. The number of visits to the physician for this pathology is 0.4 per 1,000 population; to the logopedist, 6.0 per 1,000 population.

The speech of deaf-mutes may become sufficiently understandable to those around them through sessions with the logopedist. However, this work is protracted and is conducted in special schools; therefore, for this form of speech pathology we did not plan either outpatient visits to logopedists or hospital treatment.

Feeble-minded patients need essentially treatment and observation by neuropathologists and psychiatrists, but sessions with such patients (usually mental defectives) are sometimes effective. We did not plan visits to the speech therapist for this pathology, considering that the examination by the psychiatrist would be sufficient. Six visits to the logopedist were planned per 1,000 population examined.

For cluttering, outpatient visits to the physician and logopedist were recommended only in those cases in which this cluttering showed a tendency to turn into stammering. The number of such visits is 0.2 per 1,000 population to the physician and six per 1,000 population to the logopedist.

From what has been stated, it follows that the total number of visits necessary for speech pathology is 67.6 per 1,000 population to the physician and 1,445.7 per 1,000 population to the logopedist.

The largest amount of outpatient-polyclinic care is for those with pathology of the stammering and simple dyslalia types (864 and 319.2 visits per 1,000 population, respectively).

At present, the therapeutic visits to the physician for speech pathology are distributed among the neuropathologist, otorhinolaryngologist, and pediatrician. Apparently, it would be more practical even at present to have speech therapists who would concentrate particularly on the treatment of persons with various forms of speech pathology. Work experience with patients with speech pathology emphasizes the idea that speech therapy staffs are best trained from the group of neuropsychiatrists.

Through medical examinations we demonstrated the fact that of the group of patients with various forms of speech pathology 0.8 per 1,000 population need hospital treatment; this includes 0.5 per 1,000 population for stammering and 0.3 per 1,000 population for alalia (Table 177).

Table 177
STANDARDS FOR THE URBAN POPULATION
REQUIREMENT OF HOSPITALIZATION IN THE SPEECH
THERAPY DEPARTMENT FOR 1965–1970
(per 1,000 population)

Name of disease	No. of cases of speech pathology	Hospitalization requirement	Average number of bed-days
Stammering	15.5	0.5	60
Alalia	0.4	0.3	60
Total	15.9	0.8	60

These figures are perfectly feasible for calculations for the next few years (1965–1970). Subsequently, by virtue of the more extensive development of dispensary care of the healthy population, the hospitalization requirement for speech pathology will apparently decrease, because the less marked forms of speech disorders can usually be eliminated by outpatient care if they are diagnosed in time.

It should be stated, however, that the standards of therapeutic-prophylactic care of the population proposed for logopedics for 1965–1970 will be practical in the event of organization of mass medical checkups of the population in the next few years, during the course of which all forms of speech disorders can be demonstrated.

Even at present organized groups of preschool children (nurseries and kindergartens) as well as schoolchildren undergo regular medical checkups, and the speech disorders can be detected in the majority of the children. Because the largest number of persons with various speech disorders is seen specifically in the children's age groups, the standards proposed for therapeutic-prophylactic care in the field of logopedics will not be an overestimate to any great degree.

Standards of Sanatorium–Health Resort Care
of the Urban Population

Sanatorium-health resorts occupy one of the most important places in the system of measures for the prevention and treatment of various diseases. The efficacy of treatment at sanatorium-health resorts is not inferior and in many cases is even superior to hospital treatment, and for this reason the number of sanatorium-health resorts in the USSR is steadily increasing.

Before the revolution, Russia had only 60 sanatoriums with a total of 3,000 places, but by 1964 the Soviet Union already had over 4,000 sanatorium-health resorts used annually by as many as 5,500,000 people. The health resorts of the Caucasian Mineral Waters alone annually provide treatment for some 500,000 persons.

The CPSU program adopted by the 22nd Party Congress calls for complete fulfillment of the needs of the USSR population in all kinds of medical services including sanatorium-health resorts. The CPSU calls for free sanatoriums and free medicines in addition to the already existing free medical services, *Materialy XXII s"ezda KPSS (Proceedings of the 22nd Congress of the CPSU)*, p. 392, Gospolitizdat, 1961.

Therefore, elaboration of various aspects of long-range planning of sanatorium-health resort services is of prime importance.

The most difficult aspect of long-range planning lies in working out the standards of the population's requirement of this kind of service, and yet the efficient use of the existing and planned sanatoriums is dependent upon these standards.

The question of these standards has been discussed in the literature by G. A. Nevraev, M. V. Ovchinskii, G. M. Danishevskii, M. M. Mazur, G. A. Novgorodtsev, G. A. Popov and others.

The earliest proposals concerning the sanatorium-health resort requirements for workers in the textile, chemical, and metallurgical industries in relation to different diseases were elaborated by G. A. Nevraev and M. V. Ovchinskii, *Osnovy sotsial'noi kurortologii (Principles of Social Theory of Health Resorts)*, Vol. 1, 1932. The standards calculated by these authors were based on data furnished by commissions for

326

selection of patients for health resorts, outpatient investigations, and published morbidity data for Moscow.

On the basis of selection frequency of patients for sanatorium-health resorts and from among laborers and employees in major industrial cities of the RSFSR who were on dispensary record (some 60,000), M. M. Mazur, "Potrebnost' naseleniya RSFSR v sanatorno-kurortnoi pomoshchi" (RSFSR Population's Requirement of Sanatorium-Health Resort Services), *Zdravookhranenie Rossiiskoi Federatsii,* No. 2, 1959, concluded that sanatorium-health resort treatment was needed by 65.5 persons per 1,000 adult population on the average for the RSFSR.

Providing such services called for 4.76 beds per 1,000 urban population, including 1.07 beds for patients suffering from circulatory diseases, 0.66 for those with digestive diseases, 0.33 for those with nervous diseases, 0.33 for those with diseases of the locomotive-supporting systems, and 0.27 for patients with respiratory diseases (of nontuberculous etiology).

According to G. A. Novgorodtsev and G. A. Popov "Ocherednye zadachi planirovaniya zdravookhraneniya" (Current Tasks in the Planning of Health Services), *Sovetskoe Zdravookhranenie,* No. 8, 1933, 3 sanatorium beds are required per 1,000 population.

The 20-year long-range plan for the development of the health services devised by the Hungarian Ministry of Health recommends 2.2 beds in sanatorium-health resorts for chronic patients (Laszlo Czerba, "Nekotorye voprosy 20-letnego perspektivnogo plana razvitiya bol'nits v Vengrii" (Some Aspects of the 20-Year Long-Range Plan for Chronic Patients), *VI Soveshchanie ministrov zdravookhraneniya sotsialisticheskikh stran.* Budapest. 1963).

A. Ya. Kurakov "Organizatsiya sanatorno-kurortnoi pomoshchi v Voronezhskoi oblasti" (Sanatorium-Health Resort Services in the Voronezh Region), *Sovetskoe Zdravookhranenie,* No. 11, 1963, on the basis of morbidity data for the adult population in the Voronezh Region in 1960, calculated the requirements for treatment at sanatorium-health resorts for cardiovascular patients (22.5 per 1,000 population) and those with digestive diseases (13.2).

According to Mazur and Kurakov, the differences in the population's requirement of sanatorium-health resort services are apparently due to the authors' different approaches to indications for sanatorium-health resort treatment and nonhomogeneous data on the population's morbidity at these authors' disposal.

We used data on the frequency of the population's requests for medical aid, supplemented with data from medical examinations of the population, as our starting data for working out standards of sanatorium-health resort services for the urban population.

The city of Stupino was chosen as the experimental base for determination of corrective factors for the larger body of data collected in five cities located in different climatic and geographical zones.

Primary records of medical institutions cannot be used to the full extent in determining the population's requirement of sanatorium-health resort services. The existing records are limited to information (far from complete) on the frequency of patients' visits to physicians for filling out sanatorium-health resort cards. This is obviously an inadequate basis for the determination. Case histories of patients who received treatment at health resorts are likewise unsuitable, because at present the vouchers for sanatoriums are not always used by those really in need of treatment at health resorts. Therefore, the need for sanatorium-health resort services was determined by experienced clinicians who continuously consulted an expert on health resorts. The examination took into account the data on the incidence of hospitalization and outpatient visits, which permitted determination of the severity of a disease in each specific case.

The need for sanatorium-health resort services was determined simultaneously with the requirement of hospitalization and treatment at night preventoria, since these types of medical aid are to a certain extent interchangeable.

Those in need of sanatorium treatment were distributed according to the specialization of sanatoriums and their location (local sanatoriums or health resorts with special curative agents, such as mineral waters, muds, etc.). All patients needing (in the experts' opinion) treatment at sanatoriums and health resorts were divided into the following groups:

1) follow-up treatment of tuberculosis;
2) treatment of chronic gastrointestinal diseases;
3) treatment of chronic cardiovascular diseases in sanatoriums with special balneological facilities;
4) treatment of chronic and cardiovascular diseases in local sanatoriums;
5) follow-up treatment of children following acute forms of rheumatic fever;
6) treatment of children suffering from chronic pneumonia and suppurative diseases of the lungs;
7) treatment of children with rheumatic heart defects;
8) treatment of patients with neuroses, neurosthenias and other functional diseases of the nervous system, including children suffering with logoneuroses, at sanatoriums with special balneological facilities;
9) treatment of patients with neuroses, neurosthenias, and other functional diseases of the nervous system, including children suffering from logoneuroses at local sanatoriums;
10) treatment of urolithiasis, chronic cystitis, and other urinary tract diseases;
11) diseases of the locomotive-supporting systems;
12) women with chronic genital diseases;
13) treatment at other kinds of sanatoriums.

In their selection of patients for treatment at sanatorium-health resorts, the physicians serving as experts assumed that the following groups of patients were in need of these services:

1) many of the patients who had been hospitalized for protracted (chronic) disease except in cases of complete recovery following operation;

2) patients suffering from protracted (chronic) diseases without a clear clinical picture, who did not require hospitalization (chronic gastritis, chronic, sluggish cholecystitis, early stages of hypertension, cardiovascular neurosis, etc.).

All these patients recognized by the experts to be in need of treatment at health resorts were distributed among various sanatoriums according to their location (local sanatoriums or those with special therapeutic facilities) and specialization. This is especially important for cardiovascular patients, for many of whom balneological treatment is contraindicated or on whom the journey to the resort and the change of climate may have a detrimental effect. In these cases the experts recommended treatment at local (surburban) sanatoriums providing the necessary physiotherapy and medicaments in addition to diet and curative physical exercises.

The local sanatoriums have been recommended primarily for patients following a myocardial infarction, those suffering from angina pectoris with frequent attacks, patients recently recovering from stomach operations, those suffering from early stages of rheumatic fever following an attack, rheumatic heart failure with circulatory disturbance, or other diseases.

The requirement of sanatorium-health resort treatment for patients suffering from different diseases was based on existing instructions for selection of patients for sanatorium-health resorts and indications and contraindications for treatment there, *Rukovodstvo dlya vrachei po sanatorno-kurortnomu otboru* (*Physicians' Manual for Selection of Patients for Treatment at Sanatorim-Health Resorts*), L.G. Gol'dfail, Editor, Medgiz. 1961.

The need for treatment at sanatorium-health resorts was determined by the clinical experts in collaboration with experts on health resorts, based on the cards collected for each patient providing information on sickness rate, hospitalization, outpatient visits, and comprehensive medical examinations.

The information thus collected enabled us to determine the number of patients in need of sanatorium-health resort treatment (according to the disease and the type and location of sanatoriums) per 1,000 population of different age and social grouping.

According to our data, the need for sanatorium-health resort services (sanatoriums and polyclinics at health resorts) is 91.7 per 1,000 population.

For patients suffering from different diseases (per 1,000 population) this requirement is shown in Table 178, based on the data for Stupino.

The highest requirement of such treatment was determined among patients with various digestive complaints, 28.7 per 1,000 population, and the largest proportion of these patients suffered from various forms of chronic gastritis (19.7‰), gastric and duodenal ulcers (4.3‰), and diseases of the liver and biliary tracts (3.6‰).

Table 178

REQUIREMENT OF SANATORIUM-HEALTH RESORT TREATMENTS IN THE CASE OF DIFFERENT DISEASES (per 1,000 population)

Disease	Incidence of chronic diseases	No. of patients in need of sanatorium-health resort services
1. Infectious diseases	10.3	6.2
These include:		
tuberculosis of respiratory and other organs	8.5	5.8
2. Rheumatic fever	13.2	7.1
This includes:		
rheumatic heart failure	10.9	5.9
rheumatic polyarthritis	1.2	0.5
3. Metabolic and allergic diseases	2.4	1.0
These include:		
diabetes mellitus	0.5	0.3
4. Endocrine diseases	11.3	0.4
These include:		
thyroid diseases	10.9	0.4
5. Diseases of the nervous system	42.9	14.3
These include:		
cerebral atherosclerosis and other vascular lesions, with the exception of hypertension and cerebral hemorrhage	1.5	0.2
lumbosacral radiculitis and sciatica	14.9	6.2
neuroses	22.8	7.1
6. Eye diseases	2.6	0.3
These include:		
glaucoma	0.5	0.3
7. Otorhinolaryngological diseases	50.9	0.6
8. Respiratory diseases	12.9	2.3
These include:		
chronic suppurative diseases of the lungs (chronic pneumonia, bronchoectatic disease)	1.8	1.0
pulmonary fibrosis, emphysema	5.3	0.5
9. Circulatory diseases	67.4	19.9
These include:		
cardiac valvular defects	1.8	1.0
myocardial fibrosis from atherosclerosis	14.3	2.8
hypertension in stages I, II, III	14.2	9.1
varicose veins	2.9	0.1
cardiovascular neurosis	8.5	3.0
10. Digestive diseases	57.0	28.7
These include:		
chronic gastritis	32.2	19.7
gastric and duodenal ulcers	6.1	4.3
intestinal diseases	4.3	0.9
chronic hepatitis and hepatic cirrhosis	0.9	0.6
other diseases of the liver and biliary tracts	9.3	3.0
11. Diseases of the bones, muscles and joints	21.3	3.1
12. Skin diseases	7.5	1.0
These include:		
eczema	3.4	0.8
psoriasis	1.0	0.2
13. Renal and urinary diseases	6.0	2.2
14. Women's diseases	47.2	3.1

Circulatory diseases follow diseases of the digestive organs (19.9 cases per 1,000 population) in importance with regard to the need for sanitorium-health resort treatment.

Patients with various stages of hypertension (9.1‰) account for about 50% of all persons suffering from circulatory diseases and requiring sanatorium-health resort treatment. Of these, 8.4 per 1,000 population show stages I and II of hypertension and only 0.7 per 1,000 population stage III (most of these need treatment at local sanatoriums).

The need for sanatorium treatment among cases of myocardial fibrosis from atherosclerosis amounts to 2.8 cases per 1,000 population, and 3 cases per 1,000 population among persons suffering from cardiovascular neuroses.

Sanatorium-health resort treatments were recommended for 14.3 cases of nervous diseases per 1,000 population, including 7.1‰ neurotic patients and 6.2‰ patients suffering from diseases of the peripheral nervous system.

Determination of the relative proportion of patients in need of sanatorium-health resort treatment is of special interest in the case of some common diseases.

Table 179 provides comparative data on relative requirement of sanatorium-health resort services for some individual diseases according to Mazur and our own material obtained at Stupino (Moscow Region).

Table 179 shows there is agreement between Mazur's and our data, or else only negligible discrepancies with respect to the requirement of sanatorium-health resort

Table 179

COMPARATIVE DATA ON THE RELATIVE REQUIREMENT OF SANATORIUM-
HEALTH RESORT SERVICES FOR INDIVIDUAL DISEASES ACCORDING TO MAZUR
AND OUR OWN MATERIAL ON STUPINO IN THE MOSCOW REGION
(percentages of the number of cases)

Disease	Mazur's data	Our data on Stupino
Hypertension, myocardial fibrosis and other cardiovascular diseases	34	29.5
Peptic ulcers	48	70.4
Chronic gastritis	44	61.1
Chronic colitis	32	20.9
Diseases of the liver and biliary tracts	30	30.2
Nervous diseases	15	33.1
Diabetes mellitus	35	60
Rheumatic diseases	37	53.7
Diseases of bones and joints	30	14.5
Chronic bronchitis and other protracted diseases of the respiratory organs, of nontuberculous etiology	32	17.4
Renal and urinary diseases	33	36.6
Women's diseases	30	6.5
Skin diseases	12	13.3
Average	31.5	34.4

treatment for different diseases (cardiovascular, hepatic renal, urinary, etc.). There are significant discrepancies in only a few groups of diseases, and this can be attributed to different ways of selecting patients for treatment.

However, notwithstanding the differences in our data toward larger or smaller values, the relative percentages of the need for sanatorium-health resort services in the listed group of diseases are almost the same, 31.5% according to Mazur and 34.4% according to data for Stupino. The requirements by the different age and sex groups in the population are listed in Table 180.

Table 180

REQUIREMENT OF SANATORIUM-HEALTH RESORT
TREATMENT IN THE DIFFERENT AGE AND SEX
POPULATION GROUPS

Age group	No. of persons requiring treatment (per 1,000 population)		
	both sexes	men	women
Under 1 year	—	—	—
1–2 years	8.1	7.7	8.5
3–6 years	17.2	10.0	23.5
7–12 years	18.7	18.4	19.0
13–15 years	12.8	8.8	17.7
16–19 years	35.3	32.5	38.3
20–29 years	61.2	59.3	62.6
30–39 years	134.7	135.0	134.5
40–49 years	165.1	164.1	165.7
50–59 years	183.8	191.3	178.4
60 years and over	52.9	96.8	34.2
Total	91.7	88.6	94.6

The table shows that the highest relative requirement of sanatorium-health resort services occurred in the age groups 30-39 years (134.5‰), 40-49 years (165.7‰ and 50-59 years (178.4‰). This is readily understood in view of the increased incidence of cardiovascular (myocardial fibrosis from atherosclerosis, hypertension, etc.), digestive (chronic gastritis, colitis, etc.), nervous (atherosclerosis of cerebral vessels), and other classes of disease in the middle and older age groups. All these diseases can be successfully treated either in specialized balneological or in suburban sanatoriums.

The need for sanatorium-health resort treatment is approximately the same for both sexes, 38.6 per 1,000 men, 94.6 per 1,000 women.

Table 181 shows the distribution of patients in need of sanatorium-health resort treatment according to types of sanatorium.

Table 181

DISTRIBUTION OF PATIENTS IN NEED OF SANATORIUM-HEALTH RESORT TREAT-
MENT ACCORDING TO TYPES OF SANATORIUM

Type of sanatorium	No. of patients requiring treatment per 1,000 population			Percentage of total		
	both sexes	men	women	both sexes	men	women
1. For follow-up treatment of tuberculosis cases	6.0	7.3	5.0	6.5	8.2	5.2
2. For chronic gastrointestinal diseases	28.4	31.3	26.4	31.0	35.3	27.9
3. For chronic cardiovascular diseases (of general significance)	20.9	18.4	22.9	22.9	20.7	24.1
4. For follow-up treatment of children following acute rheumatic fever	0.4	0.2	0.5	0.4	0.2	0.6
5. For children with rheumatic heart defects	1.1	0.9	1.3	1.2	1.0	1.3
6. For children with chronic pneumonia and suppurative diseases of the lungs	1.4	1.1	1.6	1.5	1.3	1.7
7. For patients with neuroses, neurasthenias and other nervous diseases (of general significance)	6.8	3.6	9.2	7.4	4.1	9.7
8. For patients with urolithiasis and other urinary diseases	2.2	2.0	2.3	2.4	2.3	2.4
9. For patients with diseased locomotive-supporting system	10.6	12.7	9.0	11.6	14.3	9.5
10. For women with chronic genital diseases	3.0	—	5.3	3.2	—	5.6
11. Other	5.5	6.8	4.4	5.9	7.7	4.7
12. For chronic cardiovascular diseases (of local significance)	5.0	3.6	6.0	5.4	4.1	6.6
13. For patients with local neuroses, neurasthenias and other nervous diseases (of local significance)	0.7	0.7	0.7	0.8	0.8	0.7
Total	91.7	88.6	94.6	100.0	100.0	100.0

Of the total number of patients in need of sanatorium-health resort treatment, 31%
are assigned to sanatoriums for chronic gastrointestinal diseases.

Another 28.1% go to sanatoriums for chronic cardiovascular diseases, and 5.4% of
these to local sanatoriums specializing in these diseases. Similar percentages for
sanatoriums providing treatment for neuroses, neurasthenia, and other functional
diseases of the nervous system are 8.2 and 0.8%, respectively.

A relatively large number of patients are sent to sanatoriums for chronic diseases
of the locomotive-supporting systems (11.6%) and follow-up treatment of tuberculosis.

Of the total number of patients with circularory diseases that must be sent to sanatoriums (20.4 per 1,000 population) 14.8‰ are assigned to cardiological sanatoriums

providing balneological treatment, 4.7‰ to suburban sanatoriums for cardiovascular diseases without specific balneological facilities, 0.6‰ to sanatoriums designed for the treatment of neuroses and neurasthenias in cases of cardiovascular diseases closely related to nervous disturbances, and only 0.3‰ to sanatoriums of other specializations.

Sanatorium treatment for digestive diseases is needed by 28.9 cases per 1,000 population. Of these, 28.5‰ go to sanatoriums specializing in gastrointestinal diseases, while the rest may be treated at cardiological or other sanatoriums. This is understandable since, in most cases, the treatment of gastrointestinal diseases is only possible at specialized balneological institutions with the necessary equipment and personnel.

Sanatorium-health resort treatment was provided for 14.3‰ of patients with nervous diseases, of whom 5.8‰ needed special sanatoriums for the treatment of neuroses, neurasthenias, and other functional nervous disorders, while cardiovascular sanatoriums were recommended for 1.1‰ of cases in which the nervous disease affected the cardiovascular system. A fairly high percentage (6.4‰) of patients with nervous diseases must be treated at sanatoriums designed for diseases of the locomotive-supporting systems. These are patients with diseases of the peripheral nervous system (lumbosacral radiculitis, neuritis and sciatica, etc.).

The distribution of rheumatic patients requiring sanatorium-health resort services is of interest.

Of the 7.1‰ cases in need of sanatorium treatment, 4.1‰ were recommended to sanatoriums specializing in cardiovascular diseases, 0.4‰ to sanatoriums designed for follow-up treatment of children following rheumatic fever, 1‰ to sanatoriums for children with rheumatic heart defects, 0.6‰ to sanatoriums for patients suffering from diseases of the locomotive-supporting system, while the remainder of such cases were sent to other sanatoriums for prophylactic purposes.

Of the 6.2‰ suffering from diseases classed as infectious, 5.3‰ require treatment sanatoriums for tuberculosis of the respiratory and other organs, 0.6‰ in sanatoriums for diseases of the locomotive-supporting system, and the remainder of such cases in sanatoriums of other specializations.

The data on the percentage of cases in need of sanatorium health resort services determined by the experts at Stupino are essentially figures that can be used for determining the standards of requirement for this kind of medical service when applied to large-scale data on urban population morbidity.

Calculations of the requirement of sanatorium-health resort services were based on morbidity data for five cities with a total population of about 1.5 million, situated in different climatic and geographical zones of the USSR (Rubezhnoe, Dneprodzerzhinsk, Kopeisk, Stupino, Chelyabinsk).

The urban population's requirement of sanatorium-health resort services, based on the morbidity (calculated from sickness rate) of inhabitants of the five cities according to the different groups of chronic diseases, is shown in Table 182.

Table 182
AVERAGE INDEXES OF THE REQUIREMENT OF THE POPULATION OF FIVE CITIES
FOR SANATORIUM-HEALTH RESORT TREATMENT FOR DIFFERENT DISEASES

Disease	Average (per 1,000 population) of diseases in 5 cities	Percentage of cases calling for sanatorium-health resort treatment	No. of cases requiring treatment (per 1,000 population)
VII. Rheumatic fever	9.9	53.7	5.3
VIII. Metabolic and allergic disorders	5.1	41.6	2.2
X. Endocrine diseases	6.5	3.5	0.2
XIII. Nervous diseases	53.4	33.1	17.6
XIV. Eye diseases	32.1	11.6	3.7
XV. Otorhinolaryngological diseases	194.1	1.1	2.1
XVI. Respiratory diseases	53.0	1.7	9.3
XVIII. Circulatory diseases	58.2	29.5	17.7
XIX Digestive diseases	85.7	50.3	43.3
XX. Diseases of bones, muscles and joints	32.8	14.5	4.7
XXI. Skin diseases	46.4	13.3	6.1
XXII. Renal and urinary diseases	10.9	36.6	3.9
XXIV. Women's diseases	44.1	6.5	2.8

Our data on requirement standards for sanatorium-health resort services for patients suffering from different diseases, based on the sickness rate, cannot be considered absolutely reliable. In each case the need for sanatorium-health resort services is determined by the nature and course of the disease; therefore as the population becomes increasingly better provided with all kinds of medical services, detection of disease in the early stages will improve, thus raising the requirements. On the other hand, the requirement of sanatorium-health resort services will be somewhat reduced owing to the increasing volume of hospitalization.

However, our data may provide a basis for calculation since they are based on objective patterns of the population's morbidity.

In our determination of the need for sanatorium-health resort services, we bore in mind that not all patients needing this kind of medical care have to be treated at sanatoriums. Many of them can undergo successful outpatient treatment at health resorts with balneological facilities.

To illustrate this, information is provided below on the requirement rate for admission to sanatoriums and polyclinic treatment for cases of circulatory and digestive diseases.

Some circulatory diseases, such as first-stage hypertension, cardiovascular neuroses, etc., can be successfully treated at polyclinics located at health resorts.

Young and middle-aged patients suffering from chronic gastritis, chronic cholecystitis and certain other digestive diseases can also be treated on an outpatient basis.

Therefore, of the total 17.6‰ patients sent for treatment at sanatorium-health resorts for circulatory diseases and 43.3‰ suffering from diseases of the digestive organs, 6.6 and 21.9‰, respectively, can be treated at health resort polyclinics.

For complete fulfillment of patients' requirements regarding sanatorium-health resort treatments, prompt attention must be paid to expanding health resort facilities, espicially polyclinics and guest houses.

The working experience of health resort polyclinics at the Caucasian Mineral Waters has demonstrated that the number of persons treated at health resorts could be nearly doubled within a short time. The polyclinics at the health resorts of Kislovodsk, Essentuki and Zheleznovodsk treat the same number of cases as the sanatoriums.

For further expansion of outpatient treatment at health resorts more guest houses and hotels must be built and the capacity of health resort polyclinics increased. In expanding the outpatient facilities, the balneological amenities (clinics, bathhouses, drinking springs, etc.) should be improved first and foremost.

Another important measure for increasing the number of persons treated at health resorts is the utilization of pioneer camps as guest houses for patients in autumn and winter.

At the same time, the construction of new sanatoriums and the reconstruction of existing ones should be further promoted. The majority of working patients wish to undergo treatment during the summer vacation, and therefore inexpensive summer buildings should be erected at sanatoriums, with modern materials (plastics, etc.), in order to increase the summertime capacity of sanatoriums.

Implementation of these measures will make it possible to satisfy fully the population's requirement of treatment at sanatorium-health resorts.

Standards of Therapeutic-Prophylactic Care of the Urban Population in the Field of Physiotherapy

As in other sections of this work, the starting data for determining standards of physiotherapeutic services for the urban population were the data on general morbidity (from sickness rate), hospitalization, and attendance at outpatient institutions collected in Stupino, Rubezhnoe, Kopeisk, Dneprodzerzhinsk and Chelyabinsk.

Moreover, comprehensive medical examinations of 10,000 inhabitants were carried out at Stupino for detection of diseases for which the subjects had not requested medical aid. The result of these examinations introduced corrections in the morbidity data and the scope of physiotherapeutic services.

However, methods of determining standards of physiotherapeutic service for the population should reckon with a specific feature of this kind of medical aid, i.e., that the level of utilization of physical methods, determined by copying out pertinent data from the primary records, is not fully dependent upon the population's morbidity.

The scope of application of physiotherapy is most commonly determined by the treating physicians who, in sending their patients to physiotherapeutic offices and departments, should consider numerous factors, including the capacity and equipment of physiotherapeutic offices and the numbers and qualifications of their staff. The qualifications of the treating physicians themselves and their acquaintance with the correct use of physical treatment methods also are contributing factors.

Another specific feature in determining the standard of physiotherapeutic care is the impossibility of proposing any standards based on data collected in an individual outpatient polyclinic or hospital.

The extent of application of physiotherapy markedly differs for different diseases treated in an outpatient clinic or in a hospital, and therefore the utilization of this kind of medical aid varies in hospitals with a different range of departments and in outpatient polyclinics differing in their degree of specialization. For instance, if a hospital includes a large oncological department and a department for abortions, which use scarcely any physiotherapy, the use of physiotherapy in the hospital as a whole will be low.

As is known, in the majority of towns (as opposed to large cities), outpatient services in several specialized fields, such as dermatovenereological diseases, oncology, psychoneurology, and phthisiology, are provided by corresponding departments of territorial hospitals, whereas special dispensaries are available in cities.

Because of these methodological peculiarities, the town of Stupino was chosen as a special base for determining volume factors of the services. The work there was preceded by administrative measures designed to improve the equipment and operation of the Stupino Municipal Hospital. These measures were necessary to ensure the optimal conditions to provide physiotherapeutic services for the population.

The data specially copied from outpatients' cards and cards of physiotherapeutic offices, characterizing the frequency of prescriptions for physical methods of treatment, were then subjected to expert evaluation. Experienced clinicians who were thoroughly acquainted with practical outpatient-polyclinic services were invited to serve as the experts. They introduced corrections in the volume and manner of use of physiotherapy, in accordance with current knowledge and the achievements of medical science, in every case treated as an outpatient or inpatient. In this way the data collected at Stupino made it possible to determine the degree of application of physiotherapy to different diseases treated in a polyclinic or in a hospital.

These indexes are important essentially because they make it possible to determine the requirement for physiotherapeutic aid on larger-scale morbidity data for the urban population.

Volume of Physiotherapeutic Care of the Urban Population

Our determination of the volume of physiotherapeutic care was based on the following principles:

The unit we adopted for recording (observation) purposes was a prescription for physiotherapy—given by the treating physicians of all specialties in connection with the patient's visit to the polyclinic or hospital for the disease in question—at various therapeutic-prophylactic institutions.

The population's requirement for physiotherapy was calculated for the entire city population, with differentiation of the requirement for treatment in the hospital or polyclinic. A separate record was kept for the volume of physiotherapeutic care in various prophylactic services.

Simultaneously, we determined the number of physiotherapeutic prescriptions per case (request for medical aid in connection with the disease) at the polyclinic and the hospital, and per hospitalized case by classes of diseases and the most common individual nosologic entities. Furthermore, we considered the characteristic features of physiotherapeutic services for different age and sex groups of the population.

The volume of physiotherapeutic services at the morbidity and hospitalization levels current in Stupino is shown in Table 183. At the existing morbidity level there were actually 231.12 physiotherapeutic prescriptions per 1,000 population in the course of a year, 207.97 of them in the polyclinic and 23.15 in the hospital.

The experts' recommendations resulted in a certain increase in these indexes, to 277.23 prescriptions per 1,000 inhabitants, including 251.36 in the polyclinic and 25.87 in the hospital.

It is seen from Table 183 that with the existing level of total morbidity and hospitalization, the largest number of physiotherapeutic prescriptions was in connection with diseases of the bones, muscles and joints, i.e., 48.17 per 1,000 population.

Following in importance were otorhinolaryngological diseases, viz., 45.13 per 1,000 population, including 12.07 in cases of acute inflammation of the upper respiratory tract, 11.66 for otitis, and 8.11 for rhinitis.

The requirement for physiotherapeutic services for nervous diseases is high, 43.97 per 1,000 population, including 18.81 for lumbosacral radiculitis.

The fourth place with respect to volume of physiotherapeutic care is occupied by skin diseases, i.e., 23.61 prescriptions per 1,000 population, including 12.29 for pyodermitis.

These are followed by the class of infectious diseases, with 18.72 prescriptions per 1,000 population, including 5.97 for influenza.

Then come diseases of the digestive organs, i.e., 16.48 prescriptions per 1,000 population, of which 4.63 are for chronic gastritis, 3.2 for gastric and duodenal ulcers.

These are closely followed by circulatory diseases with 16.08 prescriptions per 1,000 population.

Then come oral and dental diseases (12.48), traumata (10.84), respiratory diseases (6.77), and women's diseases (7.42).

These 11 classes of diseases account for 90% of all physiotherapeutic prescriptions.

The differentiation of physiotherapeutic services for the different age and sex groups is shown in Table 184.

The highest utilization of physiotherapy occurs in the age group from 40–49 years, 407.24 prescriptions per 1,000 population. The index is lower in younger age groups, but rises to 230.93 prescriptions per 1,000 members of the age group in children up to and including 2 years. The frequency of physiotherapeutic prescriptions in the different age groups is mainly dependent upon the total morbidity level.

However, the relationship between morbidity level and use of physiotherapy is

Table 183

INTENSIVE INDEXES OF TOTAL MORBIDITY, HOSPITALIZATION AND PRESCRIPTIONS FOR PHYSIOTHERAPY IN THE POLYCLINIC AND HOSPITAL
(per 1,000 population)

Disease	No. of cases	No. of hospitalized cases	No. of physiotherapeutic prescriptions					
			actual			actual plus additions by the experts		
			total	these include		total	these include	
				in poly-clinic	in hospi-tal		in poly-clinic	in hospi-tal
I. Infectious diseases	245.7	17.3	17.52	14.75	2.77	18.72	15.95	2.77
These include:								
tonsillitis	61.6	0.7	2.18	1.95	0.22	2.22	2.0	0.22
epidemic viral influenza	120.8	2.0	5.52	4.90	0.62	5.97	5.35	0.62
phlegmons and abscesses	11.1	0.4	3.30	3.21	0.09	3.66	3.57	0.09
III. Injuries	90.3	7.1	9.67	9.49	0.18	10.34	10.16	0.18
VII. Rheumatic fever	12.5	3.0	3.75	1.65	2.10	3.75	1.65	2.10
XIII. Nervous diseases	59.5	3.1	33.99	31.45	2.54	43.97	41.30	2.67
These include:								
lumbosacral radiculitis	15.6	0.8	16.18	15.2	0.98	18.81	17.83	0.98
XV. Otorhinolaryngological diseases	291.8	6.4	42.14	41.29	0.85	45.13	43.88	1.25
These include:								
acute otitis	15.9	0.3	6.77	6.68	0.09	6.99	6.90	0.09
chronic otitis	9.8	0.4	4.63	4.63		4.67	4.67	
chronic tonsillitis	28.9	3.2	5.92	5.61	0.31	6.05	5.74	0.31
rhinitis	20.3	0.3	7.31	7.31		8.11	7.89	0.22
acute inflammation of the upper respiratory tract	176.5	0.2	11.54	11.36	0.18	12.07	11.85	0.22
XVI. Respiratory diseases	45.1	7.0	6.50	4.94	1.56	6.77	5.12	1.65
These include:								
bronchopneumonia	13.6	4.9	2.32	1.34	0.98	2.36	1.34	1.02
XVII. Circulatory diseases	68.9	5.1	13.59	10.29	3.30	16.08	12.70	3.38
These include:								
hypertension	21.8	2.7	7.39	5.06	2.33	7.90	5.53	2.37
XIX. Digestive diseases	94.1	27.3	15.83	8.87	6.96	16.48	9.49	6.99
XX. Diseases of bones, muscles and joints	68.8	1.2	39.47	38.45	0.72	48.17	46.51	1.66
These include:								
diseases of joints	19.2	0.8	10.60	9.98	0.62	11.27	10.65	0.62
diseases of muscles tendons and ganglia	38.6	0.2	25.44	25.35	0.09	30.02	29.45	0.57
XI. Skin diseases	42.2	0.5	15.62	15.54	0.08	23.61	22.94	0.67
These include:								
pyoderma	14.2	0.1	9.62	9.53	0.09	12.29	11.89	0.40
XXIV. Women's diseases	59.4	4.9	7.05	6.82	0.23	7.40	7.13	0.27
These include:								
diseases of the ovaries and fallopian tubes	7.3	1.4	3.51	3.47	0.04	3.55	3.51	0.04
other classes and diseases	522.0	22.6	24.76	23.02	1.74	34.59	32.43	2.16
Total	1600.7	105.5	229.89	206.86	23.03	275.01	249.26	25.75
Over and above morbidity	58.9	46.8	1.23	1.11	0.12	2.22	2.10	0.12
Sum total	1659.6	152.3	231.12	207.97	23.15	277.23	251.36	25.87

Table 184

INDEXES OF TOTAL MORBIDITY, HOSPITALIZATION AND PHYSIOTHERAPEUTIC
PRESCRIPTIONS BY AGE AND SEX GROUPS (per 1,000 population of the corresponding age)

Age group	Sex	No. of cases	No. of hospital-ized cases	No. of physiotherapeutic prescriptions		
				total	in polyclinic	in hospital
0–2 years	Both sexes	2100.4	222.9	217.43	143.48	73.95
	Men	2080.6	227.6	230.90	159.01	71.89
	Women	212.0	218.5	203.57	127.51	76.06
3–6 years	Both sexes	2096.6	134.9	209.64	178.39	31.25
	Men	2057.2	133.7	221.09	193.14	27.95
	Women	2137.6	136.2	197.55	162.83	34.72
7–12 years	Both sexes	1333.0	97.2	117.37	96.76	20.61
	Men	1216.0	88.2	109.40	87.52	21.88
	Women	1459.8	107.2	126.07	106.85	19.22
13–15 years	Both sexes	994.4	76.6	90.85	79.69	11.16
	Men	915.3	59.4	57.84	51.75	6.04
	Women	1080.3	95.3	127.09	110.37	16.72
16–19 years	Both sexes	857.4	65.8	70.89	58.93	11.96
	Men	969.3	61.4	81.92	71.68	10.24
	Women	745.3	70.1	59.84	46.16	13.68
20–29 years	Both sexes	1341.7	108.5	160.78	149.49	11.29
	Men	1244.8	74.8	172.40	161.97	10.43
	Women	1419.1	135.7	151.52	137.83	13.69
30–39 years	Both sexes	1828.3	97.9	318.34	295.04	23.30
	Men	1603.3	90.5	312.88	276.53	36.35
	Women	2013.9	104.0	322.82	310.28	12.54
40–49 years	Both sexes	1958.2	106.9	407.24	374.88	32.36
	Men	1801.0	103.2	437.22	400.32	36.90
	Women	2064.9	109.6	386.92	357.64	29.28
50–59 years	Both sexes	1858.5	114.2	361.59	326.92	34.67
	Men	1799.3	125.8	373.64	333.74	39.90
	Women	1897.6	106.4	353.6	322.4	31.2
60 years and over	Both sexes	1191.7	72.6	146.63	125.18	21.45
	Men	1359.8	77.2	223.65	179.95	43.70
	Women	1130.1	71.4	118.27	105.02	13.25

not wholly proportional, because of the differences in the structure of total morbidity among persons of different age.

Middle-aged and elderly people suffer from a higher incidence of chronic diseases requiring a considerably more extensive use of physiotherapeutic treatment (diseases of the peripheral nervous system, diseases of the bones, muscles and joints). In contrast, children suffer mostly from acute inflammatory diseases (influenza, catarrh of the upper respiratory tract, tonsillitis), for which physiotherapy is less frequently used.

The differences in the degree of application of physiotherapy to different diseases are shown in Table 185.

Table 185

AVERAGE NUMBER OF PHYSIOTHERAPEUTIC PRESCRIPTIONS ACCORDING TO
INDIVIDUAL DISEASES AND CLASSES OF DISEASES

Disease	No. of prescriptions per request for medical aid						No. of prescriptions per hospitalized case	
	actual			actual plus added by experts			actual	actual plus added by experts
	total	including		total	including			
		in poly-clinic	in hospital		in poly-clinic	in hospital		
I. Infectious diseases	0.07	0.06	0.01	0.08	0.07	0.01	0.16	0.16
These include:								
tonsillitis	0.035	0.032	0.003	0.036	0.033	0.003	0.31	0.31
epidemic viral influenza	0.046	0.041	0.005	0.049	0.044	0.005	0.31	0.31
phlegmons and abscesses	0.3	0.29	0.01	0.33	0.32	0.01	0.22	0.22
III. Injuries	0.1	0.1		0.11	0.1	0.01	0.025	0.025
VII. Rheumatic fever	0.3	0.13	0.17	0.3	0.13	0.17	0.7	0.7
VIII. Nervous diseases	0.57	0.53	0.04	0.74	0.69	0.05	0.8	0.86
These include:								
lumbosacral radiculitis	1.04	1.0	0.04	1.2	1.16	0.04	1.2	1.2
XV. Otorhinolaryngological diseases	0.14	0.14		0.15	0.15		0.13	0.15
These include:								
otitis	0.44	0.44		0.15	0.15		0.13	0.15
chronic tonsillitis	0.21	0.20	0.01	0.21	0.2	0.01	0.09	0.1
acute and chronic rhinitis	0.36	0.36		0.40	0.39	0.01		0.5
acute inflammation of upper respiratory tract	0.066	0.065	0.001	0.069	0.067	0.002	0.16	0.19
XVI. Respiratory diseases	0.14	0.10	0.04	0.15	0.11	0.04	0.22	0.24
These include:								
bronchopneumonia	0.17	0.1	0.07	0.17	0.1	0.07	0.2	0.2
XVII. Circulatory diseases	0.2	0.15	0.05	0.23	0.18	0.05	0.64	0.66
These include:								
hypertension	0.33	0.23	0.1	0.36	0.25	0.11	0.85	0.87
XIX. Digestive diseases	0.17	0.09	0.08	0.08	0.18	0.1	0.25	0.25
These include:								
gastric and duodenal ulcers	0.6	0.3	0.3	0.65	0.34	0.31	0.75	0.75
XX. Diseases of bones, muscles and joints	0.57	0.56	0.01	0.7	0.68	0.02	0.6	1.4
These include:								
diseases of the joints	0.52	0.52		0.55	0.55		0.32	0.32
diseases of muscles, tendons and ganglia	0.66	0.66		0.78	0.76	0.02	0.45	2.8
XXI. Skin diseases	0.37	0.37		0.56	0.55	0.01	0.16	0.8
These include:								
pyoderma	0.68	0.68		0.87	0.84	0.03	0.9	2.6
XXIV. Women's diseases	0.12	0.11	0.01	0.12	0.12	0.01	0.05	0.05
These include:								
oophoritis	0.4	0.4		0.4	0.4			
Total	0.14	0.12	0.02	0.17	0.15	0.02	0.21	0.22
In addition to the above-listed diseases								
Sum total	0.14	0.12	0.02	0.17	0.15	0.02	0.15	0.16

On the average, there is 0.17 physiotherapeutic prescription for every case of disease, including 0.15 in the polyclinic and 0.02 in the hospital, and there is 0.16 physiotherapeutic prescription for every hospitalized case. If cases of hospitalization for uncomplicated climacteric, errors of refraction and accommodation, abortions and normal deliveries are excluded from the total hospitalization, there is 0.22 physiotherapeutic prescription for every hospitalized case.

There were significant differences in the frequency of physiotherapeutic application in the different hospital departments.

There was 0.7 physiotherapeutic prscription per hospitalized case in the neurological department as against 0.01 in the obstetric department (Table 186).

Table 186
USE OF PHYSIOTHERAPY IN DIFFERENT
HOSPITAL DEPARTMENTS

Department	No. of prescriptions per hospitalized case
Therapeutic	0.5
Surgical	0.07
Otorhinolaryngological	0.2
Ophthalmological	0.13
Neurological	0.7
Gynecological	0.01
Obstetric	0.01
Pediatric	0.3
Infectious (for adults)	0.1
Infectious (for children)	0.3

The second place with respect to frequency of physiotherapy application in the hospital is occupied by the therapeutic department, with 0.5 physiotherapeutic prescription per hospitalized case.

The following is a breakdown of the total number of physiotherapeutic prescriptions in the polyclinic by physicians' specialties:

	%
Therapy	40.0
Otorhinolaryngology	16.0
Surgery	12.7
Neurology	11.4
Pediatrics	6.8
Dermatovenereology	6.0
Obstetrics and gynecology	4.0
Other	3.1

In the hospital the breakdown was somewhat different:

Department	%
Internal medicine	40.9
Infectious, for children	19.3
Pediatrics	12.7
Neurological	11.5
Surgical	6.3
Otorhinolaryngological	3.6
Gynecological	2.3
Infectious, for adults	2.0
Other	1.4

Hence, among all the different specialties, the largest number of physiotherapeutic prescriptions was given by internists in both the polyclinic and hospital.

It is of interest to know the relative importance of the different kinds of physiotherapy in the polyclinic and hospital. Electrotherapy accounts for 42.6% of all prescriptions in the polyclinic and 38.5% in the hospital; phototherapy accounts for 39.5 and 26.5%, respectively; hydrotherapy for 6.2 and 3.5%; thermotherapy for 9 and 25.5%; and other treatments account for 2.7 and 6%.

Currently, electric phototherapy [e.g., heat treatments] has become the most widespread kind of physiotherapy owing to the extensive electrification of the USSR, considerable development of the electric and electronics industry, and the availability of portable equipment.

The leading role of these kinds of physiotherapy has been confirmed by several authors (A. A. Tamazov, S. Ya. Freidlin, Yu. N. Alabovskii and others), based on analysis of work done by physiotherapists at hospitals and polyclinics.

However, some recent studies have described extensive practical implementation by therapeutic-prophylactic medical institutions of such highly efficient physiotherapeutic methods as mud therapy and other types of physiotherapy that do not require any equipment.

According to V. I. Sovetov "Puti razvitiya fizioterapevticheskoi pomoshchi v SSSR" (Ways of Developing Physiotherapy in the USSR), *Vrachebnoe Delo,* 6, 1960, electric phototherapeutic procedures account for 50%, the remainder involving the use of muds, peat, paraffin, ozakerite, mineral waters, i.e., forms of physiotherapy not requiring equipment.

The number of physiotherapeutic prescriptions issued in the course of prophylactic treatment reaches 14.3 per 1,000 population.

Hence, at the existing level of sickness rate, hospitalization and prophylactic care there is a need for 291.52 physiotherapeutic prescriptions per 1,000 urban population per year, including 265.65 at the polyclinic and 25.87 at the hospital. This number does not include prescriptions for inhalation, massage and physical exercises.

Standards of Therapeutic-Prophylactic Care of the Urban Population in the Field of Physiotherapy

Calculations of the standards, based on morbidity data for the population of five cities situated in different climatic and geographical zones of the USSR, with a total population of up to 1.5 million, are presented in Table 187.

Table 187
VOLUME OF PHYSIOTHERAPEUTIC CARE OF THE URBAN POPULATION
(CALCULATED FROM THE AVERAGE MORBIDITY INDEXES FOR THE FIVE CITIES)

Disease	Average number of cases (requests for medical aid) per 1,000 inhabitants in the 5 cities	Average number of physiotherapeutic prescriptions per case at the polyclinic	Number of physiotherapeutic prescriptions at the polyclinic per 1,000 population	No. of hospitalized cases per 1,000 population in the 5 cities	Average number of physiotherapeutic prescriptions per hospitalized case	Number of physiotherapeutic prescriptions at the hospital per 1,000 population	Total physiotherapeutic prescriptions at the polyclinic and hospital
I. Infectious diseases	216.0	0.07	15.2	24.7	0.16	3.95	19.15
III. Injuries	96.6	0.1	9.66	8.8	0.25	2.20	11.86
VII. Rheumatic fever	9.9	0.13	1.29	3.2	0.7	2.24	3.53
XIII. Nervous diseases	56.8	0.69	39.10	5.8	0.8	4.64	43.83
XV. Otorhinolaryngological diseases	242.4	0.15	36.36	8.6	0.15	1.29	37.65
XVI. Respiratory diseases	59.7	0.11	6.57	16.5	0.22	3.63	10.20
XVII. Circulatory diseases	58.2	0.18	10.48	7.3	0.65	4.74	15.22
XIX. Digestive diseases	85.7	0.1	8.57	27.6	0.25	6.90	15.47
XX. Diseases of bones, muscles and joints	42.3	0.68	28.76	2.6	1.40	3.64	32.4
XXI. Skin diseases	53.3	0.55	22.31	1.7	0.8	1.36	23.67
XXIV. Women's diseases	46.6	0.11	5.13	6.3	0.05	0.31	5.44
Other classes and diseases	281.1	0.06	16.87	24.8	0.09	2.23	19.10
Total	1248.6	0.16	200.39	137.9	0.26	37.13	237.52
In addition to the total	64.5	0.034	2.58	57.0	0.003	0.17	2.75
Sum total	1315.0	0.15	202.97	195.1	0.19	37.30	240.27

It is seen from Table 187 that after recalculation at Stupino with the physiotherapeutic requirement coefficient, the results were as follows: a total of 240.27 physiotherapeutic prescriptions per 1,000 population, including 202.97 at the polyclinic and 37.30 at the hospital. There was 0.15 prescription per polyclinic patient and 0.19 per hospitalized case. This index rises to 0.26 physiotherapeutic prescription per hospitalized case after exclusion of hospitalizations for abortions and certain age-induced changes placed outside the listed total.

However, calculation of the optimal requirement for physiotherapeutic services must take into account several chronic diseases revealed by medical examinations.

We calculated the additional volume of physiotherapy required in catering for newly detected chronic diseases in those population groups already subjected to periodic examinations (preschool children, schoolchildren, adolescents, workers in industry, staff of public catering enterprises and children's institutions, etc.).

Since the structure of the newly detected chronic diseases differs from that of the total morbidity, we could not make use of the average number of physiotherapeutic prescriptions for entire classes of diseases. The supplementary volume of physiotherapy was calculated for each newly detected disease separately and then totaled by classes.

Therefore, after addition of the necessary volume of physiotherapy for treatment of newly detected chronic diseases (26.8 and 3.7 prescriptions per 1,000 population at the polyclinic and hospital, respectively), the requirement for physiotherapeutic

Table 188
STANDARDS OF THERAPEUTIC-PROPHYLACTIC CARE OF THE URBAN
POPULATION IN THE FIELD OF PHYSIOTHERAPY

Kind of prescription	No. of prescriptions per 1,000 population			Average number of treatments per prescription		No. of treatments per 1,000 population		
	in poly-clinic	in hos-pital	total	in poly-clinic	in hos-pital	in poly-clinic	in hos-pital	total
Electrotherapy								
Galvanization	23.66	4.79	28.45	9.7	9.5	229.5	45.5	275.0
Chamber bath	1.38	0.02	1.4	8.3	7.3	11.5	0.1	11.6
Diathermy	15.62	2.09	17.71	11.6	11.6	181.2	24.2	205.4
D'arsonvalization	5.06	2.00	7.06	7.8	7.6	39.5	15.2	54.7
Franklinization	0.23	0.02	0.25	9.4	9.4	2.2	0.2	2.4
Treatment with induction currents	0.23	0.04	0.27	7.8	7.2	1.8	0.3	2.1
UHF therapy	51.68	6.84	58.52	7.1	6.9	366.9	47.2	414.1
Phototherapy								
Irradiation with a quartz mercury lamp	92.86	8.81	101.67	4.9	7.5	455.0	66.1	521.1
Irradiation with other light sources	12.17	2.05	14.22	5.1	5.1	62.1	10.5	12.6
Hydrotherapy								
Baths	12.63	1.35	13.98	10.8	7.6	136.4	10.3	146.7
Showers	1.6	0.08	1.69	7.9	6.9	12.7	0.6	13.3
Thermotherapy	20.67	10.45	31.12	9.7	7.7	200.5	80.5	281.0
Other	6.20	2.46	8.66	8.2	8.0	50.8	19.8	70.6
Total	244.0	41.0	285.0			175.0	320.5	2070.6

care comes to 270.81 prescriptions per 1,000 population, including 229.75 at the polyclinic and 41.06 at the hospital.

Above, we were concerned with the use of physiotherapy in therapeutic services for the urban population; account must also be taken of the volume of work performed by the physiotherapeutic offices in various forms of prophylactic services. There is a need for 14.3 physiotherapeutic prescriptions for polyclinic outpatients in connection with prophylactic examinations of preschool children, laborers, and pregnant women; dispensary services, and other kinds of prophylactic services.

Therefore, the total volume of physiotherapeutic care becomes 285 prescriptions, of which 244 are in the polyclinic and 41 in the hospital.

The average number of treatments per prescription for different kinds of physiotherapy was determined by statistical methods based on data quoted from documentation of physiotherapeutic offices at Stupino and the physiotherapeutic department of Municipal Hospital No. 57 in Moscow. We used the physiotherapeutic cards of patients who had completed a full course of treatment. The results are presented in Table 188.

Table 188 shows the need for the following treatments per 1,000 population: 965.3 electrotherapy, 593.7 phototherapy, 160 hydrotherapy, and 281 thermotherapy. These standards are important to provide the basis for calculations of the requirements for specific kinds of equipment.

A total of 2,070.6 treatments are required for the principal kinds of physiotherapy per 1,000 population, or, in round numbers, 2 treatments per person.

Basic Patterns of
Morbidity, Sickness Rate and Hospitalization
and Composite Data on
Therapeutic-Prophylactic Care Standards

The Morbidity of the Urban Population (based on sickness rate at therapeutic-prophylactic institutions)

Detailed investigation of total morbidity (based on sickness rate) of the population of five cities showed that although the cities were situated in different climatic and geographical zones of the USSR and the studies were made in different years (1956, 1957, 1959, and 1962), there were no significant differences in the sickness rate indexes, both in general and also with reference to the chief nosological entities.

There were some differences in the incidence of certain diseases, depending upon several factors specific for each disease. Fluctuations in intensive morbidity indexes for influenza were most frequently dependent upon the differences between years with epidemic outbreaks and years that were epidemiologically quiet.

In some cases, differences in the incidence of influenza and acute catarrh of the upper respiratory tract were due to different approaches adopted by the physicians in the different cities toward the different diagnoses.

The studies showed that because of the variations involved in differential diagnostics for influenza and nasal catarrh, the diagnoses made in medical institutions of the different cities were most frequently those generally adopted by the physicians in the particular city.

These two diseases belong to different classes, and therefore the physicians' preference for one diagnosis or the other may affect the place occupied by the former or the latter disease classes in the population's total morbidity, irrespective of their actual incidence. The incidence of influenza and nasal catarrh should probably be taken into account jointly in analysis of the population's morbidity in different cities.

The fluctuations in the incidence of the population's medical aid requirements with respect to parasitic infestations depend upon the different scope of tests for helminthiases (especially in children) in the different cities. The same applies to fungus diseases.

The varying scope of prophylactic stomatological examinations in the different cities likewise resulted in significant differences in sickness rates with respect to dental and oral diseases. This was convincingly demonstrated in the case of Stupino, where the stomatologists examined the entire population for the state of the teeth and oral cavity in the year in which studies of the sickness rate by stomatologists were made, and as a consequence, the sickness rate was found to be triple that in the other cities.

Variations in the incidence of certain diseases (especially injuries) were also affected by the presence of certain industries in the different cities.

Another factor affecting the incidence of different diseases is the difference in the population structure in the different cities, because of the significant differences in the incidence of certain nosologic entities in the different age and sex groups. Nevertheless, the basic morbidity patterns of different age groups in all the investigated cities were fairly uniform as is seen from Figure 43.

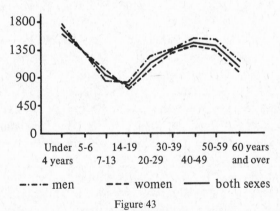

Figure 43

Average age indexes of total morbidity (based on sickness rate) of inhabitants of both sexes in the 5 cities (number of requests for medical aid per 1,000 population of the corresponding age and sex)

The morbidity indexes are comparatively high in children up to 4 years old and then decline gradually, reaching a minimum at the ages of 14–19. They gradually rise in the older age groups, again declining in the age group of inhabitants 60 years old and over.

The number of requests for medical aid per 1,000 population (excepting deliveries and abortions) varies from 1,070 to 1,236 in the different cities, with the exception of

Stupino, where there were 1,600.7 requests for medical aid per 1,000 population, but the difference was due to increased requests for medical aid with respect to dental and oral diseases (340.8‰), as already mentioned.

The intensive indexes of the population's total morbidity in the investigated cities are little different from corresponding indexes published by other authors in different years.

According to L. A. Brushlinskaya (*Sostoyanie zdorov'ya naseleniya Moskvy (State of Health of the Moscow Population)*. Moscow, 1946), the number of requests for medical aid from sick persons was 1,061.8 per 1,000 Moscow inhabitants in 1937. This index was found to be 1,112 when calculated from data collected by the same author in a large number of RSFSR cities in 1959 ("Osnovnye itogi izucheniya zdorov'ya naseleniya RSFSR za 1958g." (Principal Results of Health Studies for the RSFSR Population in 1958).—In: IV *nauchnaya sessiya Instituta organizatsii zdravookhraneniya i istorii meditsiny imeni N. A. Semashko,* Synopses of Reports. Moscow, 1961). By random investigations, the total morbidity was 1,276.6 per 1,000 population on the eve of World War II in several cities (P.M. Kozlov, *Sanitarnaya statistika (Public Health Statistics)*. Medgiz. Moscow, 1949). There were 1,225.5 requests for medical aid per 1,000 population in the city of Ivanovo without dental and oral diseases (*Materialy po zabolevaemosti naseleniya g. Ivanovo (Data on the Morbidity of the Ivanovo Population),* edited by Prof. A. M. Merkov. Moscow, 1959).

Investigations of total morbidity in many cities in 1958–1959 showed that the number of requests each year for medical aid per 1,000 population was as follows: ‡ 1,327.7 in Riga (S. Ya. Belyaeva), 1,129.1 in Kishinev (G. G. Chaiko and I. D. Gol'dberg), 1,144.8 in Kalinin (N. A. Frolova), 1,318.9 in Tallin (I.G. Levina), 1,261.5 in Vilnius, 1,153.4 in Kaunas, 1,387 in Klaipeda (L. V. Gargasas), 1,108.5 in Tbilisi (A. Korchava), 1,190 in Ugleuralsk (A. G. Vershinina)(IV *nauchnaya sessiya Instituta organizatsii zdravookhraneniya i istorii meditsiny imeni N.A. Semashko 26 iyunya–1 iyulya 1961 g. (Fourth Scientific Session of the Semashko Institute of Public Health held 26 June–1 July 1961)*. Synopses of Reports. Moscow, 1961).

Comparison of data on the total morbidity of the urban population in the USSR with analogous data published in the medical press of capitalistic countries is of some interest.

Inhabitants of capitalist countries obtain medical care mostly from private practitioners. Therefore the documentation of therapeutic-prophylactic institutions existing in such countries cannot be used as the basis for morbidity studies, and the investigators (including those in the U.S.A.) engaged in such studies are obliged to resort to rather inaccurate methods of periodic questioning of the inhabitants concerning their past medical history. In cases where no physician had been invited the investigators relied on self-diagnoses provided by the inhabitants themselves, obviously detracting from the quality of the data collected.

The high fees charged by private physicians discourage many from visiting physicians in the case of comparatively mild forms of diseases, especially chronic ones, and consequently many diseases remain undiagnosed. Therefore, the data reported for the capitalist countries are not fully comparable (especially with regard to the incidence of diseases) with analogous data obtained in the USSR, where every kind of medical care is free and fully available.

However, even under these conditions, certain main trends of the total morbidity of the urban population outside the USSR are closely similar to the Soviet data (for instance, with respect to age-contingent indexes).

According to Sydenstriker, the morbidity at Hagerstown was 1,081 cases per 1,000 population (943 per 1,000 men and 1,210 per 1,000 women), (Sydenstriker, E. "The Illness Rate among Men and Women," *Public Health Reports,* Vol. 4, No. 30. 1927.

Data collected by Collins and others show that the total morbidity of the population in selected districts of Baltimore in 1938-1943 was 1,379 per 1,000 population of both sexes (Collins, S. "Specific Causes of Illness Found in Monthly Canvasses of Families," *Public Health Reports,* Vol. 65, No. 39. 1950).

Composite data of six separate random investigations of the total morbidity of the urban population carried out in different years and in different American cities were published in the U.S.A. in 1955. According to these composite data, the total intensive index was 1,064 cases of diseases per 1,000 urban population ("Sickness Experience in Selected Areas of the United States," *Public Health Monograph,* No. 25. 1955.)

Finally, the population's total morbidity indexes (1,323 cases per 1,000 inhabitants of both sexes per annum) were also published in the report by the President's Commission on the Health Needs of the Nation (*Building America's Health.* A Report to the President by the President's Commission on the Health Needs of the Nation. Vol. 3 and Statistical Appendix. Washington, 1952–1953.

A somewhat higher total morbidity was reported for Japan. According to random investigation of 50,000 inhabitants in different areas of Japan, the total morbidity is 2,000 per 1,000 population per annum (of these, acute nasopharyngitis and the common cold account for 711 cases per 1,000 population)(*A Brief Report on Public Health Administration in Japan.* Ministry of Health and Welfare. Tokyo, 1958.)

A distinctive feature of American total morbidity data is the significantly higher index of disease for women than for men, largely depending upon the investigation methods (as was also pointed out by authors of published works).

The women, who were the ones most frequently questioned by the investigators concerning the diseases suffered by members of the family, remembered their own diseases better than those of the males in the family.

It is of considerable interest to compare the recent total morbidity data for the urban population with similar data collected in the first decade of the Soviet regime.

According to Rozhdestvenskii, the morbidity in the city of Tver [Kalinin] in 1925 was 2,034.1 cases per 1,000 population (1,857.7 for men, 2.181 for women) (M. I. Rozhdestvendkii "Zabolevaemost' rabochikh tekstil'noi promyshlennosti g. Tveri v 1925 g." (Morbidity of Textile Workers in Tver in 1925). In: *Statisticheskie issledovaniya professional'noi zabolevaemosti tekstil'shchikov,* No. 1. Moscow, Gosmedizdat. 1929.)

In 1939 Vasil'ev published morbidity data for the settlement of Motovilikha (one of the districts of the city of Perm) in 1926–1927. According to his data, the number of cases was 2,167 per 1,000 men and 1,691 per 1,000 women (N. Vasil'ev "Zabolevaemost' naseleniya poselka Motovilikha Permskogo okruga Ural'skoi oblasti v 1926–1927 gg." (Morbidity in the Settlement of Motovilikha of the Perm District in the Urals Region in 1926–1927). In: *Statisticheskie issledovaniya professional'noi zavolevaemosti,* No. 2. Moscow–Leningrad, 1930.)

A comparison of these data with recent data shows that the total morbidity of the population of industrial cities has been reduced by nearly one-half. The decrease has been especially marked in the case of rheumatic fever (by a factor of 2–3), pyodermas and suppurative diseases of subcutaneous tissue (by a factor of 4–5), diseases of the digestive organs (by a factor of 3–5), and tuberculosis (by one-half).

Certain diseases such as anemia and chlorosis, including iron deficiency anemia, which created a morbidity of up to 80 cases per 1,000 population 30 years ago, now occur only in isolated cases among the urban population.

In view of the absence of significant differences in the age and sex indexes and the sickness rate levels for the population of the different cities, on the whole for the majority of the most widespread nosologic entities, and for convenience of calculation, our determination of the standards of the urban population's need for therapeutic-prophylactic services was based on average indexes of sickness rate, hospitalization, and frequency of visits to outpatient polyclinics for the five cities.

The average intensive indexes of total morbidity (based on sickness rate) for the five cities are listed in Table 189.

Table 189 shows there was an average of 1,247.1 requests for medical aid for diseases per 1,000 population (1,265.2 for men, 1,233.5 for women).

In addition, therapeutic institutions rendered medical aid in induced abortions, deliveries, the climacteric, and errors of refraction and accommodation, which, strictly speaking, cannot be regarded as diseases and were therefore grouped separately. With the addition of requests for medical aid in cases of these physiological conditions and age-induced changes, the overall indexes become 1,315, 1,275.4 and 1,348.7‰.

Special features of the sickness rate for the population of different sexes are shown in Table 190.

There is no significant difference between the sexes with respect to the basic sickness rate patterns. However, if women's requests for medical aid for deliveries

Table 189
AVERAGE INTENSIVE INDEXES OF TOTAL MORBIDITY FOR FIVE CITIES
(based on sickness rate)

Disease	Average number of requests for medical aid per 1,000 population		
	men	women	both sexes
Class I. Infectious diseases	237.6	198.4	216.0
Class II. Parasitic diseases	15.8	14.1	14.9
Class III. Injuries	138.3	62.2	96.6
Class IV. Poisoning	2.2	1.9	2.1
Class V. Industrial and occupational diseases	0.7	0.2	0.5
Class VI. Vitamin deficiency diseases	2.3	1.8	2.0
Class VII. Rheumatic fever	6.4	12.7	9.9
This includes:			
rheumatic heart failure	2.8	5.9	4.5
Class VIII. Metabolic and allergic disorders	6.0	6.7	6.4
Class IX. Neoplasms	7.3	12.7	10.4
These include:			
malignant	2.8	3.6	3.3
benign	4.5	9.2	7.1
Class X. Endocrine diseases	0.9	7.6	4.5
These include:			
thyroid diseases	0.7	7.1	4.2
Class XI. Diseases of the hemopoietic system	0.6	1.2	0.9
Class XII. Psychic disorders	4.3	2.4	3.2
Class XIII. Nervous diseases	53.8	59.4	56.8
These include:			
cerebral atherosclerosis and other vascular cerebral lesions	4.0	6.2	5.2
lumbosacral radiculitis, neuritis and sciatica	26.0	18.5	21.8
neuroses and psychoneuroses	11.4	21.9	17.2
Class XIV. Eye diseases	40.3	37.9	39.0
These include:			
glaucoma	0.4	7.6	8.9
Class XV. Otorhinolaryngological diseases	269.6	220.8	242.4
These include:			
chronic otitis	10.4	7.6	8.9
chronic tonsillitis	11.6	12.3	11.9
Class XVI. Respiratory diseases	68.2	52.6	59.7
These include:			
bronchitis, chronic and nonspecified	12.3	8.1	10.1
pulmonary fibrosis and emphysema	3.9	1.9	2.8
Class XVII. Circulatory diseases	45.8	68.1	58.2
These include:			
myocardial fibrosis from atherosclerosis	10.2	16.8	13.9
hypertension	10.8	20.1	16.0
venous diseases	6.7	6.6	6.6
Class XVIII. Oral and dental diseases	125.6	153.1	140.7
Class XIX. Diseases of the digestive organs	91.4	81.3	85.7

Table 189 (continued)

Disease	Average number of requests for medical aid per 1,000 population		
	men	women	both sexes
These include:			
gastritis, chronic and nonspecified	22.1	20.9	21.4
gastric and duodenal ulcers	9.6	1.5	5.1
Class XX. Diseases of bones, muscles and joints	45.9	39.4	42.3
Class XXI. Skin diseases	60.7	47.4	53.3
These include:			
eczema	5.3	5.2	5.2
Class XXII. Renal and urinary diseases	8.2	17.2	13.0
Class XXIII. Diseases of the male genitals	3.9	—	1.7
Class XXIV. Diseases of the female genitals	—	84.8	46.6
Class XXV. Congenital defects	0.4	0.7	0.6
Class XXVI. Diseases of pregnancy, pathology of labor and diseases of the postnatal period	—	14.9	8.2
Class XXVII. Neonatal diseases	0.5	0.4	0.5
Class XXVIII. Diseases not included in the nomenclature and wrongly designated	28.1	33.6	31.1
Total	1265.2	1233.5	1247.1
In addition:			
Abortions	—	61.2	33.2
Deliveries	—	36.9	20.0
Climax	0.2	4.4	2.5
Errors of refraction and accommodation	10.0	13.9	12.2
Sum total	1275.4	1349.9	1315.0

Table 190

AGE INDEXES OF TOTAL MORBIDITY (according to sickness rate) FOR THE URBAN POPULATION OF BOTH SEXES (number of requests for medical aid in cases of disease per 1,000 population of the corresponding sex)

	Age groups									
	up to 4 years	5–6 years	7–13 years	14–19 years	20–29 years	30–39 years	40–49 years	50–59 years	60 and over	Total
Number of requests per 1,000 persons per annum:										
both sexes	1737.7	1339.0	940.5	762.0	1126.0	1327.4	1454.3	1405.2	1041.2	1247.1
men	1762.6	1330.5	886.5	793.9	1239.3	1353.4	1523.1	1494.4	1187.4	1265.2
women	1714.3	1349.0	996.5	728.8	1051.4	1314.3	1409.1	1348.8	976.4	1233.5

and abortions are included in the total number of requests, the intensive indexes are changed markedly toward higher values in the groups of young and middle-aged women. This circumstance had a significant bearing on the incidence of hospitalization and outpatient attendance, as will be discussed below.

**Morbidity of the Urban Population According to Data of
Complete Medical Examinations**

It has been pointed out that the chief purpose of complete medical examinations of inhabitants in the experimental districts of Stupino was detection of protracted (chronic) diseases for which no requests for medical aid had been recorded during the preceding year, when the sickness rate of the same population was investigated.

The medical examinations detected either early, clinically latent forms of chronic diseases, often unknown to either the patient himself or the medical institution, or diseases for which requests for medical aid had been made in previous years, but for which the patients had not resorted to medical aid in the year preceding the examinations because they were in a state of remission.

Simultaneously, the medical examinations detected chronic diseases for which requests for medical aid had been recorded in the preceding year, but which had not been confirmed by examination because of complete recovery or because of inaccurate diagnosis.

Data on the frequency of detection of various protracted diseases in the inhabitants examined are presented in Table 191.

Table 191 shows that the examinations revealed 839.5 cases per 1,000 examined inhabitants of protracted diseases or deviations from the norm that were not detected by sickness rate for the preceding year.

However, for our purposes it was important to detect not only all the chronic diseases or pathological deviations, but also those fairly pronounced clinically and calling for medical attention (hospitalization, outpatient treatment, treatment at sanatoriums and health resorts, dispensary observation, or night preventoria).

Detailed expert evaluation by clinicians of different specialties revealed that only 599.3‰ of chronic cases revealed in the course of examination need the above-enumerated medical services. In 195.3 cases per 1,000 population, the examinations did not confirm the presence of chronic diseases recorded in the same persons during the preceding year in initial records of medical institutions.

The methodological techniques for using data from complete medical examinations to work out standards of therapeutic-prophylactic services at different stages were described in the section on working methods and in the sections dealing with standards for different medical specialties.

Outpatient Polyclinic Care of the Urban Population

As already mentioned, data on attendance at outpatient polyclinics by the urban population were copied from cards in outpatient clinics and other initial records from all the therapeutic-prophylactic institutions in the territory of the cities investigated. The total number of therapeutic-prophylactic visits includes only visits to

Table 191
MORBIDITY OF THE URBAN POPULATION ACCORDING TO DATA YIELDED BY
THE COMPLETE MEDICAL EXAMINATIONS (No. of detected diseases per 1,000 population
examined)

Diseases	No. of previously unknown chronic cases revealed by the examinations	No. of chronic cases requiring medical aid detected upon examination	No. of previously known chronic cases not confirmed by the examinations
Class I. Infectious diseases	14.7	14.0	2.4
Class II. Parasitic infestations	2.6	0.6	1.9
Class III. Injuries	0.3	0.1	—
Class IV. Poisoning	—	—	—
Class V. Industrial and occupational diseases	0.1	0.1	—
Class VI. Vitamin deficiency diseases	0.3	0.3	—
Class VII. Rheumatic fever	11.0	10.5	2.5
This includes:			
rheumatic heart failure	7.1	6.8	1.9
Class VIII. Metabolic and allergic disorders	4.3	3.7	0.8
Class IX. Neoplasms	31.7	22.3	6.7
These include:			
malignant	2.3	2.2	1.2
benign tumors of the female genitals	5.9	5.6	2.6
benign dermal neoplasms	2.3	0.9	0.1
Class X. Endocrine diseases	20.8	19.3	6.4
These include:			
thyroid diseases	20.4	18.9	6.1
Class XI. Diseases of the hemopoietic system	0.8	0.7	—
Class XII. Psychic disorders	13.6	12.3	1.4
These include:			
pathological development of the personality (psychopathy)	8.6	7.9	0.5
Class XIII. Nervous diseases	90.9	79.1	26.4
These include:			
cerebral atherosclerosis and other vascular cerebral lesions, with the exception of hypertension with cerebral hemorrhage	9.3	7.5	0.8
lumbosacral radiculitis, neuritis and sciatica	15.1	13.7	9.2
neuroses	32.9	29.4	15.2
stammering	15.0	13.5	—
Class XIV. Eye diseases	35.8	20.4	1.1
These include:			
cataract	10.0	9.3	0.3
glaucoma	5.3	5.3	—
Class XV. Otorhinolaryngological diseases	178.1	89.5	22.3
These include:			
chronic otitis	26.8	20.8	3.2
pharyngitis	39.4	12.1	4.6
chronic tonsillitis	48.0	29.4	9.5
rhinitis	23.5	5.9	2.5

Table 191 (continued)

Diseases	No. of previously unknown chronic cases revealed by the examinations	No. of chronic cases requiring medical aid detected upon examination	No. of previously known chronic cases not confirmed by the examinations
Class XVI. Respiratory diseases	18.7	10.0	6.6
These include:			
bronchitis, chronic and nonspecified	3.9	2.4	1.9
pulmonary fibrosis, emphysema	11.5	5.0	2.5
Class XVII. Circulatory diseases	180.3	165.6	21.5
These include:			
myocardial fibrosis from atherosclerosis	35.4	32.5	5.0
hypertension (all stages)	54.6	53.7	2.9
atherosclerosis, general and			
nonspecified	12.6	12.5	1.1
hemorrhoids	16.8	13.7	1.7
varicose veins (except hemorrhoidal)	26.7	22.1	1.3
Class XIX. Diseases of the digestive organs	75.8	47.6	28.8
These include:			
gastritis, chronic and nonspecified	25.8	24.2	15.4
gastric and duodenal ulcers	6.6	6.7	2.4
uncomplicated hernia	19.0	3.7	1.1
Class XX. Diseases of bones, muscles and joints	27.8	13.7	15.8
Class XXI. Skin diseases	24.8	12.9	4.2
These include:			
eczema	7.2	6.0	1.9
neurodermitis	5.6	3.0	1.5
Class XXII. Renal and urinary tract diseases	2.7	2.4	4.6
Class XXIII. Diseases of the male genitals	1.8	1.1	0.2
Class XXIV. Diseases of the female genitals	47.2	42.3	37.6
These include:			
cervical erosion	9.9	9.6	5.8
oophoritis and salpingitis	9.6	9.1	5.5
Class XXV. Congenital defects	1.3	0.4	0.1
Class XVII. Neonatal diseases	0.1	—	—
Class XXVIII. Diseases not included in the			
nomenclature and wrongly designated	22.8	14.5	1.4
These include:			
simple stammering	6.7	3.0	—
complicated stammering	8.5	7.3	—
In addition:			
Diseases related to climax	4.1	3.2	2.0
Total	808.4	583.4	194.6
In addition:			
Presbyopia	1.4	0.1	—
Hypertrophy	1.5	1.0	0.3
Pes planus	7.7	0.1	0.1
Severe myopia	3.0	2.9	—
Concomitant strabismus	5.7	4.7	—
Sum total	839.5	599.3	195.3

Table 192

FREQUENCY OF OUTPATIENT POLYCLINIC VISITS BY DIFFERENT GROUPS OF DISEASES, PER 1,000 URBAN POPULATION

Disease	No. of requests for medical aid for the diseases (average indexes for the 5 cities)			No. of actual therapeutic-consultative visits			Added by the experts			Total data			Average number of therapeutic consultative visits per request for medical aid
	men	women	both sexes	men	women	both sexes	men	women	both sexes	men	women	both sexes	
Class I. Infectious diseases	237.6	198.4	216.0	530.9	392.0	452.6	129.2	105.2	116.0	660.1	497.2	568.6	2.63
Class II. Parasitic infestations	15.8	14.1	14.9	26.4	21.8	23.8	9.1	10.5	9.9	35.5	32.3	33.7	2.26
Class III. Injuries	138.3	62.2	96.6	285.9	112.7	187.9	29.7	18.6	23.5	315.6	131.3	211.4	2.18
Class IV. Poisoning	2.2	1.9	2.1	3.4	2.5	2.9	0.6	0.6	0.6	4.0	3.1	3.5	1.66
Class V. Industrial and occupational diseases	0.7	0.2	0.5	0.8	0.8	0.8		—		0.8	0.8	0.8	1.6
Class VI. Vitamin deficiency diseases	2.3	1.8	2.0	1.6	1.0	1.3	0.1	0.1	0.1	1.7	1.1	1.4	0.70
Class VII. Rheumatic fever	6.4	12.7	9.9	24.4	48.0	37.6	4.6	7.3	6.0	29.0	55.3	43.0	4.40
This includes:													
rheumatic heart failure	2.8	5.9	4.5	8.3	17.2	13.3	2.9	4.8	4.0	11.2	22.0	17.3	3.84
Class VIII. Metabolic and allergic disorders	6.0	6.7	6.4	11.7	15.8	14.0	3.6	3.5	3.5	15.3	19.3	17.5	2.73
Class IX. Neoplasms	7.3	12.7	10.4	26.7	43.5	36.0	2.6	5.5	4.2	29.3	49.0	40.2	3.86
These include:													
malignant	2.8	3.6	3.3	12.0	13.6	12.8	0.9	0.9	0.9	12.9	14.5	13.7	4.15
benign	4.5	9.2	7.1	14.7	29.8	23.2	1.7	4.6	3.3	16.4	34.4	26.5	3.73
Class X. Endocrine diseases	0.9	7.6	4.5	3.4	20.2	12.9	0.8	9.4	5.6	4.2	29.6	18.5	4.11
These include:													
thyroid diseases	0.7	7.1	4.2	2.1	18.9	11.4	0.7	9.3	5.4	2.8	28.2	16.8	4.00
Class XI. Diseases of the hemopoietic system	0.6	1.2	0.9	1.4	2.0	1.7	0.5	0.4	0.5	1.9	2.4	2.2	2.44
Class XII. Psychic disorders	4.3	2.4	3.2	12.0	7.0	9.2	9.4	7.6	8.4	21.4	14.6	17.6	5.50
These include:													
alcoholism	2.2	0.2	1.1	7.9	1.3	4.3	4.9	0.1	2.3	12.8	1.4	6.6	6.0
Class XIII. Nervous diseases	53.8	59.4	56.8	177.8	155.7	165.1	43.2	63.2	54.3	221.0	218.9	219.4	3.86
These include:													
cerebral arteriosclerosis and other vascular cerebral lesions, with the exception of hypertension with cerebral hemorrhage	4.0	6.2	5.2	12.5	12.5	12.5	3.3	6.1	4.9	15.8	18.6	17.4	3.34
lumbosacral radiculitis, neuritis and sciatica	26.0	18.5	21.8	109.1	65.6	84.6	15.1	16.1	15.6	124.2	81.7	100.2	4.59
neuroses and psychoneuroses	11.4	21.9	17.2	20.8	42.1	32.9	10.1	27.3	19.6	30.9	69.4	52.5	3.05
Class XIV. Eye diseases	40.3	37.9	39.0	69.3	53.7	60.4	22.7	20.1	2x.1	92.0	73.8	81.5	2.09
These include:													
glaucoma	0.4	0.6	0.5	1.3	1.2	1.2	0.4	0.6	0.5	1.7	1.8	1.7	3.40
Class XV. Otorhinolaryngological diseases	269.6	220.8	242.4	603.5	458.1	520.6	149.2	142.2	146.0	752.8	601.2	666.6	3.75

	1	2	3	4	5	6	7	8	9	10	11	12	13
These include:													
chronic otitis	10.4	7.6	8.9	15.1	9.6	12.1	9.5	8.4	8.9	24.6	18.0	21.0	2.36
chronic tonsillitis	11.6	12.3	11.9	38.6	42.0	40.5	20.8	23.5	22.3	32.4	35.8	34.2	2.87
Class XVI. Respiratory diseases	68.2	52.6	59.7	136.8	99.0	115.5	21.1	21.6	21.4	157.9	120.6	136.9	2.29
These include:													
bronchitis, chronic and nonspecified	12.3	8.1	10.1	18.8	11.0	14.5	1.8	2.0	1.9	20.6	13.0	16.4	1.62
pulmonary fibrosis, emphysema	3.9	1.9	2.8	11.4	3.2	6.8	0.2	0.2	0.2	11.6	3.4	7.0	2.50
Class XVII. Circulatory diseases	45.8	68.1	58.2	152.0	214.5	186.9	33.3	55.9	45.8	185.3	270.4	232.7	4.00
These include:													
myocardial fibrosis from atherosclerosis	10.2	16.8	13.9	36.2	46.5	42.0	6.7	12.6	10.0	42.9	59.1	52.0	3.74
hypertension	10.8	20.1	16.0	47.1	86.9	69.5	12.4	21.7	17.6	59.5	108.6	37.1	5.44
venous diseases	6.7	6.6	6.6	19.1	17.6	18.2	0.4	1.2	0.9	19.5	18.8	19.1	2.89
Class XVIII. Oral and dental diseases	125.6	153.1	140.7	373.6	447.2	414.6	31.4	36.3	34.1	405.0	483.5	448.7	3.19
Class XIX. Diseases of the digestive organs	91.4	81.3	85.7	256.4	188.5	217.9	18.4	23.1	21.0	274.8	211.6	238.9	2.78
These include:													
gastritis, chronic and nonspecified	22.1	20.9	21.4	66.4	50.5	57.5	3.8	7.4	5.8	70.2	57.9	63.3	2.95
gastric and duodenal ulcers	9.6	1.5	5.1	52.6	6.7	26.7	2.1	0.8	1.4	54.7	7.5	28.1	5.50
hernia	4.4	2.5	3.3	10.9	5.0	7.5	0.4	—	0.2	11.3	5.0	7.7	2.33
Class XX. Diseases of bones, muscles and joints	45.9	39.4	42.3	110.6	83.8	95.4	35.8	34.6	35.1	146.0	117.9	130.1	3.07
Class XXI. Skin diseases	60.7	47.4	53.3	138.0	91.2	111.3	34.9	28.8	31.5	172.9	120.0	142.8	2.67
These include:													
eczema	5.3	5.2	5.2	15.5	13.8	14.5	4.8	5.5	5.2	20.3	19.3	19.7	3.78
Class XXII. Renal and urinary diseases	8.2	17.2	13.0	24.8	39.5	33.0	2.9	8.7	6.2	27.7	48.2	39.2	3.01
Class XXIII. Diseases of the male genitals	3.9	—	1.7	12.2	—	5.3	0.9	—	0.4	13.1	—	5.7	3.35
Class XXIV. Diseases of the female genitals	—	84.8	46.6	—	194.5	108.7	—	37.8	20.8	—	232.3	129.5	2.78
These include:													
colpitis	—	15.1	8.4	—	41.6	23.2	—	12.3	6.8	—	53.9	30.0	3.57
cervical erosion	—	7.8	4.2	—	24.2	13.4	—	4.7	2.6	—	28.9	16.0	3.8
Class XXV. Congenital defects	0.4	0.7	0.6	0.5	1.3	0.9	0.1	0.1	0.1	0.6	1.4	1.0	1.66
Class XXVI. Diseases of pregnancy, pathology of labor and diseases of the postnatal period	0.4	14.9	8.2	0.6	21.7	12.7	0.4	4.2	2.5	1.6	25.9	15.2	1.85
Class XXVII. Neonatal diseases	0.5	0.4	0.5	0.6	0.1	0.3	0.2	0.1	0.2	0.8	0.2	0.5	1.0
Class XXVIII. Diseases not included in the nomenclature and wrongly designated	28.1	33.6	31.1	64.8	80.2	73.3	18.1	25.3	22.1	82.9	105.5	95.4	3.07
Total	1265.2	1233.5	1247.1	3050.9	2796.3	2903.0	602.9	671.7	640.9	3653.8	3468.0	3543.9	2.84
In addition:													
abortions	—	60.6	33.2	—	115.1	61.0	—	14.8	8.2	—	129.9	69.2	2.10
climax	0.2	4.4	2.5	—	11.2	6.1	—	3.9	2.1	—	15.1	8.2	3.28
errors of refraction and accommodation	10.0	13.9	12.2	8.2	8.8	8.6	4.2	3.0	3.5	12.4	11.8	12.1	1.0
deliveries	—	36.3	20.0	—	375.7	207.0	—	—	—	—	375.7	207.0	10.35
Total, without oral and dental diseases	1275.4	1348.7	1315.0	3059.1	3307.1	3185.7	607.1	693.4	654.7	3666.2	4000.5	3840.4	2.92
Sum total, without oral and dental diseases	1149.8	1195.6	1174.3	2685.5	2859.9	2771.1	575.7	657.1	620.6	3261.2	3517.0	3391.7	2.89

physicians dealing directly with outpatients. The total number of therapeutic-prophylactic visits does not include visits to physicians employed in clinical and biochemical laboratories, roentgenologists, physiotherapists, and physicians working in functional diagnostics offices. The patients are sent to these physicians otherwise than through the front office. The volume of their work is largely dependent upon the capacity of therapeutic-diagnostic offices and the qualifications of the treating physicians of different specialties.

A large part of the work in therapeutic-diagnostic offices (X-ray room, physiotherapeutic office, functional diagnostics room, laboratory) is performed by medical personnel other than doctors; staff posts of physicians for these offices are established following principles other than those involved in the establishment of the positions of physicians directly concerned with the reception of outpatients.

For these reasons, separate studies were made of the volume of work done by the therapeutic-diagnostic office (including work done by the physicians employed in these offices). Prophylactic visits were likewise recorded separately from the therapeutic-consultative visits.

Data on the frequency of therapeutic-consultative visits for different diseases are presented in Table 192.

It is seen from Table 192 that there was an average of 3,840.4 therapeutic-consultative visits per 1,000 urban population, 3,666.2 and 4,000.5 for men and women, respectively.

These figures include both actual visits and visits added on recommendations made by physicians of different specialties who carried out an expert evaluation of the completeness and quality of the outpatient-polyclinic services for every disease for which medical aid was requested, from the standpoint of modern clinical views.

The number of actually performed therapeutic-consultative visits per 1,000 urban population of both sexes was 3,185.7, and the clinical experts recommended further addition of 654.7 visits per 1,000 population.

Table 192 also lists information on the average number of therapeutic-consultative visits for different groups of diseases and certain nosological entities. There was an average of 2.92 outpatient visits for therapeutic-consultative purposes per case of request for treatment of a disease.

Data on the level of attendance for therapeutic-consultative purposes, by persons of both sexes and different age presented in Table 193 and Figure 44 are of considerable interest.

It is seen from Table 193 and Figure 44 that the intensive indexes of outpatients' attendance for therapeutic-consultative purposes show approximately the same features as the corresponding total morbidity indexes (based on sickness rate).

The attendance indexes are comparatively high in children up to 4 years old, after which they decline gradually in older children's age groups, reaching their minimum in the age group 14–19; they then proceed to increase with advancing age, again decreasing in the age group of 60 years and over.

Table 193

FREQUENCY OF OUTPATIENT VISITS FOR THERAPEUTIC-CONSULTATIVE PURPOSES
BY AGE GROUPS OF THE URBAN POPULATION (number of visits for therapeutic-
consultative purposes per 1,000 population in the corresponding age and sex group)

	Age groups									Total
	up to 4 years	5–6 years	7–13 years	14–19 years	20–29 years	30–39 years	40–49 years	50–59 years	60 and over	
No. of actual visits:										
both sexes	3107.3	2685.5	1982.8	1561.6	3612.7	3843.6	4070.7	3834.8	2422.9	3185.7
men	3002.0	2549.8	1788.9	1431.6	3381.5	3517.3	4186.2	4394.6	2865.0	3059.1
women	3223.0	2852.6	2181.1	1704.1	3918.9	4154.7	4011.6	3510.6	2198.8	3307.1
Visits added by the experts:										
both sexes	965.8	914.1	522.8	375.5	474.4	693.2	801.1	825.7	673.5	654.7
men	910.7	900.9	497.5	395.8	451.6	610.0	719.0	759.4	676.1	607.1
women	1022.4	926.6	550.3	354.2	491.7	761.7	856.8	869.6	668.9	693.4
Composite data:										
both sexes	4073.1	3599.6	2505.6	1937.1	4087.1	4536.8	4871.8	4660.5	3096.4	3840.4
men	3912.7	3450.7	2286.4	1827.4	3833.1	4127.3	4905.2	5064.0	3541.1	3666.2
women	4246.3	3779.2	2731.4	2058.3	4410.6	4916.4	4868.4	4380.2	2867.7	4000.5

Indexes of outpatient attendance by the urban population for therapeutic-consultative purposes by different medical specialties are shown in Table 194.

As is seen from Table 194, the first place with respect to outpatient attendance for therapeutic-consultative purposes is occupied by therapy, followed by pediatrics, stomatology, and obstetric-gynecology.

Of the total of 3,840.4 outpatient visits per 1,000 urban population, there were 313 house calls, mostly by pediatricians (192.7‰) and the therapists (106‰).

Data on distribution of therapeutic-consultative visits for different groups of diseases and separate nosologic entities among physicians of different specialties are very important for further standard-planning calculations.

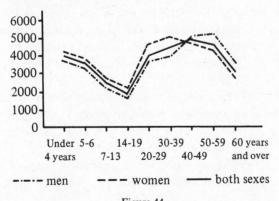

Figure 44

Frequency of outpatient visits for therapeutic-prophylactic purposes by age groups of the urban population (No. of visits per 1,000 population of the corresponding age and sex)

Table 194

INDEXES OF ATTENDANCE BY THE URBAN POPULATION AT OUTPATIENT POLY-CLINICS FOR THERAPEUTIC-CONSULTATIVE PURPOSES BY DIFFERENT MEDICAL SPECIALTIES (No. of outpatient visits per 1,000 population)

Specialty	Actual visits			Added by the experts			Composite data		
	total	at the poly-clinic	at home	total	at the poly-clinic	at home	total	at the poly-clinic	at home
Therapy	1126.0	1032.4	93.6	143.7	131.3	12.4	1269.7	1163.7	106.0
Surgery	364.0	359.5	4.5	32.8	32.4	0.4	396.8	391.9	4.9
Otorhinolaryngology	135.6	134.6	1.0	90.4	89.7	0.7	226.0	224.3	1.7
Ophthalmology	80.9	80.9	—	47.5	47.5	—	128.4	128.4	—
Dermatovenereology	108.2	106.5	1.7	37.3	36.7	0.6	145.5	143.2	2.3
Neuropathology	103.0	101.7	1.3	83.8	82.7	1.1	186.8	184.4	2.4
Phthisiology	91.8	90.9	0.9	9.6	9.5	0.1	101.4	100.4	1.0
Pediatrics	362.9	217.4	145.5	116.9	69.7	47.2	479.8	287.1	192.7
Psychiatry	6.1	5.9	0.2	16.8	16.2	0.6	22.9	22.1	0.8
Oncology	3.5	3.5	—	0.5	0.5	—	4.0	4.0	—
Stomatology	432.1	431.8	0.3	25.7	25.7	—	457.8	457.5	0.3
Obstetrics and gynecology Including:	371.6	370.8	0.8	49.7	49.6	0.1	421.3	420.4	0.9
for deliveries	207.0	207.0	—	—	—	—	207.0	207.0	—
for abortions	61.0	61.0	—	8.2	8.2	—	69.2	69.2	—
Total	3185.7	2935.9	249.8	654.7	591.5	63.2	3840.4	3527.4	313.0

These data will be helpful in establishing a more correct distribution among the different medical specialties, since physicians of many specialties participate in the services provided for outpatients suffering from certain diseases.

Data on the degree of participation of physicians of different specialties in providing medical services for outpatients suffering from various diseases were collected in the experimental districts at Stupino and used as corrective factors for the more extensive data accumulated elsewhere. These data are presented in Table 195 (according to classes of diseases).

Table 195 shows that first place belongs to therapists, who account for 35.2% of all the therapeutic-consultative visits dealt with by physicians of different specialties. Second place is occupied by dentists (18.8%), followed by pediatricians (14.3%), surgeons (10.5%), obstetrician-gynecologists (5.2%), etc.

Besides outpatient-polyclinic visits for therapeutic-consultative purposes, prophylactic visits, listed in Table 196, were also taken into account in the course of investigation.

The degree of participation of physicians of different specialties in prophylactic examinations was in accordance with the above. Pediatricians performed 34.8% of

Table 195

DISTRIBUTION OF THERAPEUTIC-CONSULTATIVE VISITS AMONG PHYSICIANS OF DIFFERENT SPECIALTIES

(percentages with respect to total for each class of diseases)

Class of disease	Therapy	Surgery	Otorhinolaryngology	Ophthalmology	Phthisiology	Neurology	Psychiatry	Stomatology	Dermatovenereology	Obstetrics-gynecology	Pediatrics	Oncology
Infectious diseases	51.3	5.6	3.7	0.2	7.3	0.8	—	0.2	1.3	0.3	29.3	—
Parasitic infestations	16.8	4.2	1.1	—	—	0.3	—	—	16.4	0.1	62.3	—
Injuries	3.6	85.5	—	4.2	—	3.0	—	0.5	0.3	—	1.3	0.1
Poisoning	68.5	2.9	—	—	—	—	—	—	—	—	28.6	—
Industrial and occupational diseases	33.4	—	—	—	—	66.6	—	—	—	—	—	—
Vitamin deficiency diseases	—	—	—	—	—	—	—	—	—	×	100.0	—
Rheumatic fever	83.1	0.6	0.4	0.5	—	2.0	—	—	7.6	—	13.9	—
Metabolic and allergic disorders	61.5	4.5	0.3	0.4	—	5.1	—	—	1.7	—	20.5	—
Neoplasms	6.4	42.4	1.1	—	0.4	3.6	—	—	—	35.6	0.9	7.5
Endocrine diseases	80.6	9.1	1.3	—	—	3.9	—	—	—	3.2	1.9	—
Psychiatric disorders	—	—	—	0.7	—	70.4	28.7	—	—	—	0.9	—
Nervous diseases	48.5	3.4	0.8	94.5	0.1	43.4	1.1	—	—	0.3	1.8	—
Eye diseases	0.8	0.2	—	0.1	0.4	0.2	—	0.5	—	—	4.2	—
Otorhinolaryngological diseases	47.6	0.1	24.3	0.1	0.4	0.2	—	—	—	—	27.3	—

Table 195 (continued)

Class of disease	Therapy	Surgery	Otorhinolaryngology	Ophthalmology	Phthisiology	Neurology	Psychiatry	Stomatology	Dermatovenereology	Obstetrics-gynecology	Pediatrics	Oncology
Respiratory diseases	49.2	0.2	1.0	0.1	2.3	—	—	—	—	—	47.2	—
Circulatory diseases	80.4	9.3	0.4	1.6	—	6.0	—	0.1	0.1	0.2	1.9	—
Oral and dental diseases	—	—	—	—	—	—	—	96.9	—	—	3.1	—
Diseases of the digestive organs	72.7	14.75	—	—	0.05	0.1	—	0.05	0.3	0.3	12.0	0.05
Diseases of the bones, muscles and joints	46.6	29.5	0.2	—	—	14.8	—	6.3	—	0.4	1.9	—
Skin diseases	6.2	14.0	1.4	0.1	0.1	0.8	—	—	69.1	0.1	8.1	0.1
Renal and urinary diseases	58.2	19.7	—	—	—	1.4	—	—	1.4	12.8	6.5	—
Diseases of the male genitals	7.7	76.9	—	—	—	3.9	—	—	—	—	11.5	—
Diseases of the female genitals	1.3	0.8	—	—	0.1	0.5	—	—	0.1	97.1	0.1	—
Congenital defects	—	42.1	—	—	5.3	5.2	—	—	—	15.8	31.6	—
Diseases of pregnancy, pathology of labor and diseases of the postnatal period	7.8	12.3	—	—	—	0.5	—	0.6	—	78.8	—	—
Neonatal diseases	—	80.0	—	—	—	—	—	—	—	—	20.0	—
Diseases not included in the nomenclature and wrongly designated	40.1	12.3	2.6	1.1	0.1	7.8	—	8.6	0.4	3.5	23.4	0.1
In addition: diseases related to climax	65.5	0.9	—	—	—	6.3	—	—	—	27.3	—	—
Total	36.2	10.5	5.0	2.0	1.3	4.3	0.2	18.8	2.1	5.2	14.3	0.1
In addition: climax												
errors of refraction and accommodation												
abortions, artificial and nonspecified deliveries												
Sum total	34.5	9.8	4.7	2.1	1.2	4.0	0.2	18.1	2.0	9.9	13.4	0.1

Table 196
FREQUENCY OF OUTPATIENT VISITS BY THE
URBAN POPULATION FOR PROPHYLACTIC PURPOSES

Kind of prophylactic visit	No. of visits per 1,000 population
Routine visits by physicians for supervision of children up to 1 year old	87.7
Examinations of preschool children	173.9
Outpatient services for 7-year-olds entering school	49.2
Examinations of schoolchildren	264.9
Occupational examinations of workers	309.6
Examinations of adolescent workers	16.3
Examinations of pregnant women	132.5
Examinations of personnel in public dining rooms and children's institutions	39.6
Issuance of various certificates and examination for further sending of the subjects to medical expert commission for evaluation of occupational fitness and for treatment at sanatoriums and health resorts	78.9
Periodic checkups during dispensary care	69.2
Other prophylactic visits	211.1
Total	1432.9

the total number of prophylactic examinations, followed by obstetrician-gyneco-logists (28.8%) and therapists (12.9%).

Hospitalization of the Urban Population

Intensive hospitalization indexes for the urban population for different groups of diseases are shown in Table 197.

It is seen from Table 197 that there were 195.1 actually hospitalized cases for 1,000 urban population of both sexes (147.6 per 1,000 men, 234 per 1,000 women); the experts added 9.9 and 10.8‰, respectively; and the composite data were 205,156.6 and 244.8‰.

The same table includes data on the average duration of hospitalization for in-patients suffering from different diseases, the composite average hospitalization period was 14.4 days.

It should be noted, however, that although the clinicians serving as experts intro-duced the necessary corrections in the frequency indexes of hospitalization require-ments, they had in their possession only data on the sickness rate of the population; therefore the listed data, like the preceding attendance data, cannot be regarded as the optimal standards of the population's requirement of hospital and outpatient-

Table 197

FREQUENCY OF HOSPITALIZATION OF THE URBAN POPULATION FOR DIFFERENT GROUPS OF DISEASES

Disease	No. of hospitalized cases per 1,000 population									Average number of days per inpatient at the hospital
	actual			added by the experts			composite data			
	men	women	both sexes	men	women	both sexes	men	women	both sexes	
Infectious diseases	29.3	20.9	24.7	0.8	1.5	1.2	30.1	22.4	25.9	15.4
Parasitic infestations	4.3	3.9	4.1	—	0.1	—	4.3	4.0	4.1	7.0
Injuries	12.6	5.6	8.8	0.3	0.2	0.3	12.9	5.8	9.1	12.7
Poisoning	1.1	0.9	1.0	0.2	—	0.1	1.3	0.9	1.1	6.7
Industrial and occupational diseases	0.1	0.1	0.1	—	—	—	0.1	0.1	0.1	18.7
Vitamin deficiency diseases	0.1	0.1	0.1	—	—	—	0.1	0.1	0.1	12.1
Rheumatic fever	2.6	3.6	3.2	0.2	0.6	0.4	2.8	4.2	3.6	28.7
This includes: rheumatic heart failure	0.7	1.2	1.0	0.1	0.5	0.3	0.8	1.7	1.3	35.6
Metabolic and allergic disorders	0.7	0.8	0.8	—	0.2	0.1	0.7	1.0	0.9	18.3
Neoplasms	2.2	4.2	3.3	0.1	0.1	0.1	2.3	4.3	3.4	26.6
These include: malignant	1.4	1.8	1.6	—	—	—	1.4	1.8	1.6	34.6
benign	0.8	2.4	1.7	0.1	0.1	0.1	0.9	2.5	1.8	20.2
Endocrine diseases	0.2	1.3	0.8	—	0.1	0.1	0.2	1.4	0.9	14.9
These include: thyroid diseases	0.1	1.0	0.6	—	0.1	0.1	0.1	1.1	0.7	15.7
Diseases of the hemopoietic system	0.3	0.4	0.4	—	—	—	0.3	0.4	0.4	18.9
Psychic disorders	2.8	3.6	3.2	0.6	0.1	0.3	3.4	3.7	3.5	80.8
Nervous diseases	7.6	4.5	5.8	0.5	0.8	0.6	8.1	5.3	6.4	16.9
These include: cerebral arteriosclerosis and other vascular cerebral lesions, with the exception of hypertension with cerebral hemorrhage	0.5	0.4	0.4	0.2	0.1	0.2	0.7	0.5	0.6	22.4
lumbosacral radiculitis, neuritis and sciatica	4.1	1.5	2.7	0.2	—	0.1	4.3	1.5	2.8	16.8
Neuroses and psychoneuroses	1.1	1.1	1.1	—	0.4	0.2	1.1	1.5	1.3	15.3
Eye diseases	1.3	1.1	1.2	0.4	0.2	0.3	1.7	1.3	1.5	13.2
These include: glaucoma	0.2	0.2	0.2	—	0.1	—	0.2	0.3	0.2	20.1
Otorhinolaryngological diseases	10.1	7.4	8.6	1.6	1.7	1.7	11.7	9.1	10.3	8.6
These include: chronic otitis	0.7	0.4	0.6	—	—	—	0.7	0.4	0.6	13.7
chronic tonsillitis	—	—	—	0.9	1.5	1.3	—	—	—	—
Respiratory diseases	20.0	13.7	16.5	1.2	0.5	0.8	12.2	14.2	17.3	13.5
These include: bronchitis, chronic and nonspecified	0.8	0.3	0.6	—	—	—	0.8	0.3	0.6	12.1
pulmonary fibrosis, emphysema	0.7	0.2	0.5	0.1	—	0.05	0.8	0.2	0.55	17.2
Circulatory diseases	7.7	7.0	7.3	0.5	1.4	1.0	8.2	8.4	8.3	19.2
These include: myocardial fibrosis from atherosclerosis	1.4	0.9	1.2	0.1	0.1	0.1	1.5	1.0	1.3	19.3
hypertension	2.3	2.6	2.5	0.4	1.0	0.8	2.7	2.6	3.3	42.0
venous diseases	1.5	1.2	1.3	—	0.1	0.05	1.5	1.3	1.35	14.2
Oral and dental diseases	0.9	0.8	0.8	0.3	—	0.1	1.2	0.8	0.9	17.3
Diseases of the digestive organs	32.0	24.0	27.6	1.5	1.3	1.4	33.5	25.3	29.0	12.5
These include: gastritis, chronic and	4.1	2.4	3.1	0.4	0.3	0.4	4.5	2.7	3.5	10.9

Table 197 (continued)

Disease	No. of hospitalized cases per 1,000 population									Average number of days per inpatient at the hospital
	actual			added by the experts			composite data			
	men	women	both sexes	men	women	both sexes	men	women	both sexes	
gastric and duodenal ulcers	5.4	0.6	2.7	0.4	0.2	0.3	5.8	0.8	3.0	18.4
hernia	1.9	0.9	1.4	—	—	—	1.9	0.9	1.4	10.7
Diseases of bones muscles and joints	3.3	1.8	2.6	—	0.1	—	3.3	1.9	2.6	17.1
Skin diseases	2.3	1.2	1.7	0.6	0.1	0.3	2.9	1.3	2.0	11.1
These include:										
eczema	0.6	0.3	0.5	0.4	0.1	0.2	1.0	0.4	0.7	12.7
Renal and urinary diseases	3.2	3.3	3.2	0.1	0.2	0.2	3.3	3.5	3.4	12.6
Diseases of the male genitals	0.9	—	0.4	—	—	—	0.9	—	0.4	11.3
Diseases of the female genitals	—	11.4	6.3	—	0.6	0.4	—	12.0	6.7	8.7
These include:										
cervical erosion	—	0.4	0.2	—	—	—	—	0.4	0.2	9.9
Congenital defects	0.1	0.1	0.1	—	—	—	0.1	0.1	0.1	17.5
Diseases of pregnancy, pathology of labor and diseases of the postnatal period	—	12.0	6.6	—	0.1	0.1	—	12.1	6.7	9.7
Neonatal diseases	0.1	0.1	0.1	—	—	—	0.1	0.1	0.1	15.0
Diseases not included in the nomenclature wrongly designated	1.8	1.9	1.8	0.1	0.4	0.2	1.9	2.3	2.0	10.0
Total	147.6	135.7	141.1	9.0	10.4	9.7	156.6	146.1	150.8	13.7
In addition:										
Abortions	—	61.6	33.8	—	0.4	0.2	—	62.0	34.0	3.7
Climax	—	0.2	0.1	—	—	—	—	0.2	0.1	9.7
Errors of refraction and accommodation	—	0.2	0.1	—	—	—	—	0.2	0.1	3.0
Deliveries	—	36.3	20.0	—	—	—	—	36.3	20.0	9.4
Sum total	147.6	234.0	195.1	9.0	10.8	9.9	156.6	244.8	205.0	11.4

polyclinic services, because of the need of corrections for diseases detected by the complete examinations.

The corrections were introduced in the sections devoted to standards of hospital services for the urban population by the different medical specialties and also in the composite table.

Characteristic features of hospitalization of the urban population of different ages and sexes are shown in Table 198 and Figure 45.

The overall composite frequency data on hospitalization of men and women of different ages (excluding abortions and deliveries) show basically the same patterns as the total morbidity indexes (based on sickness rate) of the same population.

The intensive hospitalization indexes, comparatively high for young children, gradually decline for schoolchildren and adolescents, then gradually rise with advancing age, and again decline in the age groups of 60 and over.

However, the dynamics of hospitalization indexes for women of various ages is radically altered if hospitalization for deliveries and abortions is added to the total

Table 198

INTENSIVE HOSPITALIZATION INDEXES FOR THE URBAN POPULATION OF
DIFFERENT AGES AND SEXES (No. of hospitalized cases per year per 1,000 population of the
corresponding age and sex)

	Age groups									Total
	up to 4 years	5–6 years	7–13 years	14–19 years	20–29 years	30–39 years	40–49 years	50–59 years	60 years and over	
Average hospitalization indexes:										
both sexes	262.6	133.2	104.9	112.8	277.6	268.7	185.9	157.5	120.8	195.1
men	273.6	133.0	101.4	599.9	115.8	160.3	185.0	190.9	158.1	147.6
women	251.3	133.3	108.7	126.9	419.6	353.4	186.0	136.8	103.0	234.0
Added by the experts:										
both sexes	6.6	5.2	6.6	2.8	8.2	16.6	10.5	14.4	10.4	9.9
men	4.4	5.1	3.5	2.4	8.6	16.7	10.2	15.7	7.7	9.0
women	8.9 ·	5.3	10.0	3.4	7.8	16.6	10.6	13.7	11.4	10.8
Composite data										
both sexes	269.2	138.4	111.5	115.6	285.8	285.3	196.4	171.9	131.2	205.0
men	278.0	138.1	104.9	102.3	124.4	177.0	195.2	206.6	165.8	156.6
women	260.2	138.6	118.7	130.3	427.4	370.0	196.6	150.4	114.4	244.8

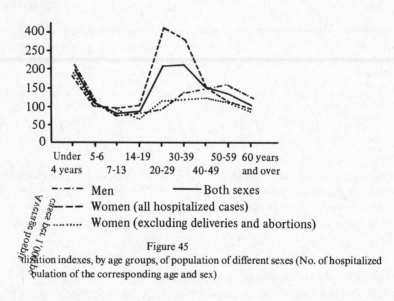

Figure 45

...lization indexes, by age groups, of population of different sexes (No. of hospitalized
...pulation of the corresponding age and sex)

number of inpatients. In this case, the hospitalization frequency indexes increase
sharply in the group of young and middle-aged women. Obviously, such additions
also have a significant effect on the age-contingent indexes calculated for the population of both sexes.

Composite Data on Standards of Therapeutic-Prophylactic Care of the Urban Population

The standards of therapeutic-prophylactic care of the urban population for the immediate future (1966–1970) were determined with a view to fairly complete fulfillment of requests for medical aid with inpatient and outpatient medical services, and also for protracted diseases newly detected by medical examinations in population groups already subjected to periodic prophylactic examinations (preschool and school-children, adolescents, draftees, certain groups of industrial workers, etc).

The planned number of outpatient visits for patients with chronic (protracted) diseases is somewhat larger than their actual number in recent years.

The volume of prophylactic services has been planned in accordance with recent methodological instructions issued by health authorities and also takes into account the working experience and personnel possibilities of therapeutic-prophylactic institutions.

The data concerning the frequency of outpatient visits for therapeutic-prophylactic services rendered to the urban population by physicians of different specialties are listed in Table 199.

It is seen from Table 199 that the plan standards per 1,000 population in 1966–1970 should include 5,277.8 visits for therapeutic purposes, 992.8 visits for dispensary care of patients suffering from protracted diseases, and 2,573.9 visits for prophylactic purposes. Furthermore, there must be 479 visits for prosthodontics per 1,000 population.

The composite table features a considerably smaller number of dental outpatient visits in comparison with the proposals of the section on Standards of Therapeutic-Prophylactic Care of the Urban Population in the Field of Stomatology (reduced from 2,300 per 1,000 population to 1,138.7). The original proposal of 2,300 visits for dental purposes was reduced because it was intended for complete satisfaction within a single year of the requirements for dental and oral care accumulated over a period of several years. Such a volume of these services was not supported by the necessary number of stomatologists and dental practitioners and the necessary equipment and it cannot be planned for one calendar year. Furthermore, one must take into account the probable absence, in the next five-year period, of dental examinations of the entire population that would detect clinically indistinct forms of dental and oral diseases which usually do not reach the stomatologists.

The working experience of stomatologists at Stupino showed that although dental examinations of the entire population of experimental districts, in the course of which all the dental and oral diseases were revealed and the subjects were recommended to resort to medical aid, resulted in a sharp increase in outpatient visits (approximately double in comparison to Moscow and Leningrad), but the number of such visits was still only 672.9 per 1,000 inhabitants examined, even though this kind of medical aid is fairly readily available.

Table 199
COMPOSITE DATA ON THE STANDARDS OF OUTPATIENT SERVICES FOR THE
URBAN POPULATION IN 1966–1970 (per 1,000 population)

Specialty	No. of visits for therapeutic purposes	No. of visits for out-patient services	Prophylactic examinations						Total visits
			industrial workers	workers, adolescents, draftees, young people aged 15–19	preschool children	schoolchildren	staff of children's institutions and public dining rooms, issuance of certificates, etc.	total prophylactic examinations	
Therapy	1427.5	271.9	122.6	61.4	—	—	261.1	410.1	2109.5
Surgery	434.5	207.3	10.7	69.0	19.7	134.1	38.6	272.1	913.9
Pediatrics	664.0	83.1	—	—	456.1	162.4	—	618.5	1365.6
Obstetrics and gynecology	421.3	116.0	223.6	—	—	—	43.3	266.9	804.2
Otorhinolaryngology	218.4	87.0	32.0	69.0	19.7	—	38.6	159.3	464.7
Ophthalmology	269.0	71.4	12.2	69.0	38.9	134.1	38.6	292.8	633.2
Neuropathology	206.6	93.6	49.7	69.0	19.7	—	6.8	145.2	445.4
Phthisiology	174.2	—	—	—	—	—	82.3	82.3	256.5
Psychiatry	126.1	—	13.8	—	—	—	25.5	39.3	165.4
Dermatovenereology	248.5	28.7	—	—	—	—	148.7	148.7	425.9
Dentistry (therapeutic)	1000.0	—	—	—	—	—	138.7	138.7	1138.7
Logopedics	67.7	—	—	—	—	—	—	—	67.7
Oncology	20.0	—	—	—	—	—	—	—	20.0
Total	5277.8	992.8	464.6	337.4	554.1	430.6	787.2	2573.9	8810.7
In addition: orthodontics	—	—	—	—	—	—	—	—	479.0
Total	—	—	—	—	—	—	—	—	9289.7

Visits to urban therapeutic-prophylactic institutions by rural inhabitants were likewise ignored. The relative importance of outpatient visits made by rural inhabitants to urban therapeutic-prophylactic institutions with reference to the total number of visits by urban inhabitants differs markedly in different Soviet cities, and therefore the indexes should be corrected for every city separately in accordance with the complex network of rural and urban medical institutions within the boundaries of the corresponding administrative territorial division.

The total number of outpatient visits by the urban population likewise does not include visits to medical offices staffed by medical assistants at industrial enterprises.

It should be noted, however, that the total number of outpatient visits per urban inhabitant (9.3 in round numbers) is somewhat too high because of the marked increase, in comparison to the existing level, in the volume of dispensary services for patients suffering from chronic diseases and also the increased number of prophylactic visits. A significant increase in the volume of outpatient services has been planned in the fields of dentistry (especially orthodontics) and logopedics.

Table 200

COMPOSITE DATA ON STANDARDS OF INPATIENT SERVICES FOR THE URBAN POPULATION IN 1966–1970

Department	Per 1,000 population		
	No. of hospitalized cases	average hospitalization period	No. of beds required
Therapeutic	44.6	17.2	2.3
Surgical	24.8	13.3	0.97
Pediatric, somatic	15.2	16.4	1.21
Obstetric	23.3	10.0	0.8
Gynecological	44.8	5.1	0.7
Otorhinolaryngological	10.6	9.2	0.29
Ophthalmological	6.2	14.5	0.26
Neuropathological	6.88	20.0	0.4
Phthisiologic	5.9	180.0	2.01
Psychiatric	7.3	80.8	1.73
Dermatovenereological	5.05	21.4	0.3
Dental	0.9	17.3	0.04
Logopedic	0.8	60.0	0.14
Infectious diseases (children)	17.6	15.5	0.9
Infectious diseases (adults)	13.1	13.5	0.6
Oncological	3.0	26.6	0.23
Total	240.03		12.87

The standards of the above-indicated sections of outpatient services for the urban population can be reduced in compilation of plans for the development of health services for the early years of the coming five-year period.

The composite data on hospitalization frequency in different departments of hospitals are provided in Table 200.

There is a need for 240.03 hospitalizations per 1,000 urban population in 1966–1970. With the average periods of hospitalization established for different departments, the total number of hospital beds should be 12.87 per 1,000 population.

A very considerable increase in the numbers of beds is planned for tuberculosis patients (2 beds per 1,000 population in hospitals and 1.1 beds in sanatoriums) with a view to a sharp reduction and gradual eradication of tuberculosis within 15–10 years.

Bibliography

PUBLICATIONS IN RUSSIAN

ALBATS, E. I. *Zdravookhranenie Rossiiskoi Federatsii,* No. 9. 1964.

ARKAD'EVA, R. I. Opyt dispansernogo nablyudeniya detei rannego i doshkol'nogo vozrasta v rabote detskoi polikliniki (Experience in the Dispensary Observation of Infants and
Preschool Children in the Work of the Pediatric Polyclinic). In: *Ambulatorno-poliklinicheskoe obsluzhivanie naseleniya.* Moscow. 1959.

AVERBUKH, L. A. Zabolevaemost' vzroslogo naseleniya goroda Kieva po dannym uglublen-
nogo izucheniya za 1958 g. (Morbidity of the Adult Population of Kiev from the Data of
Extended Studies in 1958). In: *Tezisy IV nauchnoi sessii Instituta organizatsii zdravookhraneniya i istorii meditsiny imeni N. A. Semashko.* Moscow. 1961.

BABYNIN, B. *Byulleten' Gosplana RSFSR,* Nos. 23–24. 1926.

BARSUKOV, M. I., D. V. GORFIN, S. M. DASHYUSHEVSKII, and A. K. PATRINA. Osnovnye
etapy razvitiya planirovaniya sovetskogo zdravookhraneniya za 40 let (The Main Developmental Stages in 40 Years of Soviet Public Health Planning). Abstract. In: *3-ya nauchnaya
sessiya Instituta organizatsii zdravookhraneniya i istorii meditsiny imeni N. A. Semashko,
17–22 fevralya, 1958 g.* Moscow. 1958.

BARSUKOV, M. I. and A. P. ZHUK. *Za sotsialisticheskuyu rekonstruktsiyu zdravookhraneniya.
Osnovnye polozheniya 2-go pyatiletnogo plana zdravookhraneniya SSSR (Socialist Reconstruction of Public Health. Principal Statements of the 2nd Five-Year Plan for Public Health
of the USSR).* Moscow, Medgiz. 1923.

BELITSKAYA, E. YA. *Sovetskii Vrachebnyi Zhurnal,* No. 15. 1939.

BELYAEVA, S. Zabolevaemost' naseleniya goroda Rigi v 1958 g. (Morbidity of the Population
of Riga in 1958). In: *Tezisy IV nauchnoi sessii Instituta organizatsii zdravookhraneniya i
istorii meditsiny imeni N. A. Semashko.* Moscow. 1961.

BEN, E. E. Zabolevaemost' leningradskogo naseleniya za 1928 g. (Morbidity of the Leningrad Population during 1928). In: *Statisticheskii sbornik Leningradskogo oblastnogo otdela
zdravookhraneniya za 1928 g.* Leningrad, Izdatel'stvo Lenoblizdat. 1929.

BEN, E. E. and S. A. NOVOSEL'SKII. *Zabolevaemost' naseleniya goroda Leningrada (Morbidity of the Leningrad Population).* Ogiz. 1935.

BOGATYREV, I. D. *Vrachebnoe Delo,* No. 7. 1957.

BOGATYREV, I. D. et al. O normativakh lechebno-profilakticheskogo obsluzhivaniya promyshlennykh rabochikh (Standards of Therapeutic and Prophylactic Care of Industrial

Workers). *Nauchnye trudy Instituta organizatsii zdravookhraneniya i istorii meditsiny imeni N. A. Semashko*, No. 3. Moscow. 1958.

BOGATYREV, I. D. *Sovetskoe Zdravookhranenie*, No. 1. 1959.

BOGATYREV, I. D. *Zdravookhranenie*, No. 1. 1959.

BOGATYREV, I. D. *Zabolevaemost' i lechebno-profilakticheskoe obsluzhivanie promyshlennykh rabochikh (Morbidity and Therapeutic- Prophylactic Care of Industrial Workers)*. Moscow, Medgiz. 1962.

BOGATYREV, I. D. *Zdravookhranenie*, No. 1. 1962.

BOGATYREV, I. D. O metodike nauchno-issledovatel'skoi raboty po opredeleniyu normativov potrebnosti naseleniya v lechebno-profilakticheskom obsluzhivanii (Methods of Scientific Research Work in Determining the Standards of the Population's Therapeutic-Prophylactic Care Requirements). In: *VI Soveschchanie ministrov zdravookhraneniya sotsialisticheskish stran*. Budapest. 1964.

BOGATYREV, I. D. and P. I. KAL'YU. *O metodike nauchno-issledovatel'skoi raboty po opredeleniyu potrebnosti naseleniya v meditsinskoi pomoshchi (Methods of Scientific Research in Determining the Population's Medical Care Requirements)*. Moscow, Medgiz. 1956.

BOGOSLOVSKII, S. M. *Statistika professional'noi zabolevaemosti (Statistics of Occupational Disease)*. TsSU SSSR, Part 1. Moscow. 1962.

BOGOSLOVSKII, S. M. *Zabolevaemost' (Morbidity)*. BME, Vol. 10, p. 404.

BOGOSLOVSKII, S. M., L. A. BRUSHLINSKAYA, P. I. KURKIN, and A. A. CHERTOV. *Zabolevaemost' naseleniya Moskovskoi gubernii i goroda Moskvy (Morbidity of the Population of Moscow Province and Moscow City)*. Moscow, Izdatel'stvo Mosgorzdravotdela. 1929.

BOGOSLOVSKII, S. M. and P. I. KURKIN. *Obshchestvo Vrachei*, No. 6. 1911.

BOITSOVA, O. S. *Metodika opredeleniya norm potrebnosti detskogo naseleniya v statsionarnom i sanatornom koechnom fonde (dlya lecheniya bol'nykh revmatizmom) (Methods of Determining Standards of the Child Population's Hospital and Sanatorium Bed Capacity Requirements for Treatment of Rheumatic Patients)*. Candidate Thesis. Moscow. 1960.

BOYARSKII, A. YA. and P. P. SCHUMERIN. *Demograficheskaya statistika (Demographic Statistics)*, 2nd edition. Moscow. 1955.

BRUSHLINSKAYA, L. A. Osnovnye itogi izucheniya zdorov'ya naseleniya RSFSR za 1958 g. (Main Results of the 1958 Health Examination of the Population of the RSFSR). In: *IV nauchnaya sessiya Instituta organizatsii zadravookhraneniya i istorii meditsiny*. Abstracts. Moscow. 1961.

BRUSHLINSKAYA. L. A., A. N. MEERKOV, and M. V. OVCHINSKII. *Sostoyanie zdorov'ya naseleniya goroda Moskvy (po materialam obrashchaemosti za meditsinskoi pomoshch'yu) (State of Health of the Population of Moscow City (from Data on Applications for Medical Care))*. Moscow. 1946.

CHERBA, L. Nekotorye voprosy 20-letnego perspektivnogo plana razvitiya bol'nits v Vengrii (Some Problems of the 20-Year Hospital Development Plan in Hungary). In: *VI Soveshchanie ministrov zdravookhraneniya sotsialisticheskikh stran*. Budapest. 1963.

CHERTOV, A. A. Opyt primeneniya vyborochnogo metoda k razrabotke materialov po zabolevaemosti naseleniya (Experience with the Selective Method in Processing Population Morbidity Data). In: *XIs''ezd bakteriologov, epidemiologov i sanitarnykh vrachei*. 1928.

DEICHMAN, E. I. *Gigiena i Sanitariya*, No. 10. 1955.

DEICHMAN, E. I. and Ts. N. SLAVOVA. Rasprostranennost' serdechno-sosudistykh zabolevanii sredi gorodskogo naseleniya (po materialam gg. Noginska i Chernovtsy) (Distribution of Cardiovascular Diseases among the Urban Population (from Data of the Cities of Noginsk and Chernovtsy)). In: *Tezisy IV nauchnoi sessii Instituta organizatsii zdravookhraneniya i istorii meditsiny imeni N. A. Semashko.* Moscow. 1961.

EFMAN, A. M. Normy bol'nichnoi pomoshchi rabochim metallurgii Urala (Hospital Treatment Norms for Metallurgy Workers in the Urals). *Sbornik rabot Sverdlovskogo oblastnogo gigienicheskogo instituta,* edited by V. I. VELICHKIN, No. 1, p. 43. 1936.

EL'CHIN, B. *Na fronte zdravookhraneniya,* Nos. 11–12. 1930.

ENGELS, F. *Anti-Dühring.* Gospolitizdat. 1951.

ERMAN, S. S. and S. YU. ROMANOVSKAYA. Izuchenie potrebnosti i obosnovanie normativov statsionarnoi i poliklinicheskoi pomoshchi detyam (A Study on the Need and Basis for Standards of Hospital and Polyclinic Treatment for Children). *Rukopis' instituta pediatrii AMN SSSR.* 1951.

ESIPOVICH, YA. N. Opyt organizatsii dispansernogo nablyudeniya detei i podrostkov, stradayushchikh zabolevaniyami ukha i verkhnikh dykhatel'nykh putei (Experience in Organizing Dispensary Observation of Children and Adolescents Suffering from Diseases of the Ear and the Upper Respiratory Tract). *Trudy I Vserossiiskogo s"ezda otorinolaringologov.* Moscow. 1963.

FREIDLIN, S. YA. O planirovanii vnebol'nichnoi terapevticheskoi pomoshchi v gorodakh (Planning of Outpatient Therapeutic Treatment in Cities). Abstracts. In: *3-ya nauchnaya sessiya Instituta organizatsii zdravookhraneniya i istorii meditsiny imeni I. A. Semashko, 17–22 fevralya, 1958g.* Moscow, 1958.

FREIDLIN, S. YA. *Zdravookhranenie Rossiiskoi Federatsii,* No. 8. 1958.

FREIDLIN, S. YA. *Gorodskaya poliklinika (The Urban Polyclinic).* Moscow–Leningrad. 1961.

FREIDLIN, S. YA. (editor). *Dispanserizatsiya gorodskogo naseleniya (Dispensary Systems of Urban Populations).* Meditsina. 1964.

FRIDLYAND, I. G. Znachenie professional'no-proizvodstvennykh faktotov v etiologii obshchikh zabolevanii (The Significance of Occupational Factors in the Etiology of General Diseases). In: *Tezisy doklada XIII s"ezdu infektsionistov, epidemiologov i mikrobiologov.* Moscow. 1956.

FRIDLYAND, I. G. *O tak nazyvaemom nespetsificheskom deistvii promyshlennykh yadov (The So-Called Nonspecific Effect of Industrial Poisons).* Medgiz. 1957.

FRIDZEL', E. and I. KACHAN. *Obshchaya zabolevaemost' zastrakhovannykh po gorodu Khar'kovu v 1923–1924gg. (Total Morbidity of the Insured in Kharkov in 1923–1924).* Khar'kov. 1926.

FROLOVA, N. A. Zabolevaemost' naseleniya goroda Kalinina, po dannym obrashchaemosti v 1958 g. (Morbidity of the Kalinin Population according to Sickness Rate Data for 1958). *Sovetskoe Zdravookhranenie,* No. 10. 1960.

GARGOSOV, L. V. Zabolevaemost' po dannym obrashchaemosti naseleniya gorodov Vil'nyusa, Kaunasa i Klaipedy (Population Morbidity in Vilnius, Kaunas and Klaipeda according to Data on the Sickness Rate). In: *Tezisy IV nauchnoi sessii instituta.* Moscow. 1961.

GASHIMOVA, K. A. *K metodike vyyavleniya norm potrebnosti v poliklinicheskoi pomoshchi detyam (Methods of Showing the Norms for Polyclinic Care Requirements of Children).* Candidate Thesis. Moscow. 1955.

GOL'DFAIL', L. G. (editor). *Rukovodstvo dlya vrachei po sanatorno-kurortnomu otboru (Hand-*

book for Physicians Working in Sanatorium-Health Resort Selection). Medgiz. 1961.

GOLOVANOVA, G. P. and V. YA. LEONT'EV. *Metodicheskoe posobie po otsenke fizicheskogo razvitiya detei doshkol'nogo i shkol'nogo vozrasta (Textbook on Methods of Evaluating the Physical Development of Preschool and School-Children)*, edited by A. G. TSEITLIN. Moscow. 1960.

GORFIN, D. V. Itogi i perspektivy organizatsii lechebnogo dela v gorodakh i polozhenie spetsial'nykh vidov lechebnoi pomoshchi (Results and Prospects of Therapeutic Work in Cities and the State of Specific Types of Therapeutic Treatment). In: *Lechebnoe delo v RSFSR. Materialy k dokladu V s''ezda zdravootdelov*. Moscow. 1924.

GORFIN, D. V. *Byulleten' Narodnogo Komissariata Zdravookhraneniya*, No. 20. 1927.

GOVOR, N. N. *Sovetskoe Zdravookhranenie*, No. 7. 1958.

GRIGOR'EV, M. G. Profilaktika travmatizma i lechenie povrezhdenii u rabochikh mashino-stroitel'noi i khimicheskoi promyshlennosti (Prophylaxis of Traumatism and Treatment of Injuries of Workers in Machine Construction and Chemical Industry). In: *Materialy k ob''edinennoi nauchnoi sessii, posvyashchennoi voprosam okhrany truda i profilaktiki professional'nykh boleznei i travmatizma*. Gorki. 1961.

GRININA, O. V. *Zdravookhranenie Rossiiskoi Federatsii*, No. 47. 1964.

GUREVICH, I. L. and L. B. NEPOMNYASHCHII.*Sovetskaya Vrachebnaya Gazeta*, No. 8. 1934.

ILUPINA, F. M., V. D. DUBROVINA, and L. I. GRIBKOVA. *Sovetskoe Zdravookhranenie*, No. 1. 1961.

Instruktsiya o rabote shkol'nogo vracha. Utverzhdena Ministerstvom zdravookhraneniya SSSR 10 iyulya 1954 (Instruction Pertaining to the School Physician's Work. Approved by the Ministry of Public Health of the USSR on 10 July 1954). In: *Zakonodatel'stvo po zdravookhraneniyu*, Vol. 2, No. 2, p. 512. Moscow. 1957.

Instruktsiya po organizatsii raboty poliklinicheskogo otdeleniya detskoi bol'nitsy. Utverzhdena Ministerstvom zdravookhraneniya SSSR 7 fevralya 1949 (Instruction on Organizing the Polyclinic Section of a Children's Hospital. Approved by the Ministry of Public Health of the USSR on 7 February 1949). In: *Zakonodatel'stvo po zdravookhraneniyu*, Vo. 2, No. 2, p. 487. Moscow. 1957.

Itogi vsesoyuznoi perepisi naseleniya SSSR 1959g. (Results of the 1959 All-Union General Population Census of the USSR). Composite Volume. Gosstatizdat. 1962.

KAMINSKII, L. S. *K voprosu o postroenii seti vnebol'nichnoi pomoshchi v Leningrade (The Problem of Organizing an Outpatient Service Network in Leningrad)*. Leningrad. 1934.

KAMINSKII, M. I. *Vrachebnoe Delo*, No. 2. 1955.

KAMINSKII, M. I. *Zdravookhranenie Rossiiskoi Federatsii*, No. 9. 1958.

KARCHAVA, A. I. and E. V. KIKALEISHVILI. *Zabolevaemost' vzroslogo naseleniya raiona goroda Tbilisi za 1954 g.* (Morbidity of the Adult Population of the Tbilisi District for 1954). In: *Tezisy dokladov I Gruzinskogo s''ezda gigienistov i sanitarnykh vrachei*. 1956.

KARCHAVA, A. I. Obshchaya zabolevaemost' naseleniya goroda Tbilisi v 1958 g. (Total Morbidity of the Urban Population of Tbilisi in 1958). In: *Tezisy IV nauchnoi sessii Instituta organizatsii zdravookhraneniya i istorii meditsiny imeni N. A. Semashko*.

KASSATSIER, M. YA. Serdechno-sosudistye zabolevaniya gorodskogo naseleniya RSFSR (Cardiovascular Diseases of the Urban Population of the RSFSR). *Statisticheskie materialy o serdechno-sosudistykh zabolevaniyakh*. Medgiz. 1960.

KATSENELENBAUM, M. S. O roli statisticheskikh gruppirovok v gigienicheskikh issledovaniyakh (The Role of Statistical Groupings in Hygiene Investigations). In: *Metodicheskie voprosy sanitarnoi statistiki. Informatsionnyi byulleten'*, p. 31. Moscow. 1959.

KHOTSYANOV, L. K. and G. I. PETROV. *Gigiena i Sanitariya*, No. 4. 1958.

KISELEV, S. M. *Metodologiya planirovaniya zdravookhraneniya (Methodology of Public Health Planning)*. Gosmedizdat. 1931.

KOGAN, R. B. Sotsial'no-gigienicheskaya otsenka sovremennogo urovnya zdorov'ya detei rannego vozrasta (Social-Hygiene Evaluation of the Current Health Level of Infants). In: *Sovremennye problemy organizatsii zdravookhraneniya v SSSR*. Moscow. 1964.

KOIRANSKII, B. B. and R. A. ZAKS. *Sanitariya i Gigiena*, No. 2. 1958.

KOVALEV, I. K metodologii razrabotki norm lechebno-profilakticheskoi pomoshchi gorodskomu naseleniyu (The Methodology of Working out Norms for Therapeutic-Prophylactic Care of the Urban Population). In: *Metodologicheskaya razrabotka norm lechebnoi pomoshchi gorodskomu naseleniyu*. Moscow–Leningrad. 1930.

KOZLOV, A. I. Sostoyanie travmatizma, travmatologicheskaya i ortopedicheskaya pomoshch' i perspektivy ee razvitiya v Kirovskoi oblasti (The State of Traumatism, Traumatological and Orthopedic Care and Prospects of Its Development in the Kirov Region). In: *Materialy k ob"edinennoi nauchnoi sessii, posvyashchennoi voprosam okhrany truda i profilaktiki, professional'nykh boleznei i travmatizma*. Gorki. 1961.

KOZLOV, P. M. Zabolevaemost' gorodskogo naseleniya nakanune Velikoi Otechestvennoi voiny (1939–1940) (Morbidity of the Urban Population on the Eve of World War II (1939–1940). *Rukopisnyi fond Instituta organizatsii zdravookhraneniya i istorii meditsiny imeni N. A. Semashko*. 1947.

KOZLOV, P. M. *Sanitarnaya statistika (Sanitary Statistics)*. Moscow, Medgiz. 1949.

KUDRYAVTSEVA, E. N. *Vrachebnoe Delo*, No. 10. 1955.

KURAKOV, A. YA. *Sovetskoe Zdravookhranenie*, No. 10. 1962.

KURASHOV, S. V. *Sovetskaya Meditsina*, No. 4. 1957.

KURASHOV S. V. *Sovetskoe Zdravookhranenie*, No. 3. 1957.

KURASHOV, S. V. *Organizatsiya bor'by s serdechno-sosudistymi zabolevaniyami (Organization of the Control of Cardiovascular Diseases)*. Moscow. 1960.

KURKIN, P. I. Sovremennoe polozhenie sanitarno-statisticheskikh issledovanii v Moskovskoi gubernii (Current State of Sanitary and Statistical Investigations in Moscow Province). *Trudy soveshchaniya po tekushchim voprosam sanitarnoi statistiki*. Moscow. 1910.

KURKIN, P. I. *Obshchestvennyi Vrach*, Nos. 9–10. 1917.

KURKIN, P. I. Statistika boleznennosti naseleniya v SSSR (Statistics of the Susceptibility to Disease of the USSR Population). In: S. A. NOVOSEL'SKII and G. WHIPPLE. *Osnovy demograficheskoi i sanitarnoi statistiki*. 1929.

KURKIN, P. I. Kharakteristika statisticheskogo materiala po vyrabotke norm meditsinskoi pomoshchi naseleniya (Characteristics of Statistical Data on Working out the Norms for Medical Care of the Population). In: *Metodologiya razrabotki norm lechebnoi pomoshchi gorodskomu naseleniyu*. Moscow–Leningrad. 1930.

KURKIN, P. I. *Rozhdaemost' i smertnost' v kapitalisticheskikh gosudarstvakh Evropy (Birth Rate and Mortality in the Capitalist Countries of Europe)*. 1938.

KUVSHINNIKOV, P. A. *Gigiena i Epidemiologiya*, No. 10. 1926.

KUVSHINNIKOV, P. A. *Statisticheskii metod kliniko-statisticheskikh issledovanii (The Statistical Method of Clinical Investigations)*. Medgiz. 1955.

KUVSHINNIKOV, P. A. (editor). *Voprosy izucheniya zabolevaemosti (Problems of Studying Morbidity)*. Medgiz. 1956.

Lechebno-vspomogatel'nye otdeleniya bol'nitsy obshchego tipa (Therapeutic-Supportive Sections of the General Hospital). Moscow. 1960.

LEKAREV, L. G., F. S. RYUKHOV, and V. I. TYSHETSKII. *Vrachebnoe Delo*, No. 6. 1957.

LEL'CHUK, P. L. and O. I. BARSUKOV. Zhenskaya konsul'tatsiya (osnovnye voprosy okhrany zdorov'ya zhenshchiny) (Gynecological Consultation (the Main Problem in Prophylaxis of Diseases in Women)). Rostovskoe Knizhnoe Izdatel'stvo. 1964.

LEMINEV, L. M. and YA. I. ROZOV. *Sovetskoe Zdravookhranenie*, No. 2. 1957.

LENIN, V. I. Materialy po peresmotru partiinoi programmy (Data on Revision of the Party Program). *Sochineniya (Coll. Works)*, Vol. 32. 5th edition.

LENIN, V. I. Rech' ob obmane naroda lozungami svobody i ravenstva (Speech on Delusion of the Nation by Liberty and Equality Slogans). *Sochineniya (Coll. Works)*, Vol. 38. 5th edition.

LENIN, V. I. Doklad Vserossiiskogo Tsentral'nogo Ispolnitel'nogo Komiteta i Soveta Narodnykh Komissarov o vneshnei i vnutrennei politike (Report by the All-Russian Central Executive Committee and Council of People's Commissars on Foreign and Domestic Policy). *Sochineniya (Coll. Works)*, Vol. 42. 5th edition.

LENIN, V. I. K voprosu o dialektike (The Problem of Dialectics). *Sochineniya (Coll. Works)*, Vol. 29. 5th edition.

LEVINA, I. G. Zabolevaemost' naseleniya goroda Tallina za 1958 g. (Morbidity of the Population of Tallin in 1958). In: *Tezisy IV nauchnoi sessii Instituta organizatsii zdravookhraneniya i istorii meditsiny imeni N. A. Semashko*, Moscow. 1961.

MARX, K. *Das Kapital*, Vol. 1, pp. 77, 78. [Russian edition. 1951.]

MASHKOVSKII, M. D. *Lekarstvennye sredstva (Medicaments)*. Medgiz. 1960.

MASLENKOVA, N. V. *Sovetskoe Zdravookhranenie*, No. 3. 1964.

Materialy k pyatiletnemu planu zdravookhraneniya RSFSR (Data on the Five-Year Public Health Plan of the RSFSR). Moscow. 1930.

Materialy po zabolevaemosti naseleniya goroda Ivanovo (Data on Population Morbidity in Ivanovo). Moscow. 1959.

Materialy XXII s"ezda KPSS (Materials of the XXII Congress of the Communist Party of the Soviet Union). Moscow. 1961.

MAZUR, M. M. *Zdravookhranenie Rossiiskoi Federatsii*, No. 2. 1959.

MAZUR, M. M. *Sovetskoe Zdravookhranenie*, No. 10. 1960.

MAZUR, M. M. *Voprosy kurortologii, fizioterapii i lechebnoi fizkul'tury*, No. 4. 1960.

MAZUR, M. M. *Voprosy kurortologii, fizioterapii i lechebnoi fizkul'tury*, No. 3. 1962.

MAZUR, M. M. and T. I. DOBROVOL'SKAYA. Kontingenty bol'nykh i zabolevaemost' naseleniya goroda Stupino v 1949 g. (Disease and Morbidity Rate of the Population of Stupino in 1949). In: *Voprosy izucheniya zabolevaemosti*. Medgiz. 1956.

MELLER, M. S. Zabolevaemost' detei rannego vozrasta (Infant Morbidity). In: *Sostoyanie zdorov'ya naseleniya goroda Moskvy*. Moscow. 1946.

MEL'NIKOVA, R. A. *Sovetskoe Zdravookhranenie*, No. 11. 1957.

MERKOV, A. M. *Zlokachestvennye novoobrazovaniya na Ukraine (Malignant Neoplasms in the Ukraine)*. Kharkov. 1940.

MERKOV, A. M. *Gigiena i Sanitariya*, No. 3. 1955.

MERKOV, A. M. *Sovetskoe Zdravookhranenie*, No. 7. 1957.

MERKOV, A. M. *Demografscheskaya statistika (posobie dlya vrachei) (Demographic Statistics (Textbook for Physicians))*. Moscow. 1959.

MERKOV, A. M. *Sovetskoe Zdravookhranenie*, No. 6. 1959.

Metodicheskoe pis'mo po provedeniyu massovykh profilakticheskikh ginekologicheskikh osmotrov zhenskogo naseleniya (utverzhdeno Ministerstvom zdravookhraneniya SSSR 8/IX 1956 g.) (Leaflet on the Subject of Prophylactic Gynecological Mass Examinations of the Female Population (approved by the Ministry of Public Health of the USSR on 8 September 1956)).

Metodicheskie ukazaniya po organizatsii akushersko-ginekologicheskogo obsluzhivaniya rabotnikov na promyshlennykh predpriyatiyakh. Utverzhdeno Ministerstvom zdravookhraneniya SSSR 10/I 1959. (Operating Instructions Pertaining to the Organization of an Obstetric Gynecological Service for Workers in Industrial Enterprises. Approved by the Ministry of Public Health of the USSR on 10 January 1959).

Metodicheskie materialy po organizatsii bor'by s kozhnymi i venericheskimi boleznyami (Methodical Data on the Control of Skin and Venereal Diseases). Moscow. 1962.

Metodologiya razrabotki norm lechebnoi pomoshchi gorodskomu naseleniyu (Methodology for Working Out Standards of Medical Care for the Urban Population). Moscow–Leningrad. 1930.

MIKHAILOV, S. M. K voprosu o vyrabotke norm meditsinskoi pomoshchi gorodskomu naseleniyu polupromyshlennogo goroda (The Problem of Working Out Norms for Medical Care for the Urban Population of a Semi-Industrial City). In: *Metodologiya razrabotki norm lechebnoi pomoshchi gorodskomu naseleniyu*. Moscow–Leningrad. 1930.

MINKINA, V. A. and V. I. CHEBAROVA. *Voprosy Okhrany Materinstva i Detstva*, No. 6. 1961.

MINYAEV, V. A. *Zdravookhranenie Rossiiskoi Federatsii*, No. 3. 1957.

MINYAEV, V. A. *Sovetskoe Zdravookhranenie*, No. 5. 1957.

MINYAEV, V. A. *Zdravookhranenie Rossiiskoi Federatsii*, No. 6. 1960.

MOZGLYAKOVA, V. A. Predvaritel'nye itogi izucheniya zabolevaemosti gorodskogo naseleniya SSSR v 1958–1959 gg. (Preliminary Results of a Study of the Morbidity of the Urban Population of the USSR in 1958–1959). In: *Trudy Instituta imeni N. A. Semashko i kafedr organizatsii zdravookhraneniya i istorii meditsiny*. Moscow. 1961.

Narodnoe khozyaistvo SSSR v 1961 g. (The National Economy of the USSR in 1961). Gosstatizdat. 1962.

NAZAROVA, N. S. and E. V. ABRAMOVA. O normakh potrebnosti v poliklinicheskoi i statsionarnoi pomoshchi detskogo naseleniya goroda Moskvy (Norms for Moscow's Child Population's Requirement of Polyclinic and Hospital Care). In: *Sbornik nauchnykh rabot Instituta imeni N. A. Semashko*. Moscow. 1957.

NESTEROV, V. A. *Zdravookhranenie Rossiiskoi Federatsii*, No. 11. 1963.

NESTEROV, V. A. *Materialy o vliyanii serdechno-sosudistykh zabolevanii na zdorov'e naseleniya Krasnodarskogo kraya i meditsinskom obsluzhivanii kardiologicheskikh bol'nykh (Data on the Effect of Cardiovascular Diseases on the Health of the Population of the Krasnodar Region and Medical Care of Cardiological Patients)*. Abstract of Doctoral Thesis. Leningrad. 1964.

NIKITSKII, V. S. *Sovetskoe Zdravookhranenie*, Nos. 4–5. 1945.

NIKITSKII, V. S. *Sovetskoe Zdravookhranenie*, No. 9. 1945.

Nosov, S. D. *Pediatriya*, No. 2. 1962.

Novgorodtsev, G. A. and G. A. Popov. *Sovetskoe Zdravookhranenie*, No. 8. 1963.

Novosel'skii, S. A. *Vestnik obshchestvennoi gigieny (Bulletin of Public Hygiene)*. March. 1914.

Novosel'skii, S. A. *Smertnost' i prodolzhitel'nost' zhizni v Rossii (Mortality and Life Expectancy in Russia)*. St. Peterburg. 1916.

Novosel'skii, S. A. Vliyanie voiny na estestvennoe dvizhenie naseleniya (The Effect of War on Natural Population Dynamics). *Trudy komissii po obsledovaniyu sanitarnykh posledstvii voiny.* Moscow. 1923.

Novosel'skii, S. A. and V. V. Paevskii. O svodnykh kharakteristikakh vosproizvodstva i perspektivnykh ischisleniyakh naseleniya (On Composite Characteristics of Reproduction and Future Estimates of Population). *Trudy Demograficheskogo Instituta AMN SSSR*, Vol. 1. Leningrad. 1934.

O merakh profilaktiki rasstroistv zreniya u detei doshkol'nogo vozrasta i v gody shkol'nogo obucheniya. Metodicheskie ukazaniya Ministerstva zdravookhraneniya SSSR ot 16 fevralya 1957 g. (On Measures to Prevent Visual Disturbances in Children of Preschool and School Age. Standing Instructions of the Ministry of Public Health of the USSR from 16 February 1957) Nos. 236–257. In: *Zakonodatel'stvo po zdravookhraneniyu*, Vol. 6, p. 351. Moscow. 1963.

Obshchii svod po imperii rezul'tatov razrabotki dannykh pervoi vseobshchei perepisi naseleniya, proizvedennoi 28 yanvarya 1897 goda (Summary of the Data Processed from the First General Census of the Population of the Empire, Taken on 28 January 1897), Vol. 1. St. Peterburg. 1905.

Organizatsiya meditsinskogo obsluzhivaniya detei v yaslyakh-sadu (Organization of Medical Care of Children in Kindergartens and Creches). *Metodicheskoe Pis'mo*. Moscow. 1962.

Ovcharov, V. K. *Zdravookhranenie Rossiiskoi Federatsii*, No. 5. 1964.

Ovchinskii, M. V. *Professional'naya Meditsina*, No. 8. 1928.

Paevskii, V. V. O primenenii vyborochnogo metoda i razrabotke dannykh zabolevaemosti (pervichnoi obrashchaemosti) (The Selective Method and Morbidity Data Processing (Primary Application for Treatment)). In: *XI Vsesoyuznyi s"ezd bakteriologov, epidemiologov i sanitarnykh vrachei.* Abstracts. Leningrad. 1928.

Pol'chenko, V. I. *Sovetskoe Zdravookhranenie*, No. 1. 1958.

Popov, G. A. *Vrachebnye kadry i planirovanie ikh podgotovki (Medical Personnel and the Planning of Their Training)*. Medgiz. 1963.

Preobrazhenskii, B. S. Profilaktika tugoukhosti i glukhoty (Prophlaxis of Hardness of Hearing and Deafness). In: *Programmnye doklady na V Vsesoyuznom s"ezde otorinolaringologov.* Moscow–Dushanbe. 1958.

Preobrazhenskii, B. S. *Zhurnal Ushnykh, Nosovykh i Gorlovykh Boleznei*, No. 6. 1959.

Prikaz ministra zdravookhraneniya SSSR No. 354 ot 30 iyulya 1930 g. "O merakh po dal'neishemu uluchsheniyu mediko-sanitarnogo obsluzhivaniya podrostkov" (Order of the Minister of Public Health of the USSR, No. 354 of 30 July 1930 "On Measures for Further Improvement of Medical and Sanitary Care of Adolescents"). Supplement 2.

Prikaz ministra zdravookhraneniya SSSR ot 20 iyulya 1960 g. No. 321. "O sostoyanii i merakh po dal'neishemu uluchsheniyu ambulatorno-poliklinicheskogo obsluzhivaniya gorodskogo naseleniya" (Order of the Minister of Public Health of the USSR No. 321 of 20 July 1960

"On the Current State and Measures for Further Improvement of Ambulatory and Poly-clinic Care of the Urban Population").

PRIPTSING, F. *Metod sanitarnoi statistiki (Methods of Sanitary Statistics)*. Moscow. 1925.

Programma Kommunisticheskoi partii Sovetskogo Soyuza (Program of the Communist Party of the Soviet Union). Moscow, Izd. "Pravda". 1961.

PTUKHA, M. V. *Smertnost'v Rossii i na Ukraine (Mortality in Russia and the Ukraine)*. (In Ukrainian). 1928.

PTUKHA, M. V. Osnovy ischisleniya naseleniya USSR na vtoruyu pyatiletku (Principles in the Estimation of the Population of the Ukrainian SSR in the Second Five-Year Plan. *Voprosy ekonomiki, planirovaniya i statistiki*. Moscow, Izd. AMN SSSR. 1957.

PUSTOVOI, I. V. *Sovetskoe Zdravookhranenie*, No. 6. 1956.

PUSTOVOI, I. V. *Sovetskoe Zdravookhranenie*, No. 1. 1958.

RASHIN, A. G. *Naselenie Rossii za 100 let (The Population of Russia during 100 Years)*. Moscow, Gosstatizdat. 1956.

RESLE, E. *Professional'naya Meditsina*, No. 1. 1928.

RODOV, YA. I. *Puti i perspektivy bor'by s serdechno-sosudistymi zabolevaniyami (Means and Prospects of the Control of Cardiovascular Diseases)*. Medgiz. 1960.

ROZHDESTVENSKII, M. I. Zabolevaemost' rabochikh tekstil'noi promyshlennosti goroda Tveri za 1925 g. (Morbidity of Textile Workers of the City of Tver for the Year 1925). In: *Statisticheskie issledovaniya professional'noi zabolevaemosti*, No. 1. Moscow, Gosmedizdat. 1929.

ROZHDESTVENSKII, M. I. *Professional'naya Patologiya i Gigiena*, Vol. 8. 1929.

ROZENFEL'D, D. I. *Osnovy i metodika planirovaniya zdravookhraneniya (Principles and Methods of Public Health Planning)*. Medgiz. 1954.

RUSYAEV, A. P. *Zdravookhranenie Turkmenii*, No. 6. 1957.

SAKHAROV, P. P. and E. I. GUDKOVA. *Vestnik Otorinolaringologii*, No. 2. 1955.

SHAKHGEL'DYANTS, A. E. *Zdravookhranenie Rossiiskoi Federatsii*, No. 4. 1960.

SHOSTAK, YA. E. *Zabolevaemost' tekstil'shchikov goroda Ivanovo-Voznesenska v 1927 godu (Morbidity of Textile Workers of the City of Ivanovo-Voznesensk in 1927)*. Moscow–Ivanovo–Voznesensk, GIZ. 1931.

SMULEVICH, B. YA. *Zabolevaemost' i smertnost' naseleniya gorodov i mestechek BSSR (Morbidity and Mortality of the Population of Cities and Small Towns of the Belorussian SSR)*. Minsk, Izdatel'stvo TsSU i NKZ Belorusskoi SSR. 1928.

SMULEVICH, B. YA. *Vestnik Statistiki*, No. 4. 1928.

SMULEVICH, B. YA. *Burzhuaznye teorii v svete marksistsko-leninskoi kritiki (Bourgeois Theories in the Light of Marxist–Leninist Criticism)*. 1936.

SMULEVICH, B. YA. *Sovetskoe Zdravookhranenie*, No. 2. 1947.

SMULEVICH, B. YA. *Sovetskoe Zdravookhranenie*, No. 6. 1949.

SMULEVICH, B. YA. *Sovetskoe Zdravookhranenie*, No. 1. 1953.

SOLOV'EV, Z. P. Osnovnye problemy planirovaniya zdravookhraneniya (Principal Problems of Public Health Planning). *Doklad na VI s"ezde zdravotdelov* (Manuscript.). May 1927.

SOVETOV, V. P. *Voprosy kurortologii, fizioterapii i lechebnoi fizicheskoi kul'tury*, No. 3. 1960.

SOVETOV, V. P. O novykh formakh organizatsii kurortnoi i fizioterapevticheskoi pomoshchi naseleniyu (New Forms of Organization of Health Resorts and Physiotherapy for the Population). *Uchenye Zapiski Ukrainskogo Instituta Kurortologii i Fizioterapii*. Odessa. 1961.

SSSR v tsifrakh v 1963 (The USSR in Figures for 1963). Moscow, Izd. "Statistika." 1964.

STAROVSKII, V. N. *Vestnik AN SSSR*, No. 2. 1960.

STAROVSKII, V. N. *Vestnik AN SSSR*, No. 5. 1962.

Statisticheskie issledovaniya professional'noi zabolevaemosti, No. 1. Moscow, Medgiz. 1929.

Statisticheskie issledovaniya professional'noi zabolevaemosti, No. 2. Moscow–Leningrad, Medgiz. 1930.

Statisticheskii spravochnik SSSR za 1928 g. (Statistical Handbook of the USSR for 1928).

STRUMILIN, S. G. *Nashi trudovye resursy i perspektivy (USSR—Manpower and Prospects).* Moscow. 1925.

STRUMILIN, S. G. K probleme rozhdaemosti v rabochei srede (The Birth Rate in a Working Environment). In: *Problemy ekonomiki truda*. Moscow. 1957.

STRUMILIN, S. G. *Problemy ekonomiki truda (Problems of Labor Economics)*. Moscow 1957.

SUVOROVA, E. V. Zabolevaemost' revmatizmom i serdechno-sosudistymi boleznyami v krupnykh gorodakh Belorussii za 1958 g. (Morbidity of Rheumatism and Cardiovascular Diseases in Large Cities of Belorussia during 1958). In: *Tezisy IV nauchnoi sessii Instituta organizatsii zdravookhraneniya i istorii meditsiny imeni N. A. Semashko*. Moscow. 1961.

Tablitsy smertnosti i srednei prodolzhitel'nosti zhizni naseleniya SSSR. 1958–1959 gg. (Tables of Mortality and Average Life Expectancy of the USSR Population in 1958–1959). Gosstatizdat TsSU SSSR. 1962.

TAMAZOV, A. A. *Organizatsiya fizioterapii v bol'nitsakh i poliklinikakh (Organization of Physiotherapy in Hospitals and Polyclinics)*. Medgiz. 1961.

TEKMAN, A. S. Zabolevaemost' boleznyami ukha, gorla i nosa i zadachi organizatsii otorino-laringologicheskoi pomoshchi naseleniyu (Morbidity of ENT Diseases and Problems of Organization of Otorhinolaryngological Care of the Population). Moscow. 1957.

TEPLYAKOV, B. YA. *Zdravookhranenie Rossiiskoi Federatsii*, No. 8. 1958.

TOMILIN, S. A. *Professional'naya Meditsina*, No. 12. 1924. (Supplement).

TROYAN, I. A. *Zdravookhranenie*, Nos. 1–2. 1960.

Trudy 1-i Vsesoyuznoi konferentsii po planirovaniyu zdravookhraneniya i rabochego otdykha (Proceedings of the 1st All-Union Conference on the Planning of Public Health and Vacations from Work). *Standartizatsiya i ratsionalizatsiya*, p. 79. 1933.

TRUTNEV, V. K. and P. P. SAKHAROV. Sovremennoe sostoyanie voprosa o profilaktike i lechenii angin (Current State of the Question of Prophylaxis and Treatment of Tonsillitis). *Trudy V s"ezda otorinolaringologov SSSR*. Moscow. 1959.

TUROVA, D. D. *Pediatriya*, No. 8. 1957.

TUROVA, D. D. *Detskaya bol'nitsa s poliklinikoi (Children's Hospital with Polyclinic)*. Moscow. 1964.

TUROVEROVA, N. I. *Zdravookhranenie Rossiiskoi Federatsii*, No. 1. 1964.

URLANIS, B. Ts. *Rozhdaemost' i prodolzhitel'nost' zhizni v SSSR (Birth Rate and Life Expectancy in the USSR)*. Gosstatizdat TsU SSSR. 1963.

URLANIS, B. Ts. *Dinamika i struktura naseleniya SSSR i SShA (Dynamics and Population Structure of the USSR and USA)*. Izdatel'stvo "Nauka." 1964.

VASIL'EV, V. N. Zabolevaemost' naseleniya poselka Motovilikha Permskogo okruga Ural'-skoi oblasti v 1926–1927 gg. (Morbidity of the Population of Motovilikha Village, Perm District, Ural Region in 1926–1927). In: *Statisticheskie issledovaniya professional'noi zabolevaemosti*, No. 2. Moscow–Leningrad. 1930.

VASIL'EV, V. N. Bol'nichnaya pomoshch' (Hospital Care). In: *Voprosy ucheta i planirovaniya v oblasti okhrany zdorov'ya detei i podrostkov*. Moscow. 1933.

382   MORBIDITY OF URBAN POPULATIONS

Vasil'ev, S. A. Kvoprosu o nuzhdaemosti detei v profilakticheskoi pomoshchi (The Requirement of Prophylactic Care for Children). In: *Lechebno-profilakticheskaya pomoshch' detyam i podrostkam.* Moscow—Leningrad. 1936.
Vladimirskii, M. F. *Na Fronte Zdravookhraneniya,* No. 13. 1932.
Vostrikova, A. M. *Vestnik Statistiki,* No. 12. 1962.
Vostrikova, A. M. *Vestnik Statistiki,* No. 1. 1964.
Vsesoyuznaya konferentsiya po planirovaniyu zdravookhraneniya (All-Union Conference on Public Health Planning). *Voprosy Zdravookhraneniya,* Nos. 2–3. 1933.
Vsesoyuznoe soveshchanie rabotnikov zdravookhraneniya po kadram (All-Union Conference of Public Health Workers according to Staff Categories). *Na Fronte Zdravookhraneniya,* No. 16. 1931.
Yanson, Yu. E. *Sravnitel'naya statistika naseleniya (Comparative Statistics of the Population),* Vol. 2, St. Peterburg. 1896.
Zakharova, P. I. *Zdravookhranenie Rossiiskoi Federatsii,* No. 5. 1963.
Zambrzhitskii, V. V. Zabolevaemost' naseleniya Leningradskoi gubernii v 1924 g. (Morbidity of the Population of Leningrad Province in 1924). In: *Sanitarno-statisticheskii sbornik Leningradskogo oblastnogo otdela zdravookhraneniya.* 1928.
Zdravookhranenie i rabochii otdykh vo vtoroi pyatiletke (Public Health and Vacation from Work during the Second Five-Year Plan), Vol. 1. Moscow. 1933.
Zdravookhranenie SSSR (Public Health in the USSR). Gosstatizdat. 1960.
Zhdanov, V. M. Sovremennoe sostoyanie voprosa o grippe i ostrykh katarakh verkhnikh dykhatel'nykh putei (Current State of the Problem of Influenza and Acute Nasal Catarrh). In: *Programmnye doklady na V Vsesoyuznom s"ezde otorinolaringologov.* Moscow—Dushanbe. 1958.
Zhelezov, G. Issledovanie zabolevaemosti—vazhnyi faktor planirovaniya zdravookhraneniya (Morbidity Survey—an Important Factor in Public Health Planning). In: *VI Soveshchanie ministrov zdravookhraneniya sotsialisticheskikh stran.* Budapest. 1964.
Zhuk, A. P., F. M. Ilupina, and V. D. Dubrovina. *Sovetskoe Zdravookhranenie,* No. 10. 1962.

Publications in Other Languages

Abbe, L. M. Hospital and Nursing Homes in the U.S., 1959. *Publ. Health Reports,* **74,** 1089–97. 1959.
Abbe, L. M. and A. M. Baney. *The National Health Facilities* (Ten Years of the Hill–Burton Hospital and Medical Facilities Program 1946–1956). Washington. 1958.
Abel-Smith, B. and R. M. Titmuss. *The Cost of the National Health Service in England and Wales.* Cambridge, Nat. Inst. Econ. Soc. Research. 1956.
Adams, W. Ground Rules of Specialization and Advanced Education in Medicine. *J.A.M.A.,* 185, 445–447. 1963.
Allen, G. I., L. Breslow, A. Weissman, and H. Nisselson. Interviewing versus Diary Keeping in Eliciting Information in a Morbidity Survey. *A.J.P.H.,* **44,** 917–27. 1954.
Almoners' Functions and Training. *Hosp. Soc. Serv. J.,* **66,** No. 3478. 1956.
America's Health, a Report to the National Health Assembly. New York, Harper. 1949.

Areawide Planning for Hospitals and Related Health Facilities. Washington, Public Health Monograph, No. 855. 1961.

BELLOC, N. B. *J. Am. statist. Assn.* **49**, No. 268. 1954.

BLOCK, L. Analysis of Elements of Patient Care. *Mod. Hosp.*, **86**, No. 1, 74–82; No. 2, 86–9; No. 3, 66–9; No. 4, 74–7. 1956.

BRIDGMAN, R. F. *L'hôpital rural, sa structure et son organisation*. Genève. 1-54.

BRINES, W. S. The Hospital Master Plan, Blueprint for the Future. *Hospitals*, **37**, No. 3. 41–4. 1963.

BROOKE, E. M. Factors Affecting the Demand for Psychiatric Beds. *Lancet* **2**, 1211–3. 1962.

Building America's Health (A Report to the President by the President's Commission on the Health Needs of the Nation) (Health). Washington. 1953.

BUSBY, L. Need for Infectious Disease Beds in a London Area. *Br. Med. J.*, 5359, 737–8. 1963.

Chart Book on Health Status, Health Manpower. Washington, U.S. Department of Health, Education and Welfare. 1961.

Le cinquième plan quinquenal de la construction des hôpitaux. *Techniques hospitalières*, No. 218. 1963.

COLLINS, S. D., F. R. PHILLIPS, and D. S. OLIVER. Specific Causes of Illnesses Found in Monthly Canvases of Families, Eastern Health District of Baltimore. *Public Health Rep.*, **65**, 1235–1264. 1950.

COLLINS, S. D., K. S. TRANTHAM, and J. L. LEHMAN. *Sickness Experience in Selected Areas of the U.S.*. Washington, Public Health Monograph, No. 390. 1955.

Commission on Hospital Care. Cambridge, Mass., *Hospital Care in the United States*, 1947.

La consommation médicale des Français. *Presse méd.*, **70**, 1329–30. 1962.

CRONIN, J. W. Hospital Construction, Progress and Prospects. *Hospitals*, **31**, No. 1, 28–30. 1957.

DAVIES, J. and A. BARR. The Population Served by a Hospital Group. *Lancet* **2**, 1105–8. 1957.

DAVIS, M. M. Are There Enough Beds or Too Many? *Mod. Hosp.*, **48**, 49–52. 1937.

DAVIS, M. M. *Medical Care for Tomorrow*. New York–London, Harper. 1955.

The Development of Community Care (Plan for the Health and Welfare Services of the Local Authorities in England and Wales). London. 1963.

DIJON, H. *La semaine médicale professionnelle et médico-sociale*, **31**, No. 7. 1955.

EMERSON, H. Estimating Adequate Provision for Organized Care of the Sick. *Mod. Hosp.*, **35**, 49–51. 1930.

ENTERLINE, P. E., A. E. RIKLI, H. I. SAUER, M. HYMAN, and W. H. STEWART. Death Rates for Coronary Heart Disease in Metropolitan and Other Areas. *Public Health Rep.*, **75**, 759–66. 1960.

EVANG, K. *Health Service, Society and Medicine*. London–New York–Toronto, Oxford Press. 1960.

GARDIE, A. *Les hôpitaux des grandes agglomérations urbaines—Introduction à l'étude des problèmes hospitaliers*. Paris. 1956.

GERFELDT, E. and P. TRUB. *Das Krankenhaus und seine Betriebsführung*. Stuttgart. 1959.

GODBER, G. E. Trends in Specialization and Their Effect on the Practice of Medicine. *Br. Med. J.*, 5256, 843–7. 1961.

Health Statistics—Disability Days. U.S. National Health Survey. July, 1969–July, 1960.

Health, Education and Welfare Trends. Washington, Annual Report. 1961.

HILL, A. B. *Principles of Medical Statistics.* 1937.

HILL, C. and J. WOODCOCK. *The National Health Service.* London, C. Johnson. 1949.

A Hospital Plan for England and Wales. London. 1962.

Hospital Needs and Population Trends. *Br. Med. J.,* 5201, 789–791. 1960.

How Many Beds? *Hospitals,* **36**, No. 9. 1962.

How Many General Hospital Beds Are Needed? Washington, U.S. Department of Health, Education and Welfare. 1953.

How Many Hospital Beds Are Needed? *Hosp. Soc. Serv. J.,* **66**, 1111, 1956.

How Many Maternity Beds? *Br. Med. J.,* 5337, 1963.

JONES, F. A. Length of Stay in Hospital. *Lancet,* **1**, 321–2. 1964.

LEE, R. I. and L. W. JONES. *The Fundamentals of Good Medical Care.* Committee on the Costs of Medical Care, Publication No. 22. 1933.

Length of Convalescence after Surgery. *Hospitals,* **37**, 72–3. 1963.

LINDSEY, A. *Socialized Medicine in England and Wales.* (The National Health Service, 1948–1961). Chapel Hill, Univ. of North Carolina Press. 1962.

LOGAN, W. P. D. *Lancet,* **1**, 6608. 1950.

LOGAN, W. P. D. and E. M. BROOKE. *The Survey of Sickness, 1943 to 1952.* London. 1957.

LOGAN, T. *Hospitals,* **34**, No. 6. 1960.

MACKIE, W. Planning the Hospitals of the Future. *Lancet,* **1**, 211–3. 1963.

MACKINTOSH, J. M. et al. *Lancet,* **1**, No. 7181. 1961.

McGIBONY, J. R. Hospitals—Retrospect and Prospect. *Hospitals,* **38**, 77–81. 1964.

MAGDELAINE, M. *Techniques d'étude de la fonction hospitalière.* Paris. 1959.

MAROSELLI, A. *Au service de la santé publique (18 mois d'activité).* Paris. 1957.

MENSIER, D. Contribution à l'étude statistique de l'évolution des activités médicales dans le département de l'Aube de 1948. (Dissertation). Paris. 1959.

Morbidity Statistics from General Practice—Studies on Medical and Population Subjects, Vols. 1, 7, 8, 14. London, General Register Office. 1951.

MOUNTIN, J. S. and S. P. GRAVE. *Public Health Areas and Hospital Facilities.* Washington, Public Health Monograph, No. 42. 1950.

NAGAN, P. S. *Medical Almanac.* Philadelphia–London, Saunders. 1961–1962.

National Health Survey. Interviewer's Manual. Washington. 1959.

NORRIS, V. *Br. Med. J.,* No. 19. 1952.

ODOROFF, M. E. and L. M. ABBE. Use of General Hospitals. (I), Demographic and Ecologic. *Public Health Rep.* **72**, 397–403. 1957; (II), Varieties of Payment Methods. *Ibid.,* **74**, 316–324. 1958.

PEMBERTON, J. *Br. Med. J.,* **1** No. 4598. 1949.

PEQUIGNOT, H., G. ROSCH, J. M. REMPP, and M. MAGDELAINE. *Consommation,* **9**, No. 1. 1962.

PETERSON, P. O. and M. Y. PENNELL. Physician-Population Projections; Their Causes and Implications. *A.J.P.H.,* **53**, 163–72. 1963.

QUERIDO, A. The Changing Role of the Hospital in a Changing World. *Hospitals,* **36**, 31–5. 1962.

Le Rapport de la Cour des Comptes. Les hôpitaux publics. *La semaine médicale,* **41**. 1958.

RAYNAUD, M. *Revue de l'infirmière et de l'assistante sociale*, No. 8. 1962.

ROCHAIX. M. *Essai sur l'évolution des questions hospitalières de la fin de l'Ancien Regime à nos jours*. Belfort. 1959.

ROURKE, A. J. The Circular Hospital Plan. *Hospitals*, **36**, No. 20, 34–7. 1962.

RYAN, J. T. Jr. Capital Needs of Hospitals (How Will We Be in the Next 20 Years?). *Hospitals*, , No. 6, 32–5, 1858.

SMITH, A. *J. Amer. Pharmaceut. Assn.*, **48**, No. 10. 1959.

SPENCE, J. and M. D. TAYLOR. Hospital Beds for Children. *Lancet*, No. 266, 719–21. 1954.

Studies on Medical and Population Subjects. *Hospital Morbidity Statistics*, No. 4. London, General Register Office. 1-51.

Studies in the Function and Design of Hospitals. London–New York, National Hospitals Trust. 1955.

ŠTYCH, Z. Československé zdravotnictví. Prague. 1962.

SYDENSTRICKER, E. *Public Health Rep.*, **42**, 33. 1927.

Third Session of the Staats-Medizinal Rat. *Bundesgesundheitsblatt*, No. 7. 1963.

THOILLIER, H. *L'hôpital français*. Paris. 1948.

U.S.A.—A Nationwide National Health Survey Begins. *J.A.M.A.*, **164**, No. 5a, 500–505. 1957.

VALERY-RADOT, P. *Nos hôpitaux parisiens. Histoire hospitalière*. Paris. 1948.

VERICOURT. *L'hôpital et l'aide sociale à Paris*, No. 10. 1960.

WARREN, M. D. Medical Centres. *Med. World*, **97**, 185–90. 1962.

WEST, M. D. Manpower for the Health Field: What are the Prospects? *Hospitals*, **37**, No. 5, 82–8. 1963.

WESTON, G. *Hospitals*, **37**, No. 2. 1963.

WIGGINS, W. S., G. K. LEYMASTER, et al. Medical Education in the U.S. and Canada. *J.A.M.A.*, 174, 1423–1476. 1960.

WOOLSEY, T. D. The Concept of Illness in the Household: Interest in Health in the U.S. *A.J.P.H.*, **48**, 703–712. 1958.

Name Index